AF753313

NEW DEVELOPMENTS IN MEDICAL RESEARCH

CHILDHOOD OBESITY

CAUSES, PREVENTION AND MANAGEMENT

NEW DEVELOPMENTS IN MEDICAL RESEARCH

Additional books and e-books in this series can be found on Nova's website under the Series tab.

NEW DEVELOPMENTS IN MEDICAL RESEARCH

CHILDHOOD OBESITY

CAUSES, PREVENTION AND MANAGEMENT

ROYA KELISHADI, MD
EDITOR

nova
Medicine & Health
New York

Copyright © 2020 by Nova Science Publishers, Inc.

All rights reserved. No part of this book may be reproduced, stored in a retrieval system or transmitted in any form or by any means: electronic, electrostatic, magnetic, tape, mechanical photocopying, recording or otherwise without the written permission of the Publisher.

We have partnered with Copyright Clearance Center to make it easy for you to obtain permissions to reuse content from this publication. Simply navigate to this publication's page on Nova's website and locate the "Get Permission" button below the title description. This button is linked directly to the title's permission page on copyright.com. Alternatively, you can visit copyright.com and search by title, ISBN, or ISSN.

For further questions about using the service on copyright.com, please contact:
Copyright Clearance Center
Phone: +1-(978) 750-8400 Fax: +1-(978) 750-4470 E-mail: info@copyright.com.

NOTICE TO THE READER

The Publisher has taken reasonable care in the preparation of this book, but makes no expressed or implied warranty of any kind and assumes no responsibility for any errors or omissions. No liability is assumed for incidental or consequential damages in connection with or arising out of information contained in this book. The Publisher shall not be liable for any special, consequential, or exemplary damages resulting, in whole or in part, from the readers' use of, or reliance upon, this material. Any parts of this book based on government reports are so indicated and copyright is claimed for those parts to the extent applicable to compilations of such works.

Independent verification should be sought for any data, advice or recommendations contained in this book. In addition, no responsibility is assumed by the Publisher for any injury and/or damage to persons or property arising from any methods, products, instructions, ideas or otherwise contained in this publication.

This publication is designed to provide accurate and authoritative information with regard to the subject matter covered herein. It is sold with the clear understanding that the Publisher is not engaged in rendering legal or any other professional services. If legal or any other expert assistance is required, the services of a competent person should be sought. FROM A DECLARATION OF PARTICIPANTS JOINTLY ADOPTED BY A COMMITTEE OF THE AMERICAN BAR ASSOCIATION AND A COMMITTEE OF PUBLISHERS.

Additional color graphics may be available in the e-book version of this book.

Library of Congress Cataloging-in-Publication Data

ISBN: 978-1-53618-158-6
Names: Kelishadi, Roya, editor.
Title: Childhood obesity : causes, prevention and management / Roya Kelishadil (editor), Isfahan University of Medical Sciences, Isfahan, Iran
Description: New York : Nova Science Publishers, [2020] | Series: New developments in medical research | Includes bibliographical references and index. |
Identifiers: LCCN 2020027178 (print) | LCCN 2020027179 (ebook) | ISBN 9781536181586 (hardcover) | ISBN 9781536182323 (adobe pdf)
Subjects: LCSH: Obesity in children. | Obesity in children--Treatment. | Obesity in children--Prevention.
Classification: LCC RJ399.C6 C475153 2020 (print) | LCC RJ399.C6 (ebook) | DDC 618.92/398--dc23
LC record available at https://lccn.loc.gov/2020027178
LC ebook record available at https://lccn.loc.gov/2020027179

Published by Nova Science Publishers, Inc. † New York

CONTENTS

PREFACE

Childhood obesity has become a global health problem at individual and public levels. It results from a complex interaction between genetics, lifestyle and environmental factors. Because of its adverse health effects in childhood and adulthood, it is important to expand our knowledge about its etiology, prevalence, prevention, and management.

Childhood obesity has several early-onset adverse effects on all body organs and the metabolism. Moreover, as obesity tracks from childhood to adulthood, it can be an underlying factor for the development of chronic non-communicable diseases, which are the worldwide leading cause of morbidity and mortality. Such chronic diseases can result from lifelong accumulation of some risk factors, including obesity. Therefore, sustained interventions are necessary to tackle the onset or progression of childhood obesity.

Childhood obesity is no more limited to high income countries; it has a rapid growing trend in low and middle-come countries. In addition to genetic background, environmental disruptor chemicals and their epigenetic effects are of important underlying factors for the escalating trend of childhood obesity and the trans-generational aspects of obesity. It is noteworthy to consider the early life determinants of childhood obesity, including prenatal, perinatal and post-natal factors, are usually preventable. Dietary habits are formed in the first years of life; therefore it is of crucial importance to establish healthy habits from early life.

Food industry, food environment, and social media are important factors influencing the food choices for families and their children. On the other hand, parents are the most important role models for lifestyle habits of their children.

In addition to preventative measures, it is important to know how to manage excess weight in growing children, who need enough macro- and micronutrients for their growth, but need to have controlled food intake. Various family-based and school-based interventions are suggested in this regard. In addition to energy intake, it is essential to increase the energy expenditure by regular exercise. Most healthcare providers are not aware of appropriate physical activity for weight control in the pediatric age group.

Sometimes the process of weight gain is not correctly prevented or controlled in children and adolescents, and they would suffer from morbid obesity necessitating surgical treatment. Limited evidence-based information is available about these aspects of childhood obesity.

This book is written with collaboration of international experts with different scientific backgrounds, who contributed in gathering the updates and findings from their experience on how to deal with the complex factors related to childhood obesity. The main focus of this book is on providing updated information on all above-mentioned aspects related to childhood obesity. It is expected that researchers, health care providers, physicians, health decision makers, and families would find this book as a beneficial tool for implementing widespread measures for prevention and control of childhood obesity.

Roya Kelishadi,MD
Professor of Pediatrics, Child Growth and Development Research Center,
Research Institute for Primordial Prevention of Non-Communicable Disease,
Isfahan University of Medical Sciences, Isfahan, Iran

In: Childhood Obesity
Editor: Roya Kelishadi

ISBN: 978-1-53618-158-6
© 2020 Nova Science Publishers, Inc.

Chapter 1

CHILDHOOD OBESITY IN LOWER AND MIDDLE-INCOME COUNTRIES (LMICS)

Neha Jain, Shalini Bassi and Monika Arora
Health Promotion Division, Public Health Foundation of India,
Gurugram, Haryana, India

ABSTRACT

Childhood obesity has both short term and long-term implications in one's health. It has been linked with diseases of the cardiovascular system, diabetes, cancers, mental illnesses and increased disability in adult's life. In 2010, 89% of total overweight and obese children were living in lower- and middle-income (LMICs) countries. In Africa alone, there has been a 50% rise in the number of overweight children under the age of 5 years since 2000. Asia is home to the greatest number of obese and overweight children. It has also been reported that the rate of increase has been more than 30% higher in LMICs than in developed countries. Various factors are responsible for the rampant rise in childhood obesity. Research has indicated that children from disadvantaged backgrounds or lower socio-economic groups receive lesser benefit from interventions as compared to children from affluent backgrounds or higher socio-economic background. While some of these factors relate to the socio-economic position of the children and their families. However, the surrounding environment also has a huge role to play in promoting obesity. Hence, interventions for the prevention of childhood obesity should be designed in such a manner that they do not exaggerate the existing inequalities and address it in a comprehensive and strategic manner. However, there are many challenges faced by LMICs in addressing this health concern. Lack of resources, research gaps, unavailability of data are some of the hindrances. There is no single or simple solution to the obesity epidemic. It is a complex problem and hence a multi-faceted approach, that includes a wide range of stakeholders, needs to be put in place. The childhood obesity prevention efforts must be closely integrated with other efforts to control key non-communicable diseases (NCD) risk factors, including tobacco and alcohol use, unhealthy diet and physical inactivity. Obesity prevention policies need to be inclusive and equitable, with interventions tailored to suit local contexts. This chapter details the burden of childhood obesity in LMICs, elaborates on its drivers and determinants, discusses the approaches to address childhood obesity in line with the Ottawa Charter's principles for health promotion. It also states the examples of successful childhood obesity interventions in LMICs, gives examples from high-income countries and discusses the challenges and strategic actions to combat the epidemic of childhood obesity.

INTRODUCTION

Obesity is no longer considered a concern exclusive to high-income countries. Its prevalence has reached alarming rates across the globe and poses a serious challenge in need of immediate attention. Through the health, economic and social bearings of obesity on an individual's life, it potentially counters many of the factors responsible for prolonged longevity (World Health Organization 2016). As per the World Health Organization (WHO), 2.28 billion individuals worldwide are overweight. Apart from its attribution in communicable diseases and malnutrition, obesity has also been scientifically linked to a number of diseases responsible for long term individual and social consequences. It has been attributed in a number of non-communicable diseases such as hypertension, Type II diabetes, cancer, cardiovascular diseases and even sleep apnoea (Wyatt, Winters, and Dubbert 2006). Obese individuals are also at an increased risk from depression and a lower quality of life. Direct and indirect costs (reduced work productivity, absenteeism from work etc.) and consequences of obesity pose a serious burden on the economy of a nation (Withrow and Alter 2011).

The Burden of Childhood Obesity in Lower- and Middle-Income Countries

Reportedly, 40 million young children (under the age of 5 years) around the world were overweight in 2018 (WHO, UNICEF, and The World Bank Group 2019). Earlier reports also suggested that 340 million children and adolescents (5-19year age group) were overweight or obese in 2016 (World Health Organization 2016). Furthermore, the prevalence of overweight and obesity among children and adolescents aged 5 – 19 years has risen sharply from 4 per cent in 1975 to over 18 per cent in 2016 (World Health Organization 2016). This concern is further magnified for low and middle-income countries (LMICs) which are now facing the dual burden of malnutrition (undernutrition, overweight and obesity). While the level of undernutrition still remains significant in these countries, overweight and obesity prevalence have reached an alarmingly high percentage. This phenomenon of co-existence of undernutrition and overnutrition can be explained through the fact that children living in LMICs have limited access to appropriate nutrition while growing up. They are surrounded by an environment which supports a high-fat, high-sugar, high-salt and micronutrient poor food since it is cheaper (World Health Organization 2016). Further, the economic growth of countries have led to changes in domestic retail food sector as well as agricultural sectors. This, consequently, has increased the availability of ultra-processed food in the LMICs (Reardon and Timmer 2012; Popkin, Corvalan, and Grummer-Strawn 2020). As a matter of fact, in 2010, out of the 43 million worldwide overweight children, 38 million were living in LMICs (de Onis, Blössner, and Borghi 2010). In Africa alone, there has been a 50% rise in the number of overweight children under the age of 5 years since the year 2000. World Health Organization also stated that Asia was home to almost half and Africa to a quarter of the under-5 overweight or obese children in 2018. It has also been reported that the rate of increase has been more than 30% higher in LMICs than in developed countries (World Health Organization 2019). While, it may also be possible that the prevalence of infant, child and adolescent obesity may be plateauing in some regions, however, it has been documented that in terms of absolute numbers, more overweight and obese children live in LMICs than in high income countries (World Health Organization 2016). Figure 1 shows the distribution of overweight children under the age of 5 years by country income grouping, 2018.

For children under the age of 5 years, no significant progress has been reported in terms of reduction in percentages of the overweight population since 2000. Table 1 shows the number of children under 5 years, by country income classification in 2000 and 2018.

But it has been difficult to evaluate individual childhood obesity rates in most of the countries across the globe, regardless of their income levels. Many countries do not have nationally representative surveys that measure the height and weight of school children or do not have consistent measurements over a period of time. Furthermore, different definitions of the term 'childhood obesity' by the World Health Organization, Centre for Disease Control (CDC) and International Obesity Task Force make it difficult to compare data from different regions.

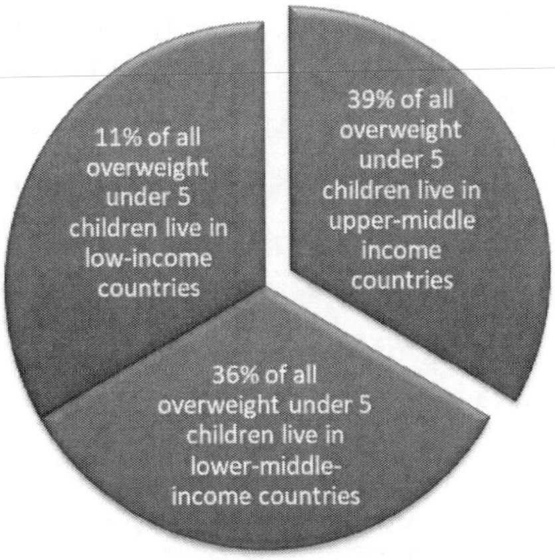

Data Source: WHO, UNICEF, and The World Bank Group 2019.

Figure 1. Distribution of overweight under 5 children in the world by country income grouping, 2018.

Table 1. Number of overweight children under 5, by country income classification, 2000 and 2018

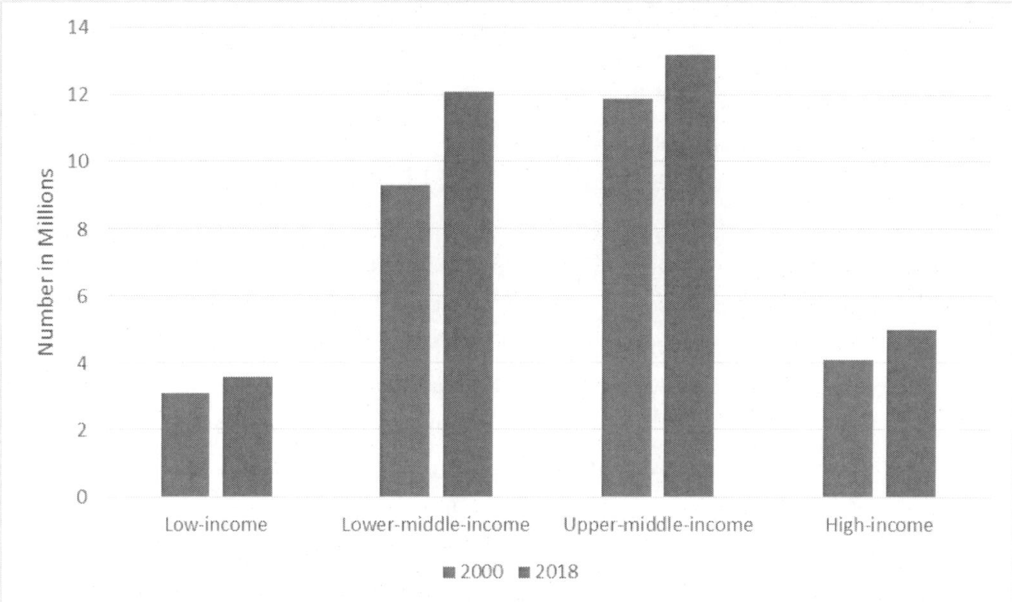

Data Source: WHO, UNICEF, and The World Bank Group 2019.

Consequences of Childhood Obesity

As mentioned before, obesity has grave consequences on the health of an individual. These consequences also stand true for overweight and obese children, who are at an increased risk from diseases such as those of the cardiovascular system, Type II diabetes, cancer, hypertension and risk of even premature mortality (Reilly and Kelly 2011). These children have consequences both in the short term (when they are an obese child or adolescent) and long term (when they are adults, but were an obese child or an adolescent). In the short term, childhood obesity has been linked with high blood pressure, dyslipidemia, abnormalities in the left ventricular mass and functions, hyperinsulinemia and/or insulin resistance (Reilly et al. 2003). Research has also linked child/adolescent overweight and obesity with significantly increased risk of disability in adult life (Neovius, Kark, and Rasmussen 2008; Karnehed, Rasmussen, and Kark 2007). While the link between childhood obesity and breast cancer could not be clearly established (Reilly and Kelly 2011), however, studies have found significant association between higher-measured Body Mass Index (BMI) in childhood with other forms of cancers (not tobacco-related) later in life (Jeffreys et al. 2004).

Determinants of Childhood Obesity in Lower- and Middle-Income Countries

Various factors are responsible for the rampant rise in childhood obesity. Some of these factors relate to the socio-economic position of the children and their families, however, the surrounding environment also has a huge role to play in promoting obesity. Determinants of childhood obesity include –

Nutrition Transition and Unhealthy Food Environment

Globalisation and urbanisation are two opposing concepts that have been partly responsible for the rise in childhood obesity in the last few decades. In this context, globalisation refers to the concept of saturating low- or middle-income country markets with inexpensive but obesity causing fast food options. On the other hand, urbanisation refers to a country's own development and Gross Domestic Product (GDP) rise leading to unhealthy food consumption (Fox, Feng, and Asal 2019). Different research and authors support either of these theories. A good example is a study conducted in Vietnam which showed that there was a significant increase in the availability of sugar-sweetened beverages (SSBs) in the country following foreign direct investments and trade liberalisation policies as compared to a control case, the country Philippines (Schram et al. 2015). Similarly, the presence of an unhealthy food environment has been found in many of the LMICs. For example, countries such as Brazil are now characterized by the presence of 'food deserts.' These gatherings were found to be prominent among urban communities and had insufficient availability and access to healthy foods such as fruits and vegetables (Davies, Frausin, and Parry 2017). In Mexico, 'food swamps,' which are similar to food deserts, were found to be prominent among LMICs communities and were characterized by the presence of unhealthy foods and drinks; food oases were common in high-income communities (Bridle-Fitzpatrick 2015).

Children and adolescents from low socio-economic backgrounds of LMICs are facing poverty and hunger and as a consequence, are deprived of nutrient-rich food. In addition, the presence of cheap fast food options and consumption of unhealthy foods due to easy availability and change in lifestyle, due to globalisation or urbanization, are encouraging the consumption of high-sugar, high-salt obesogenic food items. With urbanisation and/or globalisation facilitating easy availability of unhealthy food items, the children are now exposed to a highly obesogenic food environment.

Lack of Physical Activity

With the advent of the technological era, a shift in activity patterns have been observed among children and adolescents. Children are now more drawn to indoor activities such as television viewing, internet and computer games (Popkin 2001). A study in India found a significant association between children, who watched television for at least 90 minutes/day and being overweight as compared to those children who viewed television for no more than 45 minutes/day (Kuriyan et al. 2007). In addition, lack of simulating infrastructure is also responsible for the decrease in indulgence in physical activity by children and adolescents. Even middle-income country such as India is often synonymous with the lack of open spaces for playing, a well-developed path for walking and cycling as well as sufficient provision for other outdoor activities (Gupta et al. 2012).

Socio-Economic Position

The relationship between childhood obesity and socioeconomic position (SEP) is not uniform across different countries. It has been found that in high-income countries, the SEP is inversely related to childhood obesity (Gortmaker et al. 1993) whereas in middle-income countries or developing economies, children belonging to higher SEP have a higher prevalence of being overweight or obese (Kaur et al. 2008). This scenario in developing countries could be explained through different pathways. For instance, in India, children from higher SEP backgrounds have a relatively inactive background owing to access to smartphones, internet, indoor gaming equipment. They commute to school either by car or bus. On the other hand, children studying in government schools and belonging to lower SEP travel to school either through bicycles or walk on a daily basis. Furthermore, school cafeterias in private schools serve unhealthy and junk food which are easily available to students. This unequivocally exposes school children belonging to higher SEP in developing countries to obesogenic environments, whereas children from lower SEP, while physically active have reduced access to nutritious food, leading to undernutrition.

Marketing Tactics

Children's access to cheap, ready and obesogenic food is often linked with marketing strategies by fast-food chains and major food brands (Monteiro et al. 2013; Larson and Story 2009). Fast-food chains in high-income countries spent a significant amount of their marketing budget on targeting children (Pan American Health Organization 2011), a trend that now seems to be replicated in LMICs as well. These chains have been known to give combo meals, price incentives as well as prompt delivery as some of the marketing strategies (Epstein et al. 2006). Furthermore, a study done in six LMICs showed that strategies such as media exposure and logo recognition were predictors for the selection of foods and beverages (Borzekowski and Pires 2018).

Genetic or Endocrine Causes

Other factors and determinants of childhood obesity are genetic predispositions and family history. In some children, hormonal disorders such as hypothyroidism, Cushing syndrome, etc. can be attributed for the presence of childhood obesity (Gupta et al. 2012). Research has also linked obesity in parents to childhood obesity in their offspring (Parsons et al. 1999).

APPROACHES TO ADDRESS CHILDHOOD OBESITY

Reports suggest that while stunting, wasting and thinness have been gradually decreasing in women of LMICs, on the other hand, overweight is increasing across different age groups (Popkin, Corvalan, and Grummer-Strawn 2020). The report for the Millennium Development Goals (MDGs) stated that while hunger had almost been eradicated by half between 1990 and 2015 in LMICs, the same goals could not be met for over nutrition, the prevalence of which is higher than that of hunger (United Nations 2015b). After the MDGs were revised to form the Sustainable Development Goals (SDGs) for 2030, ending hunger and improving nutrition had been retained as a goal. The SDG report has also highlighted the importance of improving nutrition and its role in achieving other SDGs (United Nations 2015a). In this section, we discuss some of the measures that can be taken to prevent and manage childhood obesity in LMICs.

While designing any intervention for the prevention of childhood obesity (whether implemented by the government/ non-government organisation or individuals), it is imperative that these interventions consider a holistic approach to systematically manage the concern. All over the world, research in the last few decades have provided evidence that health is affected by the social, economic, political and cultural environment (Carey and Crammond 2015). In other words, several factors, beginning from personal causes to the wider environmental conditions need to be addressed in order to tackle issues such as childhood obesity.

Research has indicated that children from disadvantaged backgrounds or lower socio-economic groups receive lesser benefit from interventions as compared to children from affluent backgrounds or higher socio-economic background (Pearce et al. 2019). Hence, interventions for the prevention of childhood obesity should be designed in such a manner that they do not exaggerate the existing inequalities. The World Health Organization defined the Ottawa Charter in 1986 which defined five main strategies to address social, economic, political and environmental determinants of health (World Health Organization 1986). These strategies can be adapted to tackle childhood obesity in LMICs. These are:

- Build healthy public policy
- Create supportive environments for health
- Strengthen community action for health
- Develop personal skills
- Reorient health services

Build Healthy Public Policy

It has been found that multiple components are required in order to develop an effective and sustainable policy in any country. These include the availability of evidence to justify the policy, evidence-based advocacy by civil society organisations as well as individuals' and political will (Pérez-Escamilla et al. 2017). Fiscal policies (such as taxing unhealthy food items) can be strong tools for bringing behaviour change to address the risk factors of childhood obesity. They can play a key role in incentivizing the population to adopt healthy habits and at the same time generate revenue for the government (World Health Organization 2015). Introducing taxes and levies on unhealthy food items can increase their market price significantly, which has been evidenced to influence their purchasing. This results in a decrease in the consumption of unhealthy food and subsequently improved health outcomes (Colchero et al. 2016; Hu 2013; Sharma et al. 2014). In addition, adding taxes to food items can be an encouragement for the manufacturing companies to produce healthier food options in order to sustain the market (Briggs et al. 2016). Figure 2 shows the pathways for the effect of fiscal policies interventions (World Health Organization 2015).

Other required policies to control the risk factors for childhood obesity include control of the marketing of unhealthy food items, restriction on the sale of unhealthy foods in and around educational institutes and compulsory nutritional labelling in a manner which is easily understood by all age groups.

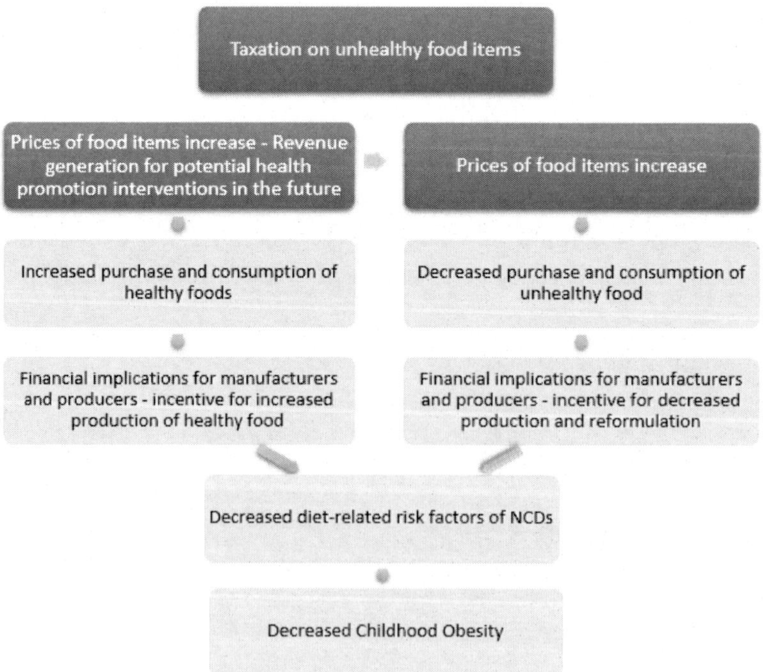

Figure 2. The pathways for the effect of fiscal policies interventions (World Health Organisation 2015).

Case Study: Taxes on Sugar-Sweetened Beverages (SSBs) and Food Items in Mexico (World Health Organization 2015)

Mexico has one of the highest prevalence of childhood obesity. 30% of all children and adolescents were estimated to be obese in Mexico. Further, the country had the highest consumption of SSBs – 160 litres per capita. 71% of the consumption of added sugar comes from SSBs (Sánchez-Pimienta et al. 2016). To combat the rising concern of obesity in the country, the Mexican government implemented two taxes in 2014:

(a) 1 peso per litre excise duty on any non-alcoholic drink with added sugar

(b) 8% ad valorem tax[1] on non-essential energy-dense food items (including snacks, confectionery products, chocolates as well as puddings, flans, ice-creams, candies and peanut butter)

Post levying of the taxes, studies have been conducted on its effectiveness to reduce the consumption of unhealthy food items. For example, a study reported that after the tax was levied in the country, 6% drop in the sale of SSBs was found (Colchero et al. 2016).

Create Supportive Environments for Health

As discussed in the earlier sections, numerous elements contribute to the presence of an obesogenic environment around a child. A variety of factors influence the environment including political and commercial factors (trade agreements, fiscal and agricultural policies and local systems), built environment (availability of unhealthy food items in school cafeterias, lack of infrastructure for physical activity), social and cultural norms of a community and knowledge, attitude and practices of other members of the family (World Health Organization 2016). Adopting measures, both upstream and downstream to change the surrounding environment will help address the rising prevalence of childhood obesity. This can be done by implementing policies which promote a healthy food environment. For example, levying a tax on SSBs, banning unhealthy food in and around schools etc.

Strengthen Community Action for Health

Community-based interventions are required in order to approach childhood obesity across all sectors of society. School-based interventions have been effective in bringing a positive behaviour change (Bassi et al. 2019). It is also imperative that stronger alliances are formed between the health and education sector to cohesively address the issue of childhood obesity (Langford et al. 2015). It is also beneficial that researchers should work with the education sector in order to develop evidence for interventions that work to

---

[1] charging a tax in proportion to the estimated value of the good.

address the concern so that it can be scaled and used in the future to inform better government policies.

Develop Personal Skills

Children and parents should be taught about nutrition and the importance of physical activities. All members of the society need to understand the importance of healthy body size, physical activity, sleep behaviours and appropriate time expenditure on indoor activities such as television watching, time spent on the internet and mobile phones, etc. (World Health Organization 2016). Community members, including parents and school children, should also be taught to read nutritional labels that accompany packaged food items.

Reorient Health Services

There is an urgent need to work across various sectors of health in order to detect and manage the underlying causes of childhood obesity at the earliest. There should be provisions for screening and management of existing cases of diabetes and hypertension in pregnant females to allow for its timely management so that the unborn child is least affected. Gestational weight gain should be properly monitored as well as managed (World Health Organization 2016). Furthermore, there should be provisions for nutritional guidance for expectant parents. This would particularly be useful in LMICs which have a lot of traditional and cultural misconceptions with respect to the diet and nutrition of infant, children as well as adolescents.

Strategies and Successful Interventions for Prevention and Management of Childhood Obesity

National Strategies and Successful Interventions from the South-East Asia Region

Bhutan

The National Adolescent Health Strategic Action Plan 2013-18 emphasized on holistic health care and development of the Bhutanese adolescents and youths by introducing healthy food items in school cafeterias; ban on sale of junk foods and soft drinks in school campuses; availability of healthier options like fresh fruits, whole grains and pulses at affordable prices, educating adolescents on importance of healthy food through life-skills training; developing separate guidelines for educating teachers and parents on healthy eating; involving adolescents, teachers, and parents to develop healthy eating behaviour through group efforts; engaging adolescents in translating healthy habits developed in schools to their homes and communities (Department of Public Health Ministry of Health Bhutan).

Thailand

The "Healthy People Healthy Thailand" strategy focused on improving diet and physical activity by combining knowledge development, social marketing campaigns, collaborative partnerships and policy changes. The strategy is coordinated and monitored by the Ministry of Health at the national level and encourages the development of supportive policies at the local level. Similar initiatives related to both food policy (e.g., providing healthy menus in children's centres, ensuring local government activities to encourage fruit and vegetable consumption) and fitness policy (e.g., awareness programs, physical activity promotion in schools) have been undertaken. These were backed by an extensive social marketing campaign in schools and workplaces using media and other communication tools (World Health Organisation 2009).

Sri Lanka

The Food-Based Dietary Guidelines 2011 issued in Sri Lanka were developed by the Nutrition Division of the Ministry of Health, in consultation with various government ministries, universities, nutrition associations and institutes, consumer and non-government organizations, and with the support from the World Health Organization and UNICEF. The guidelines emphasized on targeted catering services in educational and government institutions to ensure that fruits and vegetables are strictly included in meals (Nutrition Division Ministry of Health Sri Lanka 2011).

India

To combat the rising wave of obesity among children and adolescents, various initiatives have been taken by the central and state governments in India. Various policies and guidelines have been issued to educational institutions for providing a healthy and supportive environment to reduce consumption of unhealthy diet by students. The Ministry of Women and Child Development (WCD), Government of India addressed the issue of consumption of Foods High in Fat, Salt and Sugar (HFSS) and promotion of healthy snacks in schools of India. They gave the recommendations to reduce the availability and consumption of HFSS foods (Ministry of Women and Child Development Government of India 2015). Apart from this, the Food Safety and Standard Authority of India (FSSAI) issued the draft guidelines "*Guidelines for making available wholesome, nutritious, safe and hygienic food to school children in India*" stating that HFFS foods must be restricted in schools and within 50-meter radius of the school boundaries (FSSAI, 2015). The Central Board of Secondary Education (CBSE) issued a notice to all the schools to promote a healthy food environment. These advisories include:

1. Schools are required to ensure that there is no availability of HFFS foods in the school canteens
2. Necessary steps need to be taken by the schools to ensure non-availability of HFSS around 200 meters of the school;
3. Shops and restaurants selling proprietary foods within the vicinity of 200 meters of a school should not be permitted to sell these foods to school children in uniform;
4. Schools need to constitute the School Canteen Management Committee including teacher, parent(s), student(s) and school canteen operator(s) as members;
5. Awareness generating events regarding nutritious foods and avoidance of HFSS foods, like the celebration of Nutrition Week (1-7th September) and other such occasions may be organized throughout the year by the schools
6. Inspection of lunch boxes to rule out the consumption of unhealthy foods may be done by the schools (Central Board of Secondary Education 2018).

At the University level, after receiving a directive from the Ministry of Human Resource Development, the University Grant Commission issued an advisory to higher education institutions to ban the sale of junk food on their campuses (University Grants Commission 2018).

Case Study: School-based Obesity Reduction Programme in India

Obesity Reduction and Awareness of Non-Communicable Disease through Group Education (ORANGE) program is a school-based intervention aimed at healthy lifestyle practices for adolescents (10-13 years; n = 2345). This programme was conducted in private and government schools of Chennai (India). It involved utilizing teachers, doctors and parents to create a supportive school environment. In order to encourage behaviour modification, various awareness-raising activities for teachers and schoolchildren were introduced into the school curriculum, including diet recommendations, physical activity counselling, advice regarding lifestyle modification and yoga demonstrations. These were delivered with the help of non-government organizations and trained volunteers. The program evaluation found a decrease in waist circumference and waist-hip ratios, changes in attitudes and family habits, and levels of physical activities in students from intervention schools in comparison with students from the control schools (Ranjani et al. 2013).

Bangladesh

In Bangladesh, to raise awareness on healthy lifestyles (such as healthy eating habits among school children), strategies were adopted including publication of leaflets and special diet book, demonstrations, implementation of school board cafeteria policies, to ensure that young people consume more nutritious and less unhealthy foods (Thakur et al. 2016).

Example of Low-Cost Intervention for Managing Childhood Obesity in LMICs

A community-based controlled trial was conducted in a metropolitan city of North India. It aimed at assessing the effectiveness of a school-based, low-cost nutrition and lifestyle education intervention on behaviour modification and risk profile of Asian Indian adolescents (15–17 years) in the city. The intervention consisted of multiple components, including nutrition education lectures, promotion of physical activity, individual counselling by a trained nutritionist, increased availability of healthier food choices in the school canteen, the involvement of teachers and parents and a broad range of other activities to promote a healthy lifestyle. Subsequently, the evaluation of the programme found increased nutrition and physical activity knowledge, healthier behaviours, and improved anthropometric outcomes among children in the intervention school compared to the control group (Singhal et al. 2010).

Maldives

Multi-sectoral action plan for the prevention and control of non-communicable diseases of Maldives (2016-2020), emphasized on promotion of healthy foods and food habits in schools and the general population. This was suggested to be done through a ban on sale of unhealthy foods in school canteens or on unhealthy food brought into school by students or staff; regular monitoring of nutritional deficiencies in students by school authorities; and banning of foods high in saturated fat, sugar, and salt from school premises (Policy Planning and International Health Division Ministry of Health Maldives 2015).

Other International Efforts and Best Practices from Developed Countries

INFORMAS (International Network for Food and Obesity/Non-communicable Diseases Research, Monitoring and Action Support) is a global network of public-interest organizations and researchers aiming to monitor, benchmark and support public and private sector actions to increase healthy food environments, reduce obesity and NCDs (along with their related inequalities). INFORMAS supports the WHO's Global Action Plan for the Prevention and Control of Non-Communicable Diseases (2013-2020) ("International Network for Food and Obesity/Non-Communicable Diseases Research Monitoring and Action Support").

EPODE stands for ensemble-prévenons-lobésité-des-enfants meaning "Together Let's Prevent Childhood Obesity," a community initiative launched in 2004 in 10 towns of France, to reduce childhood obesity through a societal process. The primary EPODE target groups are children aged 0–12 years, their families, as well as a wide variety of local stakeholders who can initiate micro-changes in children and their families through local initiatives fostering better and balanced eating habits and greater physical activity in everyday life. EPODE methodology promotes the involvement of multiple stakeholders at the central level (ministries, health groups, NGOs and private partners) and at a local level (political leaders, health professionals, families, teachers, local NGOs, and the local business community) (Borys et al. 2012). Broadly, to tackle obesity in the European level, five goals including objectives and actions have been decided:

- Controlling sales in institutions to ensure that only healthy food is sold in schools and preschools
- Control on the advertising of food and drinks on television, the internet and in schools
- Mandatory nutritional information labelling that is clear and easy for the consumer to understand
- Common agricultural policy reforms and subsidies on healthy foods, i.e., fruit and vegetables
- Improve the training of health professionals so that they are able to recognize and diagnose obesity risks in infancy, childhood, and adolescence. It is also important that professionals are able to offer advice without appearing prejudiced or patronizing.

Canadian initiative to prevent childhood obesity is a framework for action comprised of three integrated strategies ("Curbing Childhood Obesity A Federal, Provincial and Territorial Framework for Action to Promote Healthy Weights"): 1) Making childhood overweight and obesity a collective priority for action for Ministers of Health and/or health promotion/healthy living. They will champion this issue and encourage shared leadership and joint and/or complementary action from government departments and other sectors of Canadian society; 2) Measuring and reporting on collective progress in reducing childhood overweight and obesity, learning from successful initiatives, and modifying approaches as appropriate and ; 3) Coordinating efforts on three key policy priorities:

- *Supportive environment*: making a social and physical environment where children live, learn and play while being more supportive of physical activity and healthy eating.
- *Early action*: identifying the risk of overweight and obesity in children and addressing it early on; and

- *Nutritious food*: looking at ways to increase the availability and accessibility of nutritious food and decrease the marketing of foods and beverages high in fat, sugar, and/or sodium to children.

The APPLE School was an innovative, school-focused health promotion initiative in Canada. The programme implemented healthy eating and active living policies, practices and strategies while engaging students, parents, schools' staff and other stakeholders. The Apple Schools programme was found to be a cost-effective intervention for obesity prevention and for the reduction of chronic disease risk over the lifetime of children (Ekwaru et al. 2017).

White House Task Force on Childhood Obesity Report ("Solving the Problem of Childhood Obesity Within a Generation: White House Task Force on Childhood Obesity Report to the President" 2010): This report presents a series of 70 specific recommendations. Summarizing them broadly herein, they include:

- Getting children, a healthy start on life, with good prenatal care for their parents; support for breastfeeding; adherence to limits on "screen time;" and quality child care settings with nutritious food and ample opportunity for young children to be physically active.
- Empowering parents and caregivers with simpler, more actionable messages about nutritional choices based on the Dietary Guidelines for Americans; improved labels on food and menus that provide clear information to help make healthy choices for children; reduced marketing of unhealthy products to children; and improved health care services, including BMI measurement for all children.
- Providing healthy food in schools, through improvements in federally-supported school lunches and breakfasts; upgrading the nutritional quality of other food sold in schools, and improving nutrition education and the overall school environment.
- Improving access to healthy, affordable food, by eliminating "food deserts" in urban and rural America; lowering the relative prices of healthier food; developing or reformulating food products to be healthier; and reducing the incidence of hunger, which has been linked to obesity.
- Getting children more physically active, through quality physical education, recess, and other opportunities in and after school; addressing aspects of the "built environment" that make it difficult for children to walk or bike safely in their communities; and improving access to safe parks, playgrounds, and indoor and outdoor recreational facilities.

New South Wales (NSW) Government plan for Preventing Overweight and Obesity in children, young people & their families to stop the growth of childhood obesity with the following aims (NSW Department of Health 2009):

- Restoring the energy balance for the NSW population, with a specific focus on children, young people, and their families;
- Reducing the factors that give rise to an obesogenic environment;
- Increasing community understanding and action around managing obesity risks; and
- Providing a platform for action through which Government can drive the change process in partnership with industry, the not-for-profit sector and communities.

Pick a Tick Initiative in Australia by National Heart Foundation nutrition experts, consumer advocacy groups, and food industry leaders are encouraging the development of simplified front-of-package nutritional labelling schemes that complement nutrition panels and also allow consumers to quickly compare the content of nutrients (e.g., energy, total/saturated fat, sugar, sodium, and fiber). The "Pick the Tick" symbols made it easier for consumers to identify healthier food choices (Young and Swinburn 2002).

Model School Tuckshop Programme (MSTP) in Singapore was developed as a way of creating a healthy and nutritional school environment, to allow for students' access to healthy food. The program intervention included restriction of unhealthy food sold in tuck shops, provision of various fruits, and indirect nutritional education with the promotion of healthy food products. The program evaluation indicated that among the students who utilized the tuck shop, about 40% purchased fruit products, showing that the availability of healthy foods in the tuck shop increased their consumption by the students. Overall, food purchase and intake patterns did not significantly change during the intervention period. However, students from the intervention schools reported higher satisfaction with the healthy food products sold in the tuck shop than did those from the control schools (all $P < 0.001$). In addition, they were highly satisfied with the educational resources provided to them. In conclusion, the healthy school tuck shop program had a positive effect on the accessibility of healthy food (Kim et al. 2012).

Challenges to Address Childhood Obesity in LMICs

The problem of childhood obesity is one that must be treated as urgent and serious in all geographic locations. It is impossible to ignore the increasing rates of childhood obesity and policy-makers need to recognize their central role as the key agents in addressing the rising epidemic. A failure to act will have major medical, social and economic consequences.

Lack of Sufficient Training

Despite increasing public health research and interventions, childhood obesity remains persistent in developed countries and a growing epidemic health problem in developing countries (Finucane et al. 2011). The WHO guidelines recommend routine assessment of height and weight for all children <5 years. For those children who are identified as overweight, provision should be made for providing counselling to parents and caregivers on nutrition and physical activity promotion. Support should be given for exclusive breastfeeding. Recommendations for children with obesity include a management plan by a referral to a local hospital or clinic (World Health Organization 2017). However, management of obesity is a challenge in LMICs, as there is no assurance that hospitals or clinics have the resources or expertise to treat childhood obesity. Even in high-income countries, it has been reported that only 20% of primary care physicians have the training, time, and resources to initiate structured lifestyle intervention for children with obesity (Kuhle et al., 2015).

Reduced Focus and Attention to Childhood Obesity

In LMIC, another challenge is that the health systems focus more on other health issues like undernutrition and infectious disease. They perceive obesity as less of a problem. Furthermore, the allocation of resources from the government for managing obesity may not be prioritized in these countries.

Research Gaps

In LMICs, there is limited research undertaken on obesity prevention and hence, more intervention trials should be conducted to build evidence-base needed to support obesity prevention and treatment. To address the needs of children in LMICs, the focus should be on a population-based diet and physical activity interventions that promote health throughout the life course.

Data Gaps

There is a lack of surveillance system data to monitor national level overweight and obesity prevalence in all genders and all ages. There is a dearth of data sources and limited access to high-quality data. This is an important gap that requires future efforts. Continued surveillance of obesity and national health outcomes is necessary to monitor and evaluate programs. Routine surveys and surveillance should be encouraged under national health programs to monitor the weight status of the population. Routine collection of data for obesity-related health outcomes through population-based surveys is not encouraged. The data on the economic consequences of childhood obesity is scarce as compared to the economic burden of adult obesity. Also, there is more focus on healthcare expenditure, ignoring other costs. There is a lack of policy-level data on designing food systems and building environment conducive to promoting healthy weight so more research is needed in this direction.

Strategic Actions to Combat Childhood Obesity

There is no single or simple solution to the obesity epidemic. It is a complex problem and hence a multi-faceted approach including a wide range of stakeholders needs to be put in place. The childhood obesity prevention efforts must be closely integrated with other efforts to control the key NCD risk factors, including tobacco and alcohol use, unhealthy diet and physical inactivity. Obesity prevention policies need to be inclusive and equitable, with interventions tailored to suit local contexts. The prevalence of overweight and obesity varies depending on the environment in which children live. The strategies and solutions to address the rising tide of overweight and obesity should focus at the community level to reach across and throughout societies.

Research Needs

Childhood obesity is a strong predictor of adult obesity, which has well-known health and economic consequences, both for the individual and society as a whole (Simmonds et al. 2016). This is strongly associated with comorbidities that contribute to cardiovascular disease and diabetes (Litwin 2014). Therefore, primordial prevention strategies are recommended to encourage children to develop healthy habits early in life and forestall the onset of obesity in later life. New scientific evidence also highlights the need to intervene even before conception and also to reduce the exposure of the pregnant woman, infant, children and adolescent to an obesogenic environment (Hanson and Gluckman 2015;

Hochberg et al. 2011). The prevention research and policy-level data should be a priority to better understand how to design an environment that promotes healthy weight in LMICs. Also, there is a need for more evaluation research on food policy, such as the implementation of taxation on SSBs, or restricted marketing of unhealthy foods to children.

School-Based Interventions

Children are the most effective target group for prevention efforts because diet-related behaviour is established early in life (Birch, Savage, and Ventura 2007; Lytle et al. 2000). Introduction of school-based education programmes and policies to improve food literacy (Hawkes et al. 2015), compulsory physical education classes or breaks (Joseph et al. 2011), availability of nutritious school meals and snacks at subsidized rates in school's canteens (Rathi, Riddell, and Worsley 2018), ban on food high in fat, sugar and salt to children (World Health Organization 2010, 2009), and promotion of locally available healthy food like fruits and vegetables (Rathi N, 2017), are cost-effective interventions to address the childhood obesity. These strategies are likely to be more effective if reinforced through curriculum-based education about healthy diets and physical activity and efforts are made to engage teachers, parents and families. A recent systematic review conducted with an aim to assess the overall effects of school-based obesity prevention interventions concluded strong evidence that supports the effectiveness of school-based interventions in reducing excessive weight gain of children (Liu et al. 2019).

Population-Wide Policies and Initiatives

Policies and initiatives, such as ban on the sale of foods high in fats, sugar and salt, nutrition labelling, increased taxes on HFFS foods, availability of healthy foods at subsidized rates, physical activity policies, and social marketing campaigns should be promoted to alter the food and physical activity environments to make healthier choices, the easier choices.

Policy Support

Obesity prevention interventions should be supported by policies at all levels of government i.e., at national, regional and local. National policies can create a supportive environment, regional policies can facilitate pooling of resources, whereas local tailoring of interventions results in more effective targeted interventions. Global support for obesity prevention can help to address transnational environmental factors, such as creating a healthier food supply.

Global efforts to control childhood obesity

The United Nations Political Declaration of the High-level Meeting of the General Assembly on the Prevention and Control of Non-Communicable Diseases and the World Health Organization (WHO) Global Strategy on Diet, Physical Activity and Health both recognized population-based prevention as essential for addressing the rising burden of NCDs, with specific emphasis on childhood obesity. The World Health Assembly (WHA) in 2004, adopted a Resolution on the Global Strategy on Diet, Physical Activity and Health (DPAS, WHA57.17) to tackle the increasing prevalence and burden of NCDs, and, in particular, global nutrition and physical activity patterns (World Health Organization, 2004). In 2008, subsequently, WHO also developed a framework to facilitate Member States to assess the implementation of DPAS at Member State level (World Health Organization, 2004). In 2011, the General Assembly of the United Nations adopted the political declaration on the prevention and control of NCDs, recognizes the burden of NCDs, including obesity ("Political Declaration of the High-Level Meeting of the General Assembly on the Prevention and Control of Non-Communicable Diseases" 2011). In 2012, the WHA endorsed Resolution (WHA65.6) on a comprehensive implementation plan on maternal and young child nutrition urging the Member States to adopt the implementation plan, including strengthening nutrition policies to tackle the double burden of malnutrition ("Sixty-Fifth World Health Assembly - Resolutions and Proceedings" 2012). The Global Action Plan for Prevention and Control of NCDs 2013-2020 developed with a "whole-population approach" to address worldwide obesity and NCD crisis (WHO 2013). The Director-General of WHO established the high-level Commission on Ending Childhood Obesity (ECHO) to develop a comprehensive, integrated package of recommendations to address childhood obesity (World Health Organization 2016).

Multi-Sectoral Partnership and Engagement

A comprehensive approach involving all relevant stakeholders including governments (national, sub-national and local level), parents, civil society, community members, academic institutions and private sectors is needed for the prevention and treatment of childhood obesity. These sectors can be identified with their clear roles and responsibilities as part of priority setting processes to address the epidemic. The sectors outside the health system, including food and agriculture, transportation, labour, trade, education, sports and mass communications should also be engaged.

Addressing Vulnerable Groups

The national policies, programmes and strategies addressing childhood obesity in LMICs should specifically address the needs of vulnerable groups. Children with disabilities and other high-risk groups, who are more susceptible to obesity should not be overlooked. Specific strategies and interventions should be designed catering to these vulnerable groups.

Monitoring and Surveillance

Surveillance, monitoring and evaluation are key to support effective action to combat the epidemic. Robust surveillance and monitoring systems should be established to understand the nature of the problem in the context of intervention and for providing data for policy development. Surveillance systems using standardized methods and tools should be developed. The current systems in the majority of the countries assess individual-level patterns of body mass index (BMI), diet, and physical activity behaviours and often lack policy and environmental-related data. The surveillance system should also incorporate environmental measures and biologic outcomes. Measures such as waist circumference, that more accurately track obesity risk, should be added. Nationwide database on trends in obesity and related comorbidities should be maintained. The surveillance system for obesity should be integrated into the existing national surveillance systems with the development of a common reporting framework.

Dedicated Funding

Implementation of childhood obesity prevention programs and initiatives require dedicated funding. The funds generated through taxes on tobacco, alcohol, unhealthy foods and non-alcoholic beverages should also be utilized for obesity prevention programs.

Conclusion

There is no doubt that childhood obesity is a serious public health concern of the 21st century. It has reached serious proportions in a lot of countries. Obesity combined with the burden of malnutrition is posing a serious challenge in the progress of lower and middle-income countries. Health impacts of childhood obesity are negating the factors that are now responsible for prolonged longevity. Health-care associated costs of childhood obesity is a serious burden on the public health systems of many of these lower and middle-income countries. In order to effectively address the causes and determinants of this health concern, it is imperative that these factors are first understood in the context of LMICs. For instance, the relationship between socio-economic position and childhood obesity is not the same in all countries. While in developed nations, there is an inverse relationship, in developing nations, this relationship differs. Children from high socio-economic position are more prone to obesity rather than children from disadvantaged backgrounds. At the same time, nutrient-deficient food eaten by low SEP children is also contributing to the increased prevalence of diseases. Hence, it is imperative that all obesity prevention policies need to be inclusive and equitable, with interventions tailored to suit local contexts. Further, moving forward, we also need to consider recent evidence and strategic methods to combat the concern as effectively as possible. For instance, the recent Lancet report on the Global Syndemic recommends tackling obesity comprehensively in the context of undernutrition, obesity as well as climate change (Swinburn et al. 2019).

To conclude, ending childhood obesity would require a collaborative and cohesive effort across various sectors of the population. Collated efforts by the government, civil society organisations, communities, parents, teachers and students would promote a positive and healthy environment for children to thrive. In line with the recommendations mentioned in the World Health Organization's Report on Ending Childhood Obesity, it is high time for the governments of LMICs to take stringent action. We need to adopt measures such as mandating proper labelling of packaged food items, implementing taxes on unhealthy food items, controlling the marketing of unhealthy food items, establishing cooperation between countries to control the impact of cross-border marketing of unhealthy food, promoting community based interventions and strengthening health systems to manage childhood obesity in an efficient manner (World Health Organization, 2016). Inspiring changes at social, economic, political and environmental level would assist the lower and middle income countries in putting an end to this epidemic.

REFERENCES

Bassi, Shalini, Vinay K. Gupta, MinHae Park, Gaurang P. Nazar, Tina Rawal, Soumyadeep Bhaumik, Kanwal Preet Kochhar, and Monika Arora. 2019. "School Policies, Built Environment and Practices for Non-Communicable Disease (NCD) Prevention and Control in Schools of Delhi, India." Edited by Santosh Kumar Tadakamadla. *PLOS ONE* 14 (4): e0215365. https://doi.org/10.1371/journal. pone.0215365.

Birch, Leann, Jennifer S Savage, and Alison Ventura. 2007. "Influences on the Development of Children's Eating Behaviours: From Infancy to Adolescence." *Canadian Journal of Dietetic Practice and Research : A Publication of Dietitians of Canada = Revue Canadienne de La Pratique et de La Recherche En Dietetique : Une*

Publication Des Dietetistes Du Canada 68 (1): s1–56. http://www.ncbi.nlm.nih.gov/pubmed/19430591.

Borys, J. M., Y. Le Bodo, S. A. Jebb, J. C. Seidell, C. Summerbell, D. Richard, S. De Henauw, et al. 2012. "EPODE Approach for Childhood Obesity Prevention: Methods, Progress and International Development." *Obesity Reviews* 13 (4): 299–315. https://doi.org/10.1111/j.1467-789X.2011.00950.x.

Borzekowski, Dina L.G., and Pedro P. Pires. 2018. "A Six Country Study of Young Children's Media Exposure, Logo Recognition, and Dietary Preferences." *Journal of Children and Media* 12 (2): 143–58. https://doi.org/10.1080/17482798.2018. 1425730.

Bridle-Fitzpatrick, Susan. 2015. "Food Deserts or Food Swamps?: A Mixed-Methods Study of Local Food Environments in a Mexican City." *Social Science and Medicine* 142 (October): 202–13. https://doi.org/10.1016/j.socscimed.2015.08.010.

Briggs, Adam D M, Oliver T. Mytton, A Kehlbacher, R Tiffin, A Elhussein, M Rayner, S Jebb, A Blakely, and P Scarborough. 2016. "A Health Impact Assessment of the UK Soft Drinks Industry Levy: A Comparative Risk Assessment Modelling Study." *Lancet Public Health* In press (1): e15–22. https://doi.org/10.1016/S2468-2667 (16)30037-8.

Carey, Gemma, and Brad Crammond. 2015. "Action on the Social Determinants of Health: Views from inside the Policy Process." *Social Science and Medicine* 128: 134–41. https://doi.org/10.1016/j.socscimed.2015.01.024.

"*Central Board of Secondary Education, Delhi Notice.*" 2018. 2018. www.cbseacademic.nic.in.

Colchero, M Arantxa, Barry M Popkin, Juan A Rivera, and Shu Wen Ng. 2016. "*Beverage Purchases from Stores in Mexico under the Excise Tax on Sugar Sweetened Beverages : Observational Study*," 1–9. https://doi.org/10.1136/bmj. h6704.

"*Curbing Childhood Obesity A Federal, Provincial and Territorial Framework for Action to Promote Healthy Weights.*" n.d. Accessed February 25, 2020. https://www.canada.ca/content/dam/phac-aspc/migration/phac-aspc/hp-ps/hl-mvs/framework-cadre/pdf/ccofw-eng.pdf.

Davies, Gemma, Gina Frausin, and Luke Parry. 2017. "Are There Food Deserts in Rainforest Cities?" *Annals of the American Association of Geographers* 107 (4): 794–811. https://doi.org/10.1080/24694452.2016.1271307.

Department of Public Health Ministry of Health Bhutan. n.d. "*National Adolescent Health Strategic Plan 2013-2018.*"

Ekwaru, John Paul, Arto Ohinmaa, Bach Xuan Tran, Solmaz Setayeshgar, Jeffrey A. Johnson, and Paul J. Veugelers. 2017. "Cost-Effectiveness of a School-Based Health Promotion Program in Canada: A Life-Course Modeling Approach." Edited by David Meyre. *PLOS ONE* 12 (5): e0177848. https://doi.org/10.1371/journal.pone.0177848.

Epstein, Leonard H, Elizabeth A Handley, Kelly K Dearing, David D Cho, James N Roemmich, Rocco A Paluch, Samina Raja, Youngju Pak, and Bonnie Spring. 2006.

"Purchases of Food in Youth. Influence of Price and Income." *Psychological Science* 17 (1): 82–89. https://doi.org/10.1111/j.1467-9280.2005.01668.x.

Finucane, Mariel M., Gretchen A. Stevens, Melanie J. Cowan, Goodarz Danaei, John K. Lin, Christopher J. Paciorek, Gitanjali M. Singh, et al. 2011. "National, Regional, and Global Trends in Body-Mass Index since 1980: Systematic Analysis of Health Examination Surveys and Epidemiological Studies with 960 Country-Years and 9·1 Million Participants." *The Lancet* 377 (9765): 557–67. https://doi.org/10.1016/ S0140-6736(10)62037-5.

Fox, Ashley, Wenhui Feng, and Victor Asal. 2019. "What Is Driving Global Obesity Trends? Globalization or 'Modernization'?" *Globalization and Health* 15 (1): 32. https://doi.org/10.1186/s12992-019-0457-y.

FSSAI. n.d. "*Guidelines for Making Available Wholesome, Nutritious, Safe and Hygienic Food to School Children in India*."

Gortmaker, Steven L., Aviva Must, James M. Perrin, Arthur M. Sobol, and William H. Dietz. 1993. "Social and Economic Consequences of Overweight in Adolescence and Young Adulthood." *New England Journal of Medicine* 329 (14): 1008–12. https://doi.org/10.1056/NEJM199309303291406.

Gupta, Nidhi, Kashish Goel, Priyali Shah, and Anoop Misra. 2012. "Childhood Obesity in Developing Countries: Epidemiology, Determinants, and Prevention." *Endocrine Reviews*. Oxford Academic. https://doi.org/10.1210/er.2010-0028.

Hanson, M. A., and P. D. Gluckman. 2015. "Developmental Origins of Health and Disease - Global Public Health Implications." *Best Practice and Research: Clinical Obstetrics and Gynaecology* 29 (1): 24–31. https://doi.org/10.1016/j.bpobgyn.2014. 06.007.

Hawkes, Corinna, Trenton G. Smith, Jo Jewell, Jane Wardle, Ross A. Hammond, Sharon Friel, Anne Marie Thow, and Juliana Kain. 2015. "Smart Food Policies for Obesity Prevention." *The Lancet*. Lancet Publishing Group. https://doi.org/10.1016/S0140-6736(14)61745-1.

Hochberg, Z., R. Feil, M. Constancia, M. Fraga, C. Junien, J. C. Carel, P. Boileau, et al. 2011. "Child Health, Developmental Plasticity, and Epigenetic Programming." *Endocrine Reviews. Endocrine Society*. https://doi.org/10.1210/er.2009-0039.

Hu, F. B. 2013. "Resolved: There Is Sufficient Scientific Evidence That Decreasing Sugar-Sweetened Beverage Consumption Will Reduce the Prevalence of Obesity and Obesity-Related Diseases." *Obesity Reviews* 14 (8): 606–19. https://doi.org/10.1111/ obr.12040.

"*International Network for Food and Obesity/Non-Communicable Diseases Research Monitoring and Action Support*." n.d. Accessed February 25, 2020. https://www. informas.org/about-informas/.

Jeffreys, Mona, George Davey Smith, Richard M. Martin, Stephen Frankel, and David Gunnell. 2004. "Childhood Body Mass Index and Later Cancer Risk: A 50-Year

Follow-up of the Boyd Orr Study." *International Journal of Cancer* 112 (2): 348–51. https://doi.org/10.1002/ijc.20423.

Joseph, R. J., M. Alonso-Alonso, D. S. Bond, A. Pascual-Leone, and G. L. Blackburn. 2011. "The Neurocognitive Connection between Physical Activity and Eating Behaviour." *Obesity Reviews* 12 (10): 800–812. https://doi.org/10.1111/j.1467-789X.2011.00893.x.

Karnehed, Nina, Finn Rasmussen, and Malin Kark. 2007. "Obesity in Young Adulthood and Later Disability Pension: A Population-Based Cohort Study of 366,929 Swedish Men." *Scandinavian Journal of Public Health* 35 (1): 48–54. https://doi.org/10.1080/14034940600858524.

Kaur S, Sachdev HP, Dwivedi SN, Lakshmy R, and Kapil U. 2008. "Prevalence of Overweight and Obesity amongst School Children in Delhi, India. - PubMed - NCBI." *Asia Pacific Journal of Clinical Nutrition* 17 (4): 526–96. https://www.ncbi.nlm.nih.gov/pubmed/19114395.

Kim, Kirang, Seo Ah Hong, Sung Ha Yun, Hyun Joo Ryou, Sang Sun Lee, and Mi Kyung Kim. 2012. "The Effect of a Healthy School Tuck Shop Program on the Access of Students to Healthy Foods." *Nutrition Research and Practice* 6 (2): 138–45. https://doi.org/10.4162/nrp.2012.6.2.138.

Kuhle, Stefan, Rachel Doucette, Helena Piccinini-Vallis, and Sara F L Kirk. 2015. "*Successful Childhood Obesity Management in Primary Care in Canada: What Are the Odds*?" https://doi.org/10.7717/peerj.1327.

Kuriyan, Rebecca, Swarnarekha Bhat, Tinku Thomas, Mario Vaz, and Anura V. Kurpad. 2007. "Television Viewing and Sleep Are Associated with Overweight among Urban and Semi-Urban South Indian Children." *Nutrition Journal* 6 (September): 25. https://doi.org/10.1186/1475-2891-6-25.

Langford, Rebecca, Christopher Bonell, Hayley Jones, and Rona Campbell. 2015. "Obesity Prevention and the Health Promoting Schools Framework: Essential Components and Barriers to Success." *International Journal of Behavioral Nutrition and Physical Activity* 12 (1): 15. https://doi.org/10.1186/s12966-015-0167-7.

Larson, Nicole, and Mary Story. 2009. "A Review of Environmental Influences on Food Choices." *Annals of Behavioral Medicine* 38 (S1): 56–73. https://doi.org/10.1007/s12160-009-9120-9.

Litwin, Sheldon E. 2014. "Childhood Obesity and Adulthood Cardiovascular Disease." *Journal of the American College of Cardiology*. Elsevier USA. https://doi.org/10.1016/j.jacc.2014.07.962.

Liu, Zheng, Han Meng Xu, Li Ming Wen, Yuan Zhou Peng, Li Zi Lin, Shuang Zhou, Wen Hao Li, and Hai Jun Wang. 2019. "A Systematic Review and Meta-Analysis of the Overall Effects of School-Based Obesity Prevention Interventions and Effect Differences by Intervention Components." *International Journal of Behavioral*

Nutrition and Physical Activity. BioMed Central Ltd. https://doi.org/10.1186/s12966-019-0848-8.

Lytle, Leslie A., Sara Seifert, Jessica Greenstein, and Paul McGovern. 2000. "How Do Children's Eating Patterns and Food Choices Change over Time? Results from a Cohort Study." *American Journal of Health Promotion* 14 (4): 222–28. https://doi.org/10.4278/0890-1171-14.4.222.

Ministry of Women and Child Development Government of India. 2015. "*Report of Working Group on Addressing Consumption of Foods High in Fat, Salt and Sugar (HFSS) and Promotion of Healthy Snacks in Schools Of.*"

Monteiro, C. A., J. C. Moubarac, G. Cannon, S. W. Ng, and B. Popkin. 2013. "Ultra-Processed Products Are Becoming Dominant in the Global Food System." *Obesity Reviews*. John Wiley & Sons, Ltd. https://doi.org/10.1111/obr.12107.

Neovius, M., M. Kark, and F. Rasmussen. 2008. "Association between Obesity Status in Young Adulthood and Disability Pension." *International Journal of Obesity* 32 (8): 1319–26. https://doi.org/10.1038/ijo.2008.70.

NSW Department of Health. 2009. *NSW Government Plan for Preventing Overweight and Obesity in Children, Young People & Their Families.*

Nutrition Division Ministry of Health Sri Lanka. 2011. "*Food Based Dietary Guidelines for Sri Lankans.*"

Onis, Mercedes de, Monika Blössner, and Elaine Borghi. 2010. "Global Prevalence and Trends of Overweight and Obesity among Preschool Children." *The American Journal of Clinical Nutrition* 92 (5): 1257–64. https://doi.org/10.3945/ajcn.2010. 29786.

Pan American Health Organization. 2011. "*Recommendations from a Pan American Health Organization Expert Consultation on the Marketing of Food and Non-Alcoholic Beverages to Children in the Americas*." Washington DC.

Parsons, T. J., C. Power, S. Logan, and C. D. Summerbell. 1999. "Childhood Predictors of Adult Obesity: A Systematic Review." *International Journal of Obesity*.

Pearce, Anna, Ruth Dundas, Margaret Whitehead, and David Taylor-Robinson. 2019. "Pathways to Inequalities in Child Health." *Archives of Disease in Childhood* 104 (10): 998–1003. https://doi.org/10.1136/archdischild-2018-314808.

Pérez-Escamilla, R., C. K. Lutter, C. Rabadan-Diehl, A. Rubinstein, A. Calvillo, C. Corvalán, C. Batis, et al. 2017. "Prevention of Childhood Obesity and Food Policies in Latin America: From Research to Practice." *Obesity Reviews* 18 (July): 28–38. https://doi.org/10.1111/obr.12574.

Policy Planning and International Health Division Ministry of Health Maldives. 2015. "*Multi-Sectoral Action Plan for the Prevention and Control of Non-Communicable Diseases in Maldives (2016-20).*" http://www.health.gov.mv/Uploads/Downloads/Informations/Informations(48).pdf.

"*Political Declaration of the High-Level Meeting of the General Assembly on the Prevention and Control of Non-Communicable Diseases*." 2011. In. https://digitallibrary.un.org/record/710899?ln=en#record-files-collapse-header.

Popkin, Barry M. 2001. "The Nutrition Transition and Obesity in the Developing World." *The Journal of Nutrition* 131 (3): 871S-873S. https://doi.org/10.1093/jn/131.3.871s.

Popkin, Barry M, Camila Corvalan, and Laurence M Grummer-Strawn. 2020. "Dynamics of the Double Burden of Malnutrition and the Changing Nutrition Reality." *www.thelancet.com* 395. https://doi.org/10.1016/S0140-6736(19)32497-3.

Ranjani, Harish, Jagadesan Sonya, Ranjit M. Anjana, and Viswanathan Mohan. 2013. "Prevalence of Glucose Intolerance Among Children and Adolescents in Urban South India (ORANGE-2)." *Diabetes Technology & Therapeutics* 15 (1): 13–19. https://doi.org/10.1089/dia.2012.0236.

Rathi, Neha, Lynn Riddell, and Anthony Worsley. 2018. "The Role of Indian School Canteens in Nutrition Promotion." *British Food Journal* 120 (1): 196–209. https://doi.org/10.1108/BFJ-05-2017-0275.

Reardon, Thomas, and C. Peter Timmer. 2012. "The Economics of the Food System Revolution." *Annual Review of Resource Economics* 4 (1): 225–64. https://doi.org/10.1146/annurev.resource.050708.144147.

Reilly, J. J., and J. Kelly. 2011. "Long-Term Impact of Overweight and Obesity in Childhood and Adolescence on Morbidity and Premature Mortality in Adulthood: Systematic Review." *International Journal of Obesity*. Nature Publishing Group. https://doi.org/10.1038/ijo.2010.222.

Reilly, J J, E Methven, Z C Mcdowell, B Hacking, D Alexander, and L Stewart. 2003. "Health Consequences of Obesity." *Arch Dis Child* 88: 748–52. https://doi.org/10.1136/adc.88.9.748.

Sánchez-Pimienta, Tania G, Carolina Batis, Chessa K Lutter, and Juan A Rivera. 2016. "Sugar-Sweetened Beverages Are the Main Sources of Added Sugar Intake in the Mexican Population." *The Journal of Nutrition* 146 (9): 1888S-1896S. https://doi.org/10.3945/jn.115.220301.

Schram, Ashley, Ronald Labonte, Phillip Baker, Sharon Friel, Aaron Reeves, and David Stuckler. 2015. "The Role of Trade and Investment Liberalization in the Sugar-Sweetened Carbonated Beverages Market: A Natural Experiment Contrasting Vietnam and the Philippines." *Globalization and Health* 11 (1): 41. https://doi.org/10.1186/s12992-015-0127-7.

Sharma, Anurag, Katharina Hauck, Bruce Hollingsworth, and Luigi Siciliani. 2014. "The Effects of Taxing Sugar-Sweetened Beverages across Different Income Groups." *Health Economics (United Kingdom)* 23 (9): 1159–84. https://doi.org/10.1002/hec.3070.

Simmonds, M., A. Llewellyn, C. G. Owen, and N. Woolacott. 2016. "Predicting Adult Obesity from Childhood Obesity: A Systematic Review and Meta-Analysis." *Obesity Reviews* 17 (2): 95–107. https://doi.org/10.1111/obr.12334.

Singhal, N., A. Misra, P. Shah, and S. Gulati. 2010. "Effects of Controlled School-Based Multi-Component Model of Nutrition and Lifestyle Interventions on Behavior Modification, Anthropometry and Metabolic Risk Profile of Urban Asian Indian Adolescents in North India." *European Journal of Clinical Nutrition* 64 (4): 364–73. https://doi.org/10.1038/ejcn.2009.150.

"*Sixty-Fifth World Health Assembly - Resolutions and Proceedings*." 2012. In.

"*Solving the Problem of Childhood Obesity within a Generation: White House Task Force on Childhood Obesity Report to the President*." 2010.

Swinburn, Boyd A, Vivica I Kraak, Steven Allender, Vincent J Atkins, Phillip I Baker, Jessica R Bogard, Hannah Brinsden, et al. 2019. "The Lancet Commissions The Global Syndemic of Obesity, Undernutrition, and Climate Change: The Lancet Commission Report." *www.thelancet.com*. Vol. 393. https://doi.org/10.1016/S0140-6736(18) 32822-8.

Thakur, JS, Neena Raina, Priya Karna, Preeti Singh, Gursimer Jeet, and Nidhi Jaswal. 2016. "Overview of National Strategies on Noncommunicable Disease and Adolescent Health in South-East Asia Region Countries." *International Journal of Noncommunicable Diseases* 1 (2): 76. https://doi.org/10.4103/2468-8827.191989.

United Nations. 2015a. "*Sustainable Development Goals*." 2015. https://www.un.org/sustainabledevelopment/sustainable-development-goals/.

United Nations . 2015b. "*The Millennium Development Goals Report*."

"*University Grants Commission August 2018. D.O No.14-24/2016 (CPP-II)*." n.d.

WHO. 2013. "Global Action Plan for the Prevention and Control of Noncommunicable Diseases 2013-2020." *World Health Organization*, 102. https://doi.org/9789241506236.

WHO, UNICEF, and The World Bank Group. 2019. "*Joint Child Malnutrition Estimates - Levels and Trends (2019 Edition)*."

Withrow, D., and D. A. Alter. 2011. "The Economic Burden of Obesity Worldwide: A Systematic Review of the Direct Costs of Obesity." *Obesity Reviews*. John Wiley & Sons, Ltd. https://doi.org/10.1111/j.1467-789X.2009.00712.x.

World Health Organisation. n.d. "*Global Strategy on Diet, Physical Activity and Health*."

World Health Organization. 1986. *The Ottawa Charter for Health Promotion*.

World Health Organization. 2009. *Population-Based Prevention Strategies for Childhood Obesity: Report of a WHO Forum and Technical Meeting*, Geneva, 15-17.

Set of Recommendations on the Marketing of Food and Non-Alcoholic Beverages to Children. 2010.

World Health Organization. 2015. *Fiscal Policies for Diet and Prevention of Noncommunicable Diseases: Technical Meeting Report*. Geneva. https://apps.who.int/iris/bitstream/handle/10665/250131/9789241511247-eng.pdf?sequence=1.

World Health Organization. 2015. *Obesity and Overweight Factsheet*. https://www.who.int/news-room/fact-sheets/detail/obesity-and-overweight.

World Health Organization. 2016. *Report of the Commission on Ending Childhood Obesity*. Geneva. https://apps.who.int/iris/bitstream/handle/10665/204176/9789241510066_eng.pdf?sequence=1.

Guidelines for Assessing and Managing Children at Primary Health-Care Facilities to Prevent Overweight and Obesity in the Context of the Double Burden of Malnutrition: Update for the Integrated Management of Childhood Illness Guidelines. 2017.

World Health Organization. 2019. *Facts and Figures on Childhood Obesity*.

Wyatt, Sharon B., Karen P. Winters, and Patricia M. Dubbert. 2006. "Overweight and Obesity: Prevalence, Consequences, and Causes of a Growing Public Health Problem." *American Journal of the Medical Sciences* 331 (4): 166–74. https://doi.org/10.1097/00000441-200604000-00002.

Young, Leanne, and Boyd Swinburn. 2002. "Impact of the Pick the Tick Food Information Programme on the Salt Content of Food in New Zealand." *Health Promotion International* 17 (1): 13–19. https://doi.org/10.1093/heapro/17.1.13.

In: Childhood Obesity
Editor: Roya Kelishadi

ISBN: 978-1-53618-158-6
© 2020 Nova Science Publishers, Inc.

Chapter 2

EPIGENETICS AND CHILDHOOD OBESITY

Sharifeh Khosravi[1], PhD, Sima Jafarpour[2], PhD, Rasoul Salehi[1,*], Motahar Heidari-Beni[3] and Roya Kelishadi[4]

[1]Pediatric Inherited Diseases Research Center, Research Institute for Primordial Prevention of Non-Communicable Disease and Department of Genetics and Molecular Biology, School of Medicine, Isfahan University of Medical Science, Isfahan, Iran

[2]Department of Genetics and Molecular Biology, School of Medicine, Isfahan University of Medical Science, Isfahan, Iran

[3]Department of Nutrition, Child Growth and Development Research Center, Research Institute for Primordial Prevention of Non-Communicable Disease, Isfahan University of Medical Sciences, Isfahan, Iran

[4]Department of Pediatrics, Child Growth and Development Research Center, Research Institute for Primordial Prevention of Non-Communicable Disease, Isfahan University of Medical Sciences, Isfahan, Iran

ABSTRACT

Childhood obesity is a major global health issue which is expected to play a pivotal role in a large number of complications associated with the overweight later in life. Obesity is a complex disease that involves interactions between environmental and genetic factors from early life. However, increasing the prevalence of obesity cannot be only explained by genetic factors so it is possibly mediated by epigenetic processes, a potential factor that

* Corresponding Author's Email: r_salehi@med.mui.ac.ir; rasol_s@yahoo.com.

might explain individual differences in obesity risk. Epigenetic alternations include genomic DNA methylation, changes in chromatic structure through histone modifications and gene expression alternation due to the non-coding RNAs among which DNA methylation and microRNAs have been studied extensively.

Because of the role of epigenetics in childhood obesity, awareness of epigenetic mechanisms may provide the chance of understanding its pathogenesis in more detaile, finding novel diagnostic markers and provide us with robust prevention and treatment modalities.

Keywords: epigenetic, obesity, children

ABBREVIATIONS

CpGs	CG dinucleotides
DNAm	DNA methylation
Dnmts	DNA methyl transferases
BMI	Body Mass Index
CGIs	CpG islands
EWAS	Epigenome wide association studies
IGT	Impaired glucose tolerance
NcRNAs	Non-coding RNA
LncRNAs	Long noncoding RNAs
miRNAs	Micro RNAs
UTR	Untranslated region

INTRODUCTION

Childhood obesity is a major global health issue which is affecting many countries, particularly in urban regions and expanding at an alarming speed. Currently developing countries experiencing the rate of childhood obesity 30% more than the developed ones (1). Early intervention and preventive measures are essential because untreated obese infant and children are more likely to persist in adulthood and come up with sevear metabolic diseases (2). Complications associated with metabolic disorders which itself rooted from childhood obesity affecting many vital organs including cardiovascular, neurological, endocrine, musculoskeletal, renal, gastrointestinal, respiratory systems and reproductive dysfunction later in life (3).

Obesity is a complex disease involving interactions between the genetic and environmental factors. Additionally epigenetic regulators are important determinants of gene regulation as well as integrating environmental signals into the genomic functionality. Dysregulation of epigenetic markings either through inheritance or under influence of environmental factors would end up with aberrant signaling pathways that could explain individual differences in obesity risk (4). Epigenetics can be identified as heritable changes that are mitotically stable and affect gene expression without any changes in the DNA sequence (5). At the molecular level, epigenetic markers include genomic DNA methylation, changes in chromatic structure through histone modifications and alteration of non-coding RNAs expression (6). Because epigenetics is reversible and susceptible to environmental factors with more readily amenable to intervention than genetic factors, therefore underesting of epigenetic phenomena related to initioation and progression of childhood obesity early in infancy and its subsequent effects throughout the individual life span opening up new windows prevent and manage the disease at its very early stage. Since among epigenetic alternations, DNA methylation and microRNAs mediated mechanisms have been studied in more details, here we discuss the epigenetic mechanisms of these two modalities in relation to susceptibility and development of childhood obesity.

DNA Methylation

DNA methylation, the most studied epigenetic modification in human subjects, refers to transfer a methyl group from S-adenosy1-L-methionine (SAM) to the C5 position of cytosine residue, forming 5-methyl-cytosine (5mC) (7).

The processes catalyzed by a family of DNA methyltransferases (Dnmts) including DNMT1, DNMT2, DNMT3A, DNMT3B.

The majority of DNA methylation occurs at the particular dinucleotide sites called CpGs islands (CGIs). These CGIs composed of short sequences of DNA with a high linear frequency of 5′-CpG-3′ sequences and are often abundant in promoters region or enhancer elements. Evidence has revealed that hypermethylation of CpG islands is related to epigenetic silencing; conversely, DNA hypomethylation leads to gene transcription (8). DNA methylations function in gene regulation is dependent on the genomic CpG context. DNA methylation in the gene promoters has different effects on gene silencing (9), and gene body regions methylation is highly correlated with gene transcription (10).

DNA Methylation and Childhood Obesity

There is growing evidence that DNA methylation might contribute to adiposity and obesity. Indeed, several studies in animal and human models have shown methylation changes in promoters of various genes that are involved in appetite control, metabolism, obesity and growth. In other words the association between DNA methylation and childhood obesity has been proven potent for several pathways and genes (11). However the mechanisms of epigenetic changes may be altered by a variety of exposures, and evidence suggests that they function at several points of time prior to conception, during pregnancy, postnatal period and during childhood. Epigenetic alternation, have also been linked with birth weight, early childhood, and adolescent obesity (12).

Like other fields, several studies of limited candidate loci have revealed associations between DNA methylation and obesity. Association of DNA methylation status at particular loci have been assessed with a range of environmental exposures and obesity. Given this, epigenetic modification is likely to occur at a network or pathway level, analyzing of an isolated gene is unlikely to give a complete picture. Focusing on one locus, however, allowed a thorough evaluation of the potential causal pathway. However epigenome wide association studies (EWAS) are of more interest due to identifying novel genes and pathways related to childhood obesity and obesity-induced complications (13).

DNA Methylation during Prenatal and Postnatal Period and Childhood Obesity

Epigenetic changes usually occurs during prenatal development (often called "fetal metabolic programming) or postnatal period. Several studies based on pre-conceptual, in utero, and postnatal developmental environment showed an impact on the long term risk in adult-onset obesity through a set point of epigenetic changes. It could be understood as a "vital period" where exposure to adverse conditions during this period may greatly impacted later adiposity and metabolic risk (14).

Maternal overweight and excessive gestational weight gain are considered risk factors for many adverse offspring outcomes over the short and long term. Sharp GC et al. (15) evaluated epigenome-wide DNA methylation in relation to maternal and offspring adiposity in 1018 participants. They found that comparing with offspring of mothers with normal weight several differentially methylated CpG sites (28 and 1621 CpG sites) were differentially methylated in cord blood of offspring of obese and underweight mothers, respectively with no overlap in the sites. Associations of maternal obesity with offspring methylation were stronger than associations of paternal obesity, supporting importance of intrauterine mechanisms. In this study there were no consistent associations of gestational weight gain with offspring DNA methylation. In general, sites that were hypermethylated in association with maternal obesity or hypomethylated in association with maternal underweight tended to be positively associated with offspring adiposity, and sites hypomethylated in association with maternal obesity or hypermethylatedin association with maternal underweight tended to be inversely associated with offspring adiposity (15).

These findings support previously postulated effect of maternal adiposity on the offspring epigenome which leading to the induction of obesity (16).

Maternal malnutrition exposure in utero may also lead to greater adiposity in later life which epigenetic modification is suggested as a probable mediating mechanism (17). Among candidate genes, one of the main genes of interest investigated in more than one report regarding maternal under nutrition and DNA methylation in the offspring which has been associated with risk of early-onset obesity is *IGF2*. This gene is maternally imprinted and is a key factor in human growth and development (18).

Maternal diet could also alter offspring body composition, accompanied by epigenetic changes in metabolic control genes. Godfrey KM et al. study findings suggest a substantial components of metabolic disease risk has a prenatal developmental basis. In this study after measuring the methylation status of CpGs from five candidate genes in umbilical cord tissue DNA from healthy neonates, it was found that greater methylation of *RXRA* at birth was strongly correlated with greater adiposity in later childhood. *RXRA* encodes retinoid X receptor A, which regulates the transcription of many genes involved in energy metabolism, adipocyte differentiation, and adipogenes is to a large extent via heterodimerization with the nuclear receptor *PPARG* (19).

Maternal glycemia can also affect DNA methylation in the offspring; this seems to be locus and/or site specific and also might differ depending on the level of hyperglycemic exposure (20). Gestational impaired glucose tolerance (IGT) during pregnancy is associated with leptin gene DNA methylation modification in offspring. These epigenetic variations supply novel mechanisms contributing to explaining the adverse health effects associated with long term programming, such as increased risk of excessive adiposity and developing obesity (21). Leptin is an adipokine which is mainly produced by the adipose tissue and it has a key role in regulating energy balance. Leptin increasing in the perinatal period has an important role in programming long-term risk of obesity. Further it has been made clear that leptin levels in cord blood were associated with adiposity at 3 y of age (22).

Low birth-weight, premature birth, intrauterine growth retardation has been also related to increased risk of obesity later in life. After evaluation of fetal weight association and methylation status of *LINE-1*, a highly repeated and widely interspersed human retrotransposon, in 319 fetal cord blood samples, it was found that newborns with low or high birth-weight had significantly lower *LINE-1* methylation levels in their cord blood compared to normal weight infants as well as among prematurely born infants. A decrease in *LINE-1* methylation may contribute to retro-transposition events mediated by this repetitive element which lead to mutagenesis by insertion, result in gene dysregulation or even alteration of gene coding sequences (23).

Nutritional, growth and weight gain status in early neonatal life have been shown to affect metabolic health across the lifespan. Postnatal rapid weight gain is associated with a subsequent increase in the risk of obesity and cardiovascular disease in later in life. As a result of study which focused on a single locus, postnatal growth and childhood adiposity were associated with altered *TACSTD2* gene expression and its promoter methylation (24). The *TACSTD2* gene encodes a cell-surface glycoprotein that is implicated in cell proliferation (25).

Association of DNA methylation states at particular loci have been assessed with a range of environmental exposures and obesity. One of locus which is repeated positively associated with BMI in several studies is hypoxia inducible factor 3A (*HIF3A*). Determination of *HIF3A* genotype and DNA methylation patterns in DNA extracted from umbilical cords of 991 infants has been shown that higher methylation levels at three CpGs in the *HIF3A at* first intron were associated with infant greater weight and adiposity. However the prenatal environmental variables which were examined in this study including exercise during pregnancy, alcohol usage before and during pregnancy, smoking patterns before and during pregnancy and maternal pregnancy BMI were not consistently associated with *HIF3A* methylation and birth weight (26).

It is noteworthy that in several EWAS-based studies it was detected differential methylation at *HIF3A* gene locus that has been detected in obese adults and children (27). However in a large EWAS in obese adults and children, it was not detected differential methylation at *HIF3A* gene locus.

There is increasing evidence that breastfeeding and its duration also has short and long-term benefits on human health. The peculiar components of human breast milk are thought to induce epigenetic changes and mediated lowering risk of a range of phenotypes including obesity (28).

To date, several studies have examined the association between breastfeeding and DNAm levels but a few studies have reported a significant association between breastfeeding and its duration and childhood obesity later. In one of these studies, Obermann-Borst et al. found that breastfeeding duration was significantly associated with a reduction in methylation of the leptin gene (*LEP*) in whole blood DNA in young children (29)]. However it has been proven that leptin is a breast milk component which prevents of obesity so that decreased production of *LEP* is associated with obesity (30, 31).

In another study, after evaluation of the effect of breastfeeding duration on infant growth and methylation in obesity-related genes (*RXRA, LEP, IGF2,* and *DNMT1)*, a significant difference was found between infant growth and buccal *RXRA* and *LEP* methylation at 12 months of breastfeeding. It is noted that selection of genes in this study was based on previous studies and their role in fat metabolism, appetite control, growth, and maintenance of DNA methylation status (32). These results support the hypothesis that epigenetic changes could induce by breastfeeding and particularly duration of it in infants.

Other genes has been suggested that breastfeeding might be associated with promoter methylation of them is *Pomc*, *Npy* and *Slc2a4* genes which higher gene expression levels of *Pomc* and *Slc2a4* genes and lower levels of the *Npy* gene in breastfed individuals might protect against obesity and diabetes (33).

Epigenome Wide Association Studies (EWAS) and Childhood Obesity

Ding et al. performed comprehensive DNA methylation profiling of gene promoters at CGIs and showed that specific DNA methylation profiles in blood differ between obese and control subjects (34). They found 251 promoters and 575 CGIs were demethylated, and 141 promoters and 277 CGIs were hypermethylated in obese children.

They analyzed the top promoters or CGIs that had significant differences in the degree of methylation between obese and lean children and found that out of these promoter and CGIs-related genes, only a few (*CDH15, GAD2, MAF, ESRRG, RXFP3, ASAM*, and *ZIC4*) were reported to be associated with the regulation of insulin and satiety or adipocyte differentiation and among these epigenetic markers, there were 10 demethylated and 15 hypermethylated gene promoters that have been previously studied, almost all of which are involved in the pathogenesis of cancers.

In another study DNA methylation profiles in whole blood from 78 obese children and 71 age- and sex-matched controls were assessed. Comparison of the methylation profiles between obese and control subjects revealed 129 differentially methylated CpG (DMCpG) loci associated with 80 unique genes that had a greater than 10% difference in methylation. The top pathways enriched among the DMCpGs included developmental processes, regulation of cell signaling, immune system regulation, and small GTPase-mediated signal transduction. In the following associations between the methylation of CpGs that were differentially methylated with respect to obesity with having a difference of methylation of above 10%, were validated across loci within the *FYN, PIWIL4*, and *TAOK3* genes. *FYN* is a member of the family of non-receptor tyrosine kinases and plays an important role in inflammation, adipocyte differentiation and function, energy consumption, and insulin signaling. *PIWIL4*, which belongs to the Argonaute protein family, may be a regulator of $p16^{INK4a}$, a known regulator of adipocyte proliferation and differentiation and it seems that *TAOK3* is involved in glucose tolerance and insulin sensitivity, at least in part through adipose tissue (35).

In another study body composition and genome-wide DNAm in whole blood were assessed in 374 pre-school children from four European countries. Specific DNAm variants were identified to be associated with BMI (212), fat-mass (230), and fat-free-mass (120). Among them methylation in 13 genes including *SNED1* (*IRE-BP1*), *KLHL6*, *WDR51A* (*POC1A*), *CYTH4-ELFN2*, *CFLAR*, *PRDM14*, *SOS1*, *ZNF643*(*ZFP69B*), *ST6GAL1*, *C3orf70*, *CILP2*, *MLLT4* and ncRNA *LOC101929268* remained significantly associated with altered lipid and glucose metabolism and differential body size and body composition measures in children (36)]. None of the identified differently methylated positions in this study were found in respective EWAS in children and adolescence (35, 37). But several genes in this study have also been found differentially methylated in relation to BMI and obesity in previous EWAS in adults (27, 38). It is noted that, this EWAS study is one of the first to compare genome-wide DNAm among several body size and body composition measures including BMI, fat-mass, fat free mass in pre-school children with a reasonably large sample size.

DNA methylation profiles in whole blood cells from 20 obese children and 17 controls was evaluated and it was found that 31 CpGs were differentially methylated in obese children compared to control subjects; 10 were hypermethylated, and 21 were hypomethylated in obese compared to control children (39).

Compare to several studies in children and adults, the association between DNA methylation level and obesity at 10 gene loci was replicated: (*ANKRD11, AVPI1, CDK19, FOXK2, HDAC4, IFT140, KIAA0753, LTBP1, MYOM2, TBC1D8*). Among these genes, *HDAC4* is an interesting candidate gene since Abu-Farha et al. showed a decreased expression of its mRNA and protein both in blood cells and adipose tissue in human obese subjects (40)]. In addition numerous genes found in severe obese analysis have also been associated with cancer.

Micro RNAs

Non-coding RNA (ncRNAs) are non-translated RNAs in many organisms that act as gene expression regulator in cellular functions (41)]. NcRNAs are classified based on their nucleotide length in two groups: long ncRNAs (lncRNAs) (>200 nts) and short ncRNAs (42)]. micro RNAs (miRNAs) are a class of short non-coding RNAs with 18-24 nucleotides long (43)]. In 1993, *Lin-4* as the first miRNA was reported in *Caenorhabditis elegans* (44)], then the second miRNA (*let-7*) was discovered in 2000 (45)]. After a while, much microRNAs were reported in varies species and human. They work as regulators of gene expression in many physiological processes at the post-transcriptional level. When the miRNA bind to their seed sequence in the 3' untranslated region (UTR) of the target mRNA, translation suppressed or mRNA degradation take place (46, 47).

Micro RNAs and Childhood Obesity

MicroRNA involve in many biological functions of the human, they are produced in different cells of the various tissues (48). Changes in miRNAs levels cause dysregulation in gene expression that eventually causes many human diseases including obesity (49). MicroRNAs can regulate many signaling pathways related to the obesity, including fatty acid metabolism, adipogenesis, metabolism of lipids and insulin pathway (50-52). Cui et al. stated that miR-486, miR-146b and miR-15b upregulated in diabetic and obese children and circulating miRNA scan indicated the future risk of type 2 diabeties (T2D) in obese children (53). Table 1 shows some important miRNAs that dysregulated in obes children.

Microarray analysis of DNA methylation in CpG sites of miRNAs coding sequences in Spanish children showed that three CpG sites related to miR-1203, miR-412 and miR-216A were differentially methylated in obese children and their controls. Changes in the epigenetic regulation of microRNAs may appear to influence in childhood obesity (54). In addition, Chen et al. identified two long non-coding RNAs (*LINC00839* and *lncRNA HCP5*) as the key regulator in children with obesity based on an *in silico* analysis. lncRNA *HCP5* act as regulator in miR17-5p and miR-27a/b expression that involve in the pathogenesis of childhood obesity (55).

Recently Flórez et al. published a systematic review about the relation of microRNAs with obesity in childhood (52). In this systematic review the articles have been carefully reviewed and 65 miRNAs were reported in this field. All studies were found the association between miRNAs and childhood obesity. In this study, they have focused on microRNAs as biomarkers and concluded that microRNAs especially miR-15b-5p, miR-486-5p, and hsa-miR-122-5p can be regarded as good biomarkers for obesity in children. Similarly, in another systematic review the miRNA expression was reviewed by considering some diseases like metabolic abnormalities in children. According to the articles reviewed in this study, four circulating miRNAs, miR-143, miR-142-3 miR-222 and 140-5p miR-222 upregulated in children with obesity and in obese children with nonalcoholic fatty liver disease (NAFLD) and/or insulin resistance two miRNAs (miR-122 and miR-34a) were upregulated same as adolescents (56).

Although there are many studies on the relationship of microRNAs in adult obesity, there are still few studies about the children obesity and microRNAs. Most studies have focused on the use of microRNAs as biomarkers, and further studies are needed to understand the mechanisms of these microRNAs and their relationship to childhood obesity.

Table 1. Circulating miRNAs with significant alterations in obese children

Author	Sample	miRNAs		Case/control	Method	Aim
Iacomino G 2019 (57)	Plasma	↑miR-551a, ↓miR-10b-5p, ↓miR-215-5p, ↑miR-486,	↑miR-501-5p ↓miR-191-3p ↓miR-874-3p ↑miR-146b	149/159	RT-qPCR	To Investigate the differential circulating miRNAs signature in early childhood obesity
Cui X 2018 (53)	Serum	↑miR-15b, ↑miR-146a, ↑miR-26b,	↑miR-222, ↑miR-20a ↓miR-197	100/146 T2D 101/82	RT-qPCR	To Investigated the possibility of predicting the future risk of adult T2D in obese children by using circulating miRNAs.
Thompson MD 2017 (58)	Plasma	↑miR-199a, ↑miR-191, ↑miR-27b, ↑mir199a-5p, ↑mir181b-5p, ↑mir122-5p, ↑mir27b-3p, ↑mir34a-5p, ↑mir192-5p, ↑mir29a-3p, ↑mir214-5p, ↑mir155-5p, NS (MiR-451, miR-16, miR-150 or miR375)	↑ miR-122 ↑ mir222-3p ↑ mir15b-5p ↑ mir223-3p ↑mir103a-5p ↑ mir23a-3p ↑ mir21-5p ↑mir451-5p ↑mir16-5p ↑ mir150-5p ↑ mir375 ↑ mir191-5p ↑mir103a-5p	20/10	ExiLENT Master Mix	To evaluate a panel of selected circulating miRNAs in obese children compared to healthy controls.
Ouyang S 2017 (59)	PBMC (peripheral blood mononuclear cells)	↓let-7g-5p, ↑miR-301a-3p, ↑miR -199b-3p, ↑miR-130a-3p, ↑miR-126-3p	↓miR-4454 ↑miR-199a-3p ↑miR-191-5p ↑miR-361-5p	6/6	Multiplexed NanoStringnCounter system	To characterize the miRNA profile associated with early childhood obesity in peripheral blood mononuclear cells (PBMCs).
Author	Sample	miRNAs		Case/control	Method	Aim

Iacomino G 2016 (60)	Plasma	↑ miR-31-5p ↑miR-2355-5p ↓miR-206		10/10	RT-qPCR	To assess the profile of circulating miRNAs expressed in plasma samples of overweight or obese (OW/Ob) and normal weight (NW) prepubertal children from a European cohort
Can U 2016 (61)	Whole blood	↓ miR-335, ↓ miR-758 ↑ miR-27, ↑miR-370 miR-33(NS)	↓miR-143 ↑miR-378,	45/41	RT-qPCR	To Evaluate the association between circulating miRNA levels and lipid metabolism
Prats-Puig A 2013 (62)	Plasma	↓miR-221, ↓miR-125b, ↑miR-486-5p, ↑miR-142-3p, ↑miR-532-5p, ↑miR-140-5p, ↑miR-222, ↑miR-122	↓miR-28-3p ↓miR-328 ↑miR-486-3p ↑miR-130b ↑miR-423-5p ↑miR-16- ↑miR-363	5/5	TaqManmiRNA low-density arrays (TLDAs)	Define the circulating pattern of miRNAs in childhood obesity

NS:not significant.

CONCLUSION

Increasing overweight and obesity among children and adolescents implies more attention to primary prevention. Obesity is a multifactorial disease with interaction between genetic variation and environmental factors from early life that possibly is mediated by genetics and epigenetic processes. Identification of methylation changes in specific genes will provide important targets for further studies for finding potential mechanisms of childhood obesity. The important feature of epigenetic phenomina is their reversible nature. Therefor by accumulation of more information regarding DNA methylation and other epigenetic alterations, novel therapeutic targets, predictive early detection biomarkers and new drug development would come to reality. Having these advancements accessible, we hope to limit the prevalence of childhood obesity and its related complications throughout individual's life span.

REFERENCES

[1] Khadaee GH, Saeidi M. Increases of Obesity and Overweight in Children: an Alarm for Parents and Policymakers %J *International Journal of Pediatrics*. 2016;4(4): 1591-601.

[2] Singh AS, Mulder C, Twisk JW, van Mechelen W, Chinapaw MJ. Tracking of childhood overweight into adulthood: a systematic review of the literature. *Obesity reviews : an official journal of the International Association for the Study of Obesity*. 2008;9(5):474-88.

[3] Kinlen D, Cody D, O'Shea D. Complications of obesity. *QJM: An International Journal of Medicine*. 2017;111(7):437-43.

[4] Campion J, Milagro FI, Martinez JA. Individuality and epigenetics in obesity. *Obesity reviews : an official journal of the International Association for the Study of Obesity*. 2009;10(4):383-92.

[5] Junien C, Nathanielsz P. Report on the IASO Stock Conference 2006: early and lifelong environmental epigenomic programming of metabolic syndrome, obesity and type II diabetes. *Obesity reviews : an official journal of the International Association for the Study of Obesity*. 2007;8(6):487-502.

[6] Kim DH, Saetrom P, Snove O, Jr., Rossi JJ. *MicroRNA-directed transcriptional gene silencing in mammalian cells*. Proceedings of the National Academy of Sciences of the United States of America. 2008;105(42):16230-5.

[7] Miranda TB, Jones PA. DNA methylation: the nuts and bolts of repression. *Journal of cellular physiology*. 2007;213(2):384-90.

[8] Raftopoulos L, Katsi V, Makris T, Tousoulis D, Stefanadis C, Kallikazaros I. Epigenetics, the missing link in hypertension. *Life sciences*. 2015;129:22-6.

[9] Boyes J, Bird A. Repression of genes by DNA methylation depends on CpG density and promoter strength: evidence for involvement of a methyl-CpG binding protein. *The EMBO journal*. 1992;11(1):327-33.

[10] Yang X, Han H, De Carvalho DD, Lay FD, Jones PA, Liang G. Gene body methylation can alter gene expression and is a therapeutic target in cancer. *Cancer cell*. 2014;26(4):577-90.

[11] Samblas M, Milagro FI, Martinez A. DNA methylation markers in obesity, metabolic syndrome, and weight loss. *Epigenetics*. 2019;14(5):421-44.

[12] Moholdt T, Hawley JA. Maternal Lifestyle Interventions: Targeting Preconception Health. *Trends in endocrinology and metabolism: TEM*. 2020.

[13] He F, Berg A, Imamura Kawasawa Y, Bixler EO, Fernandez-Mendoza J, Whitsel EA, et al. Association between DNA methylation in obesity-related genes and body mass index percentile in adolescents. *Scientific reports*. 2019;9(1):2079.

[14] Zhu Z, Cao F, Li X. *Epigenetic Programming and Fetal Metabolic Programming. Front Endocrinol (Lausanne)*. 2019;10:764.

[15] Sharp GC, Lawlor DA, Richmond RC, Fraser A, Simpkin A, Suderman M, et al. Maternal pre-pregnancy BMI and gestational weight gain, offspring DNA methylation and later offspring adiposity: findings from the Avon Longitudinal Study of Parents and Children. *International journal of epidemiology*. 2015; 44(4):1288-304.

[16] Li CC, Maloney CA, Cropley JE, Suter CM. Epigenetic programming by maternal nutrition: shaping future generations. *Epigenomics*. 2010;2(4):539-49.

[17] Vickers MH. Early life nutrition, epigenetics and programming of later life disease. *Nutrients*. 2014;6(6):2165-78.

[18] Tobi EW, Slagboom PE, van Dongen J, Kremer D, Stein AD, Putter H, et al. Prenatal famine and genetic variation are independently and additively associated with DNA methylation at regulatory loci within IGF2/H19. *PloS one*. 2012;7(5):e37933.

[19] Godfrey KM, Sheppard A, Gluckman PD, Lillycrop KA, Burdge GC, McLean C, et al. Epigenetic gene promoter methylation at birth is associated with child's later adiposity. *Diabetes*. 2011;60(5):1528-34.

[20] Bouchard L, Hivert MF, Guay SP, St-Pierre J, Perron P, Brisson D. Placental adiponectin gene DNA methylation levels are associated with mothers' blood glucose concentration. *Diabetes*. 2012;61(5):1272-80.

[21] Bouchard L, Thibault S, Guay SP, Santure M, Monpetit A, St-Pierre J, et al. Leptin gene epigenetic adaptation to impaired glucose metabolism during pregnancy. *Diabetes care*. 2010;33(11):2436-41.

[22] Mantzoros CS, Rifas-Shiman SL, Williams CJ, Fargnoli JL, Kelesidis T, Gillman MW. Cord blood leptin and adiponectin as predictors of adiposity in children at 3 years of age: a prospective cohort study. *Pediatrics*. 2009;123(2):682-9.

[23] Michels KB, Harris HR, Barault L. Birthweight, maternal weight trajectories and global DNA methylation of LINE-1 repetitive elements. *PloS one*. 2011; 6(9):e25254.

[24] Groom A, Potter C, Swan DC, Fatemifar G, Evans DM, Ring SM, et al. Postnatal growth and DNA methylation are associated with differential gene expression of the TACSTD2 gene and childhood fat mass. *Diabetes*. 2012;61(2):391-400.

[25] Cubas R, Zhang S, Li M, Chen C, Yao Q. Trop2 expression contributes to tumor pathogenesis by activating the ERK MAPK pathway. *Molecular cancer*. 2010;9:253.

[26] Pan H, Lin X, Wu Y, Chen L, Teh AL, Soh SE, et al. HIF3A association with adiposity: the story begins before birth. *Epigenomics*. 2015;7(6):937-50.

[27] Demerath EW, Guan W, Grove ML, Aslibekyan S, Mendelson M, Zhou YH, et al. Epigenome-wide association study (EWAS) of BMI, BMI change and waist circumference in African American adults identifies multiple replicated loci. *Human molecular genetics*. 2015;24(15):4464-79.

[28] Verduci E, Banderali G, Barberi S, Radaelli G, Lops A, Betti F, et al. Epigenetic effects of human breast milk. *Nutrients*. 2014;6(4):1711-24.

[29] Obermann-Borst SA, Eilers PH, Tobi EW, de Jong FH, Slagboom PE, Heijmans BT, et al. Duration of breastfeeding and gender are associated with methylation of the LEPTIN gene in very young children. *Pediatric research*. 2013;74(3):344-9.

[30] Al Maskari MY, Alnaqdy AA. Correlation between Serum Leptin Levels, Body Mass Index and Obesity in Omanis. *Sultan Qaboos University medical journal*. 2006;6(2):27-31.

[31] Palou M, Pico C, Palou A. Leptin as a breast milk component for the prevention of obesity. *Nutrition reviews*. 2018;76(12):875-92.

[32] Pauwels S, Symons L, Vanautgaerden EL, Ghosh M, Duca RC, Bekaert B, et al. The Influence of the Duration of Breastfeeding on the Infant's Metabolic Epigenome. *Nutrients*. 2019;11(6).

[33] Hartwig FP, Loret de Mola C, Davies NM, Victora CG, Relton CL. Breastfeeding effects on DNA methylation in the offspring: A systematic literature review. *PloS one*. 2017;12(3):e0173070.

[34] Ding X, Zheng D, Fan C, Liu Z, Dong H, Lu Y, et al. Genome-wide screen of DNA methylation identifies novel markers in childhood obesity. *Gene*. 2015;566(1):74-83.

[35] Huang RC, Garratt ES, Pan H, Wu Y, Davis EA, Barton SJ, et al. Genome-wide methylation analysis identifies differentially methylated CpG loci associated with severe obesity in childhood. *Epigenetics*. 2015;10(11):995-1005.

[36] Rzehak P, Covic M, Saffery R, Reischl E, Wahl S, Grote V, et al. DNA-Methylation and Body Composition in Preschool Children: Epigenome-Wide-Analysis in the European Childhood Obesity Project (CHOP)-Study. *Scientific reports*. 2017;7(1): 14349.

[37] Rounge TB, Page CM, Lepisto M, Ellonen P, Andreassen BK, Weiderpass E. Genome-wide DNA methylation in saliva and body size of adolescent girls. *Epigenomics*. 2016;8(11):1495-505.

[38] Al Muftah WA, Al-Shafai M, Zaghlool SB, Visconti A, Tsai PC, Kumar P, et al. Epigenetic associations of type 2 diabetes and BMI in an Arab population. *Clinical epigenetics*. 2016;8:13.

[39] Fradin D, Boelle PY, Belot MP, Lachaux F, Tost J, Besse C, et al. Genome-Wide Methylation Analysis Identifies Specific Epigenetic Marks In Severely Obese Children. *Scientific reports*. 2017;7:46311.

[40] Abu-Farha M, Tiss A, Abubaker J, Khadir A, Al-Ghimlas F, Al-Khairi I, et al. Proteomics analysis of human obesity reveals the epigenetic factor HDAC4 as a potential target for obesity. *PloS one*. 2013;8(9):e75342.

[41] Wei S, Du M, Jiang Z, Hausman GJ, Zhang L, Dodson MV. Long noncoding RNAs in regulating adipogenesis: new RNAs shed lights on obesity. *Cellular and molecular life sciences : CMLS*. 2016;73(10):2079-87.

[42] Marchese FP, Raimondi I, Huarte M. The multidimensional mechanisms of long noncoding RNA function. *Genome biology*. 2017;18(1):206.

[43] Bartel DP. MicroRNAs: genomics, biogenesis, mechanism, and function. *Cell*. 2004;116(2):281-97.

[44] Lee RC, Feinbaum RL, Ambros V. The C. elegans heterochronic gene lin-4 encodes small RNAs with antisense complementarity to lin-14. *Cell*. 1993;75(5):843-54.

[45] Reinhart BJ, Slack FJ, Basson M, Pasquinelli AE, Bettinger JC, Rougvie AE, et al. The 21-nucleotide let-7 RNA regulates developmental timing in Caenorhabditis elegans. *Nature*. 2000;403(6772):901-6.

[46] Guo H, Ingolia NT, Weissman JS, Bartel DP. Mammalian microRNAs predominantly act to decrease target mRNA levels. *Nature*. 2010;466(7308):835-40.

[47] Filipowicz W, Bhattacharyya SN, Sonenberg N. Mechanisms of post-transcriptional regulation by microRNAs: are the answers in sight? *Nature reviews Genetics*. 2008;9(2):102-14.

[48] Chen X, Ba Y, Ma L, Cai X, Yin Y, Wang K, et al. Characterization of microRNAs in serum: a novel class of biomarkers for diagnosis of cancer and other diseases. *Cell research*. 2008;18(10):997-1006.

[49] Hammond SM. An overview of microRNAs. *Advanced drug delivery reviews*. 2015;87:3-14.

[50] Castano C, Kalko S, Novials A, Parrizas M. Obesity-associated exosomal miRNAs modulate glucose and lipid metabolism in mice. *Proceedings of the National Academy of Sciences of the United States of America*. 2018;115(48):12158-63.

[51] Arner P, Kulyte A. MicroRNA regulatory networks in human adipose tissue and obesity. *Nature reviews Endocrinology*. 2015;11(5):276-88.

[52] Florez CAR, Garcia-Perdomo HA, Escudero MM. MicroRNAs associated with overweight and obesity in childhood. Systematic review. *MicroRNA* (Shariqah, United Arab Emirates). 2019.

[53] Cui X, You L, Zhu L, Wang X, Zhou Y, Li Y, et al. Change in circulating microRNA profile of obese children indicates future risk of adult diabetes. *Metabolism: clinical and experimental*. 2018;78:95-105.

[54] Mansego ML, Garcia-Lacarte M, Milagro FI, Marti A, Martinez JA. DNA methylation of miRNA coding sequences putatively associated with childhood obesity. *Pediatric obesity*. 2017;12(1):19-27.

[55] Chen R, Xin G, Zhang X. Long non-coding RNA HCP5 serves as a ceRNA sponging miR-17-5p and miR-27a/b to regulate the pathogenesis of childhood obesity via the MAPK signaling pathway. *Journal of pediatric endocrinology & metabolism : JPEM*. 2019;32(12):1327-39.

[56] Oses M, Margareto Sanchez J, Portillo MP, Aguilera CM, Labayen I. Circulating miRNAs as Biomarkers of Obesity and Obesity-Associated Comorbidities in Children and Adolescents: A Systematic Review. *Nutrients*. 2019;11(12).

[57] Iacomino G, Russo P, Marena P, Lauria F, Venezia A, Ahrens W, et al. Circulating microRNAs are associated with early childhood obesity: results of the I.Family Study. *Genes & nutrition*. 2019;14:2.

[58] Thompson MD, Cismowski MJ, Serpico M, Pusateri A, Brigstock DR. Elevation of circulating microRNA levels in obese children compared to healthy controls. *Clinical obesity*. 2017;7(4):216-21.

[59] Ouyang S, Tang R, Liu Z, Ma F, Li Y, Wu J. Characterization and predicted role of microRNA expression profiles associated with early childhood obesity. *Molecular medicine reports*. 2017;16(4):3799-806.

[60] Iacomino G, Russo P, Stillitano I, Lauria F, Marena P, Ahrens W, et al. Circulating microRNAs are deregulated in overweight/obese children: preliminary results of the I.Family study. *Genes & nutrition*. 2016;11:7.

[61] Can U, Buyukinan M, Yerlikaya FH. The investigation of circulating microRNAs associated with lipid metabolism in childhood obesity. *Pediatric obesity*. 2016;11(3):228-34.

[62] Prats-Puig A, Ortega FJ, Mercader JM, Moreno-Navarrete JM, Moreno M, Bonet N, et al. Changes in circulating microRNAs are associated with childhood obesity. *The Journal of clinical endocrinology and metabolism*. 2013;98(10):E1655-60.

In: Childhood Obesity
Editor: Roya Kelishadi
ISBN: 978-1-53618-158-6
© 2020 Nova Science Publishers, Inc.

Chapter 3

FOOD ENVIRONMENT AND CHILDHOOD OVERWEIGHT AND OBESITY

Nasrin Omidvar* and Mina Babashahi
Department of Community Nutrition, National Nutrition and Food Technology, Research Institute, Faculty of Nutrition Sciences and Food Technology, Shahid Beheshti University of Medical Sciences, Tehran, Iran

ABSTRACT

Childhood obesity is a multifactorial public health problem that is associated with a variety of adverse health, social and psychological consequences. A range of complex genetic, social and environmental influences is implicated in the development of obesity that goes beyond the notion of individual choice. A population-level approach recognizes the importance of access to and availability of healthy foods in child living environment, i.e., food environment. Food environment refers to 'the collective physical, economic, policy and sociocultural surroundings, opportunities and conditions that influence people's food and beverage choices and nutritional status'. It comprises two personal and external domains. The *personal food environment* domain includes endogenous dimensions, such as accessibility, affordability, convenience, and desirability at the individual and household levels. The *external food environment* reflects exogenous dimensions related to availability, food price, marketing and advertisements, schools, and informal vendors, among similar others, where consumers interface with the food. The socio-ecological interaction between the external and personal food environment domains shapes food acquisition and eating choices.

Therefore, food environment plays an important role in encouraging individuals to low quality food patterns by increasing and facilitating access to unhealthy food choices that can lead to overweight and obesity. Individual consumers, specifically children often have less control over their food environment. This has stimulated the need for development and

* Corresponding Author's Email: omidvar.nasrin@gmail.com.

validation of various tools to measure one or more dimensions of the food environment in different places (e.g., home, school, stores and restaurants). These tools can be helpful for providing evidence for the policymakers in any policy process. There are a number of food policies and interventions to modify obesogenic food environment. Some examples of such policies and regulations, include taxation of unhealthy foods and sugar-sweetened beverages and marketing restrictions on low-nutrient-density products typically sold to children, package redesign to eliminate cartoon characters and other appealing features on junk foods, menu labeling, school food and beverage policies, food pricing, school and community gardens/greenhouses, and point-of-purchase prompts for healthy eating.

Keywords: food environment, children, overweight, obesity

INTRODUCTION

Obesity, specifically in children and adolescents, is one of the main challenges of the new millennium [1, 2]. Overweight and obesity are multifactorial public health problems associated with a variety of adverse health, social and psychological consequences. A range of complex genetic, social and environmental influences is implicated in the development of obesity that goes beyond the notion of individual choice. Based on current health behavior theories, behaviors related to obesity, e.g., eating and physical activity, are determined by an interrelated set of personal and environmental factors. The interdependence of personal (biological and behavioral), as well as environmental influences on obesity have been conceptualized through ecological models (Figure 1) [3]. In this regard, the differences observed between individuals when they are placed in different environments [4] has drawn attention towards the importance of environment in causation, management and treatment of obesity. Subsequently, the term 'obesogenic environment' has been proposed to express 'the sum of influences, opportunities, or conditions" that can have effect on promoting obesity in individuals or populations' [3].

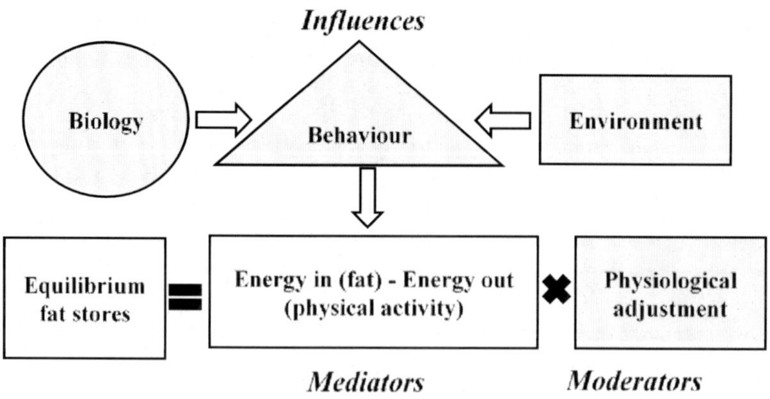

Figure 1. Conceptual model for understanding how the physical environment influences obesity [3].

One of the most important aspects of an obesogenic environment is the food environment. In today's world, food environments are characterized by energy-dense, nutrient-poor processed food products. High availability, relatively lower price and wide promotion of these foods has created a 'push' effect on unhealthy diets from the supply side which has been a predominant food system driver of population weight gain [5]. Yet, research that links food choices to the food environment is still relatively undeveloped.

This chapter reviews definitions, measurement methods, as well as policy and intervention approaches to food environmental with regard to child obesity.

FOOD ENVIRONMENT DEFINITIONS

Early research on the dimensions of the food environment began without a precise definition of the food environment. The basic origins of investigating dimensions of food environment go back to Penchansky and Thomas research in 1981 [6] who described a multidimensional conceptualization of access. They defined "access" as "a concept representing the degree of "fit" between the clients and the system." Considering the need for well-defined concepts as the key to any significant progress, several researchers have tried to expand the definition of food environment and its dimensions. Glanz et al. (2005) portrayed the food environment through the 'community nutrition environment model' (Figure 2), based on an ecological model of health behavior [7]. This model presents four aspects of the food environment: the community environment (type and location of food outlet), the consumer nutrition environment (availability of healthy options, price, promotion and nutritional information), organizational nutrition environments (home, school, and workplace) and information environment (media and advertising) [7].

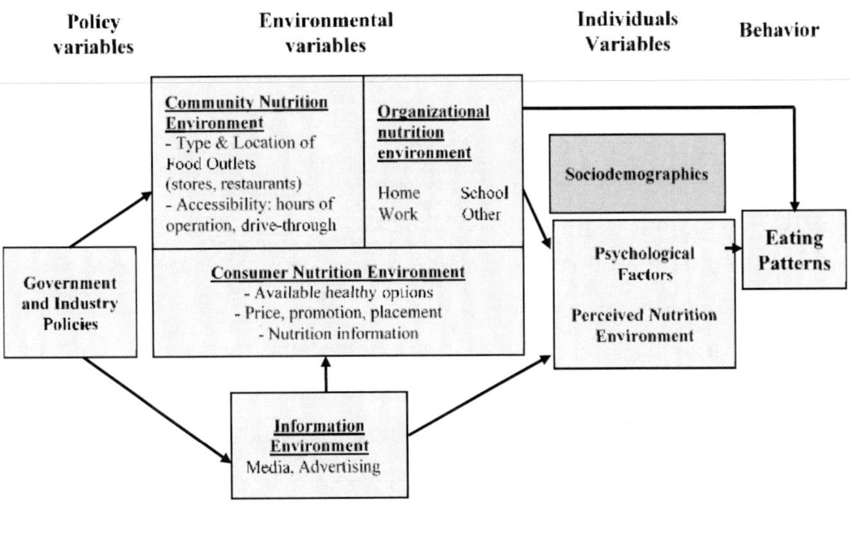

Figure 2. Model of community nutrition environments [7].

Based on Townshend and Lake, food environment is any opportunity to obtain food which includes physical, socio- cultural, economic and policy factors at both micro and macro-levels which involves food availability and accessibility in addition to food advertising and marketing [8]. In line with these definitions, The International Network for Food and Obesity/NCDs Research, Monitoring and Action Support (INFORMAS) (2013), has defined food environment as "collective physical, economic, policy and sociocultural surroundings, opportunities and conditions that influence people's food and beverage choices and nutritional status" (Figure 3) [9].

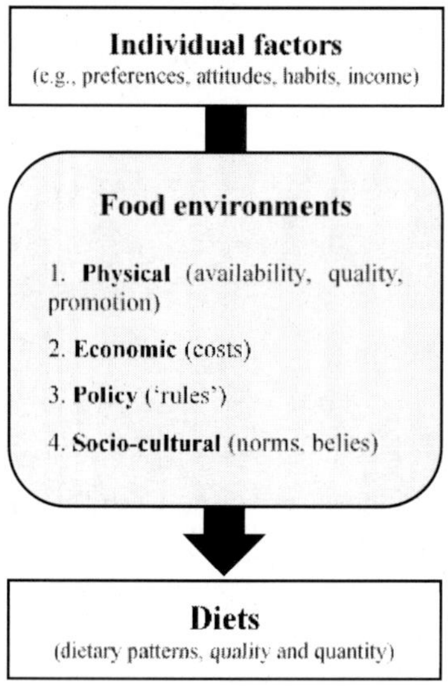

Figure 3. Food environment and its four components; and the interaction between individual factors and food environments to shape diets [9].

The Global Panel on Agriculture and Food Systems for Nutrition (GPAFSN, 2016) and the Food and Agriculture Organization of the United Nations (FAO, 2016) elaborate the INFORMAS definition by introducing the role of Food environments or the foods available to people in their everyday lives and the nutritional quality, safety, price, convenience, labelling and promotion of these foods" [10]. In addition, framing the food environments as the 'interface' or 'link' between food systems and diets is an important contribution of FAO to this definition [10, 11]. The 'interface' concept and the focus on 'interactions' helps to ground the food environment construct in relation to people's daily lives and activities that shape their diet(s). Political, economic and socio-cultural factors act as macro-level influences on the food environment and the broader food system [12, 9]. This concept is particularly valuable as it helps situate the food environment construct within the wider 'farm to fork' concept of the food system as it is defined by the United Nations Standing Committee on Nutrition (UNSCN, 2016) helping to distinguish between these related concepts [13].

A key commonality amongst the existing definitions is the conceptualization of the food environment in terms of the spaces within which food acquisition occurs, and the series of market-based opportunities and constraints that influence people's food acquisition and consumption. However, clear differences exist with regard to the articulation of dimensions. These differences likely reflect not only the diversity of food environments globally, but also the wide array of academic disciplines undertaking research, each with their respective areas of interest and expertise (e.g., public health nutrition, economics, epidemiology, geography, sociology, urban planning). The need to harmonize definitions with theoretical concepts and measurable dimensions of food environments in order to guide empirical research have been emphasized [14].

On the basis of food environments definition, as the interface where people interact with the wider food system to acquire and consume foods [15, 16], UNICEF has proposed a framework for children and adolescents' food environment (Figure 4). Based on their framework, food build environment consists of two external and personal domains, where children and their caregivers interact with the food system. The *external food environment* domain includes the retail and commercial markets, schools, and informal vendors, among similar others, where consumers interface with the food [17]. In other words, external food environments includes all the physical places where people go to purchase or consume food. It reflects exogenous dimensions related to availability, food price, marketing and advertisements, vendor and product properties (e.g., food quality and safety). Though individual consumers often have less control over their external food environment, they can influence it through demand and advocacy [16].

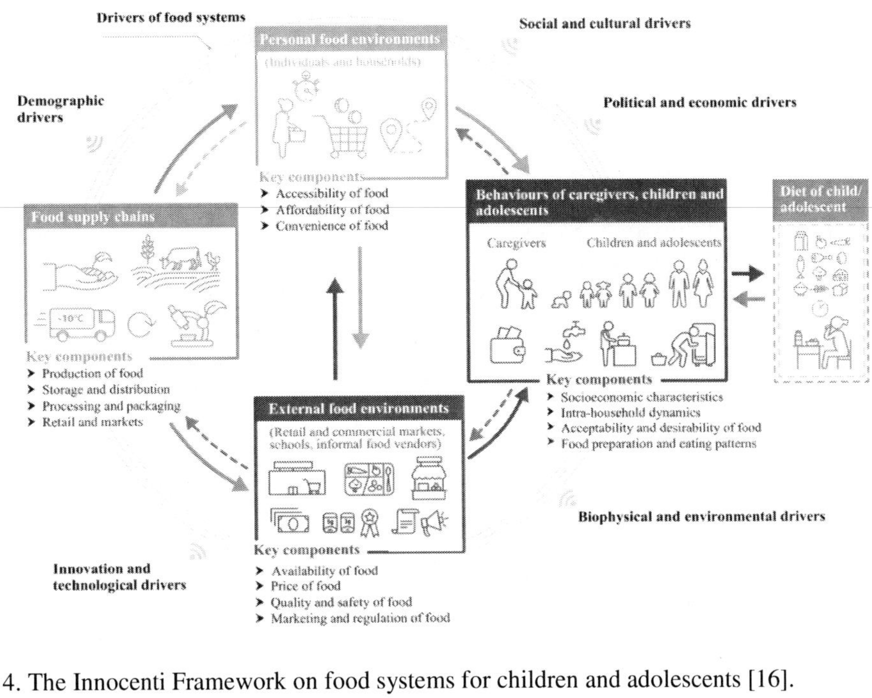

Figure 4. The Innocenti Framework on food systems for children and adolescents [16].

The *personal food environment* domain includes endogenous dimensions, such as accessibility, affordability, convenience, and desirability at the individual and household levels [15, 17]. Personal food environments depict the individual and household level factors that consumers bring to the food environment, such as purchasing power, access, convenience and desirability, and inform why people choose to procure the foods that they do. They complement dimensions of price, availability, and vendor properties in the external food environment [18]. For example, families and individuals' access to shops and markets and their purchasing power will determine the affordability and convenience of foods, while a lack of income or time is a significant burden. Rural women, in particular must often balance unpaid farm work with their role as primary caregivers [18].

Overall, the socio-ecological interaction between the external and personal food environment domains shapes food acquisition and eating choices of our children [15].

FOOD ENVIRONMENT AND CHILD OBESITY

According to the World Health Organization (WHO) report, the global prevalence of overweight and obesity among children and adolescents aged 5-19 years has dramatically increased from 4% in 1975 to over 18% in 2016 [10]. In other word, in 2016, over 340 million of this age group were overweight or obese [10]. It is estimated that by 2025, the prevalence of overweight just in preschool children will increase to 11% worldwide [19, 20].

Food environments are likely more effective to the increasing epidemic of obesity and chronic diseases, over and above individual factors such as knowledge, skills, and incentive(s) [21]. Unhealthy food environments encourage individuals to low quality food patterns by increasing and facilitating access to unhealthy food choices [22]. Over the past decades, major changes in the food system and food and eating environments have been driven by technological advances, urbanization, food and agricultural policies, and economic, social, and lifestyle changes. Food products is now readily available and accessible in multiple settings throughout the day. More processed and convenience foods are available in larger portion sizes and at relatively low prices [23]. The set of the above factors has resulted in unhealthy dietary pattern and increased rate of overweight and obesity [24, 25]. Several studies have examined the relationship between living environment and food establishments with child food intake, weight or BMI. The result of these studies indicated that environmental changes contribute to changing eating behaviors, food choices and the prevalence of obesity, especially in children.

Family environment provide children's early experiences with food and eating. Existing literature, consistently confirm the association between parental influences (parental food intake and education) and obesity in children and adolescents [26]. However, epidemiological and nutrition transitions have led to major changes in families' eating and activity pattern, including longer work hours of parents, fewer family meals, and more meals eaten away from home [27]. On the other hand, growth and enlargement of unhealthy food marketing has become an important environmental factor affecting the purchasing and consumption behaviors of families, as well as children which automatically triggers childhood obesity [28, 29]. Moreover, the increase of inactive indoor lifestyles within the families, including watching TV, playing video games, and using the internet supports the possibility of more energy-dense nutrient-poor dietary intakes underlying the sharp increase in childhood obesity [30, 31].

Schools, as one of the main settings of everyday life of children, are now remarkably different than a few decades ago. In today's schools, high-calorie, low-nutrition processed foods are available in multiple venues throughout the school day [32]. A study in the United States showed that a 10 percentage point increase in potential exposure of unhealthy (junk) foods available was associated with about one percent increase in students' BMI [33]. Health status of surrounding environment of schools affect eating behavior and weight of students. One study in the area of East Harlem, New York City, reported that children aged 6-8 years in schools with a higher convenience store density had a higher BMI (OR=1.90, 95% CI=1.15, 3.15) than those living in neighborhoods with a lower concentration of this type of stores [34]. Finding of a survey on 60 elementary schools in two Mexican cities also showed that children attending schools within the highest tertile of food stores had 4.7% higher BMI units than children from schools in the lowest tertile [35]. Similar findings have been reported about public schools in California where a higher density of convenience stores in an 800-m buffer was associated with a higher prevalence of overweight in school children, compared with the weight of those attending schools with no convenience stores in their surroundings [36].

The socioeconomic status (SES) of living area also affects household and child food eating behaviors. The results of Storr's study (2019) in Australia, indicated that the food environment of the high-SES suburb supported from healthful eating more than the low-SES suburb. Despite having a significantly lower population density in high-SES suburb, these areas had more food markets, with more open time and higher levels of healthful foods [21]. In recent decades, there has been one departure of grocery stores and an incursion of fast-food outlets in low-income neighbourhoods, which has contributed to the income and racial/ethnic disparities in access to healthy foods [23].

Environmental variables in the neighborhood of the schoolchildren's homes, including distance from and the density of restaurants and/or supermarkets have been reported to be associated with overweight/obesity or frequency intake of healthy foods in children. Correa et al. found a positive association between the presence of restaurants around the homes of 2195 students (buffer=400 m) and overweight/obesity in school children (OR=1·52; 95% CI 1·13, 2·06) in the city of Florianópolis, Brazil [37]. Another study on 3,507,542 student conducted from 2009 to 2013 in the New York City public school system showed an association between the nearest food outlets (i.e., fast-food outlets, wait-service restaurants, corner stores, and supermarkets) to children's homes and their weight outcomes [38]. Overall, living farther than 0.025 mile from the nearest fast-food restaurant was associated with lower obesity and obesity/overweight risk and lower BMI-*z*-scores. Results ranged from 2.5% to 4.4% decrease in obesity. Additionally, the investigation of data from 438 children, ages 2–6.9 years with a BMI≥85th percentile participating in "the High Five for Kids" study in Eastern Massachusetts from 2006 to 2009, showed that children who lived within 1 mile from a large supermarket had a BMI 1.06 (kg/m^2) higher compared to those living >2 miles distance [39]. Adjustment for socioeconomic characteristics and distance to fast-food restaurants attenuated this estimate to 0.77 kg/m^2.

On the other hand, Skidmore et al. [40], in a study on 1721 children aged 9-10 years in the county of Norfolk, England, showed that living further away from a supermarket increased portions of fruit (0.11 portions/ week per 1 km increase in distance to nearest supermarket, $P<0.05$) and vegetables (0.11 portions/week, $P<0.05$) consumed. Living closer to convenience stores was also associated with an increased consumption of crisps, chocolate and white bread. Density of supermarkets was associated with both an increase in vegetable intake (0.13 portions/week, $P<0.05$) and unhealthy foods. Similar findings have been reported by Timperio et al. who found higher density of fast-food retailers and convenience stores was associated with lower levels of fruit and vegetable intake in Australian children. An inverse association was between density of convenience stores and the likelihood of consuming vegetables ≥3 times/day (OR=0.84, 95%CI=0.74–0.95) [41]. The likelihood of consuming vegetables ≥3 times/day was greater, the farther children lived from a supermarket (OR=1.27, 95% CI=1.07–1.51) or a fast food outlet (OR=1.19, 95%CI=1.06–1.35) [41].

Another important environmental factor contributing to obesity in children and adolescents is screen media exposure. Recent evidence suggests that children screen time is associated with increased eating while viewing; exposure to high-calorie, low-nutrient food and beverage marketing that influences children's preferences, purchase requests, consumption habits; and reduced sleep duration [42]. Also, food advertisements for nutrient-poor, high-calorie foods stimulate food intake and television viewing is associated with "mindless" eating [43]. In addition to decreasing physical activity and increasing the consumption of highly palatable foods, television viewing can also promote weight gain in indirect ways, such as through the use of targeted product placements in television shows; by influencing social perceptions of body image; and airing programs that portray cooking, eating and losing weight as entertainment [43]. Numerous studies have demonstrated that energy intake increases during television viewing [44, 45]. Crespo et al. (2001) found that girls who watched 5 or more hours of television a day, consumed an extra 175 kcal per day on average compared to those watching 1 h or less of television daily [44]. Obese children, in particular, appear to be highly susceptible to food advertisements. For example, while both lean and obese children consumed significantly more calories and energy dense foods when watching television shows containing food advertisements than when watching similar shows without advertisements, obese children increased caloric intake to a greater degree than lean children [46, 47].

After all, TV food advertisements translates into actual buying behavior, as research indicates that the frequency with which children request foods at the grocery store is directly related to the amount of television they watch. Requests are most often made for cereals, snacks, and sweetened drinks, and frequently result in a successful purchase [48, 49, 43, 50, 51]. The television viewing was inversely associated with intake of fruit and vegetables [52, 53]. In the other hand, exposure to television food advertisement from any brand increases food intake in younger children [47] and can produce an obesogenic food preference response even in normal weight children [54]. Children who habitually watch more television are also more susceptible to the effects of television food advertising, showing an enhanced preference (particularly for branded foods) following food advert exposure compared to children who watch less television [55]. Robinson et al. reported that children preferred the taste of food and drink items displaying the McDonalds branded packaging to identical products in matched, but unbranded, packaging. This was true even of items that were not available for purchase at McDonalds at the time, such as carrot sticks [56]. Thus, adopting the rules to monitor television advertising is essential to prevent childhood obesity.

MEASURING FOOD ENVIRONMENT

A wide variety of tools have been designed to measure the food environment, many of which have been developed since the attention of health researchers and policy makers to investigate factors contributing to the increase in chronic diseases [57, 58]. Each of these tools focuses on one of different food environments that children deal with and on one or more dimensions of these food environments, from availability to accessibility, convenience or price. Some of them are observational tools and can objectively measure the aspects, although qualitative tools are also used that measure individuals' perceptions of their food [58, 59].

The following describes some of the common tools for measuring food environments and their practical aspects.

Home Food Environment Measures

Considering the direct role of home food environment, i.e., the availability and accessibility of foods in home, in eating habits of children and adolescents, researchers have attempted to develop measurement approaches of home food environment. Also, several models informed by social-cognitive and socio-ecological theories have been developed to measure family environment influences, in addition to availability of food. Based on these models, home food environment as well as family environment influences, including parenting practices and other aspects of the home will shape dietary behaviors of children in the family [60, 61]. Parenting practices, known as social aspect of food environment, have been measured through assessing different factors, e.g., parent role modeling, parenting style, mealtime routines, socio-demographic and economic characteristics, while physical aspects have been evaluated by assessing foods and beverages available and easily accessible at home environment [62]. The interplay between them have been associated with adolescent diet [63-65].

Early studies on home food environment has typically used self-report inventories to measure food availability in the home [66-68, 64]. Ideally, instruments measuring the foods in a home should take into account what is actually available at the time of the inventory, as well as foods that are usually available over a certain time period (e.g., 30 days), which will reflect the variation in shopping episodes [66]. The followings are some of the available tools for measuring home food environment:

The Exhaustive Home Food Inventory (EHFI)

EHFI was developed by Stevens et al. [69] to measures foods in the home by creating a data entry program designed to link scanning results of the universal product code (UPC) to a reference database containing food identification and nutrient information. The database facilitated the entry of foods that were not packaged with a UPC. Therefore, all foods in the home could be entered. An exhaustive inventory of all foods in the home can provide data that allow the investigator to describe the total amount of foods and nutrients available in the home and provide a denominator for relative assessments (e.g., percentage of household energy available from fruits and vegetables). Thus, the amount of a targeted food in a home is put into the context of the total amount of food in that home.

The Home Food Assessment Tool (HFA)

Nepper et al. [70] developed HFA tool to assess the availability, accessibility and visibility (readiness to eat) of healthy and unhealthy foods and beverages in the home based on the instrument previously developed by Boles et al. [71]. The tool included 23 food and beverages classified as "healthy" and "unhealthy", including 18 items of fresh fruits and 14 items of fresh vegetables. A "yes/no" format was used to indicate availability, accessibility and visibility of these foods over a thirty-day period. They showed applicability and reliability of the tool to be used for pre-adolescents.

Home Health Environment (HHE) Assessment

HHE is a questionnaire developed through modification of previously validated tools that includes 4 areas of assessment [71]: 1) healthy and unhealthy foods and drinks (23 items), 2) fresh fruits (18 items) and vegetables (14 items), 3) electronic media devices

(TV, computers, etc.), and 4) devices or physical areas in or around the home that promote physical activity. Aspects of food/drink items evaluated included availability (food or drink physically located within the home), accessibility (whether the child could reach the food), and readiness to be consumed (the food could be immediately eaten without preparation or opening a container). For example, if a fruit drink had a straw inserted in the pouch or a chips bag was already opened, these were considered "ready to consume," because a parent was not needed to prepare it for drinking or eating. Assessment of inter-rater reliability and discriminant validity showed that the tool can successfully discriminate between the home food and activity environments of preschoolers with different weight status and caregivers.

Home-Inventory Describing Eating and Activity (Home-IDEA)

Based on the validated Home Health Environment (HHE) assessment [71], Home-IDEA questionnaire was developed [72]. In the Home-IDEA, the item pool was expanded to capture foods potentially purchased by families with geographical and SES diversity. The new food items were taken from the food lists of several food frequency questionnaires being used in the US (i.e., WIC Program) [73, 74]. Also, additional food and activity items were created based on the opinions of an expert panel and families from diverse backgrounds. The final pool of items included 126 foods and drinks, 16 physical activity devices, and 12 electronic devices. The instrument was successfully validated, and was able to discriminate between characteristics of the home environments that were related to obesity-related behaviors with those that promoted healthy eating and activity behaviors.

Healthy Eating Index (HEI)

HEI was initially designed by the USDA for individual diets based on the Dietary Guidelines for Americans [75]. It has the potential to be extended beyond individual diets to survey the quality of foods available in a given food supply [76, 77]. The HEI is based on a score from 0 to 100 of ten equally weighted dietary components. A higher score demonstrating that the food availability is closer to the recommended amounts.

School Food Environment Measures

Given the influence of the school environment on children's diet and physical activity, the need for valid tools to measure characteristics of school environment have been expressed. Most population based assessments of school environment, including school food environment have been based on surveys (paper or telephone interview) from School Principal or Administrators [78, 79], and some have evaluated the schools by direct observation [80]. Some of the available tools developed in the last decade to measure school food environment are as follows:

School Cafeteria Nutrition Assessment (SCNA)

The School Cafeteria Nutrition Assessment (SCNA) was developed as part of the Evaluation of Arkansas Act 1220 of 2003, specifically to support the completion of more in-depth assessments of school food environments in Arkansas schools [81]. Two separate but complementary measures were developed to evaluate monthly school lunch menus (SCNA-M) and to observe foods offered in school cafeterias during the lunch time (SCNA-O). These measures provide versatility in assessing cafeterias serving pre-kindergarten through 12th-grade students. Both the SCNA-M and SCNA-O are observational tools to assess availability of fruit, vegetables, grains (whole or white), chips (reduced-fat or regular), side dishes, main dishes, `a la carte selections, and desserts. Side dishes, main dishes and `a la carte items are categorized into protein, vegetable, added fat, and whole or white grain sources.

School Environment Assessment Tool (SEAT)

SEAT was developed by *Nathan* et al. [82], by conducting a systematic review of the literature to identify school environmental factors associated with student diet, physical activity, sedentary behavior or excessive weight gain followed by an expert panel evaluation of the drafted tool. It was further refined and pilot tested among primary school principals to check for acceptability and comprehension. The final tool is consisted of 65 food and drink items. Principals are asked to report (yes/ no/ don't know/ refused) the availability of foods and drinks at the school a) canteen, b) vending machines or c) via fundraisers. The validity of the tool was assessed by comparing the principals' responses to the telephone survey items with those reported by an observer.

Stores and Restaurants Food Environment Measures

Due to the global trend of convergence of eating out and shopping from smaller stores towards large supermarkets that offer a wide range of products, assessing the consumer nutrition environment is of great importance. Consumer food choices are influenced by the way the products are sold (brand, package, etc.), their prices, promotional strategies used and even where they are placed in the store. Several tools have been developed to assess the consumer nutrition environment. Most of these tools measure two factors: availability and price [83-85]. However, some of the tools are developed to assess factors such as variety and/or quality [86], in-store advertising and/or product placement [87, 88]. In this section, some examples of these tools have been introduced:

The Nutrition Environment Measures Survey for Stores (NEMS-S)

NEMS-S was developed and validated by Glanz et al. (2007) to measure the food environment of stores [86]. The NEMS-S checklist is constructed based on the availability and affordability (price) of 10 food categories/indicators, including fruit, vegetables, milk, ground beef, hot dogs, frozen dinners, baked goods, beverages (soda/juice), whole grain bread, and baked chips. The healthfulness scores of NEMS-S combine factors of variety, price, quality, shelf placement, promotions, store placement, nutrition information, and healthier alternatives for each of the healthy and unhealthy foods included [89]. Researchers have variably changed NEMS-S for context specificity in various localities and countries. For example, Andreyeva et al. designed Revised Nutrition Environment Measures Survey (R-NEMS) for neighborhoods of low socio-economic status [90]. Also, NEMS-S has been modified for food environments of Guatemala in the form of a mobile phone application by Kanter et al. (2014) [91]. This could be applied for food environment survey in other rural settings and low-income. Reliability of NEMS-S is comparative advantage over other tools that has been tested for inter-rater and test-retest nationally in neighborhoods of various socioeconomic status [86].

Also, the Nutrition Environment Measures Survey for restaurants (NEMS-R) assay was developed to assess the relative healthfulness of foods and beverages available on the main menu and child's menus, considering availability, facilitators, and supports for healthful eating, barriers to healthful eating, pricing, and promotion to food consumption in restaurants [92].

Shelf-Space/Shelf Length Measurement

Measuring the linear shelf space of specific healthy and unhealthy foods in food stores within a given distance of an individual's home is another approach being used for evaluating food environment [84, 85]. In this method, basically Shelf length of healthy foods (mostly fresh fruits and vegetables), as well as unhealthy/energy–dense snacks are measured. The shelf-space measure shows the level of food availability of area that can be related to residents' homes. Accumulative shelf-space availability of specific unhealthy foods, particularly energy-dense snack foods, has been positively associated with weight status of the residents [85].

The GroPromo instrument

This tool is developed to assess the placement and promotional environment in grocery stores [88]. Seven product categories were selected for observation, based on their nutritional value and associations with childhood obesity. Also, nine types of locations in grocery stores were identified for assessment.

Store Survey Instrument

Store survey instrument is a tool developed to evaluate food environment with weighted scoring as an indicator. The instrument measures exterior and interior marketing conditions, availability, quality and price of produce, and availability of other healthful food [87].

Retail Food Environment Index (RFEI)

The *Retail Food Environment Index (RFEI),* is a ratio of the number of convenience stores and fast food restaurants and supermarkets in a certain area that measures relative access to healthy food sources. Based on the assumption that fast food restaurants and convenience stores contribute to a toxic food environment compared to grocery stores, a higher RFEI shows a more "toxic" food environment. In Canada and U.S. this index has been associated with residents' weight status [93, 94].

Subjective Measures of Food Availability

Perception of availability predicts consumption; greater perceived access to fruits and vegetables has shown to be significantly correlated with higher fruit and vegetable consumption [95]. While some studies have shown that self-reported perceptions of food access associated well with objective assessments of the local food environment [96], others conclude that the two are not directly related and this assumption does not apply everywhere [97-99]. Interviews and questionnaires provide an ordinarily applied approach with more subjective data, including consumer perceptions of the food environment such as the Perceived Availability of Healthy Food Questions [59]. Subjective measurements are thus important to take into consideration when evaluating how people interact with their environments to purchase and consume food [100].

Each of the above tools has its advantages and limitations. Therefore, depending on the purpose of the research, one or more tools can be used simultaneously for a more comprehensive view of the food environment. Measuring the food environment is hampered by several factors. First, the complexity of food environment, for instance, the variation in portion sizes at restaurants makes it difficult to assess nutritional value. Also, there is a lack of common metrics for measuring many of the features of the food environment. There is also a lack of validated environmental measures [25]. Accelerating multilevel ecological research in this area is quite a challenge.

INTERVENTIONS FOR IMPROVING THE FOOD ENVIRONMENT

Based on the community nutrition environments model [10], supportive food environments can be highly effective in improving dietary behavior and preventing chronic diseases [101]. Environmental and policy interventions have been identified as the most promising strategies for creating population-wide improvements in eating, physical activity, and weight status by a number of authors and international agencies [14, 18, 9, 15]. However, it is well accepted that creating a healthy food environment require involvement of various sectors of society to take action [102, 18, 15], as presented in Figure 5. Based on the figure, food environment is highly influenced by the society and its socio-cultural practices, government policies and regulations and the food industry.

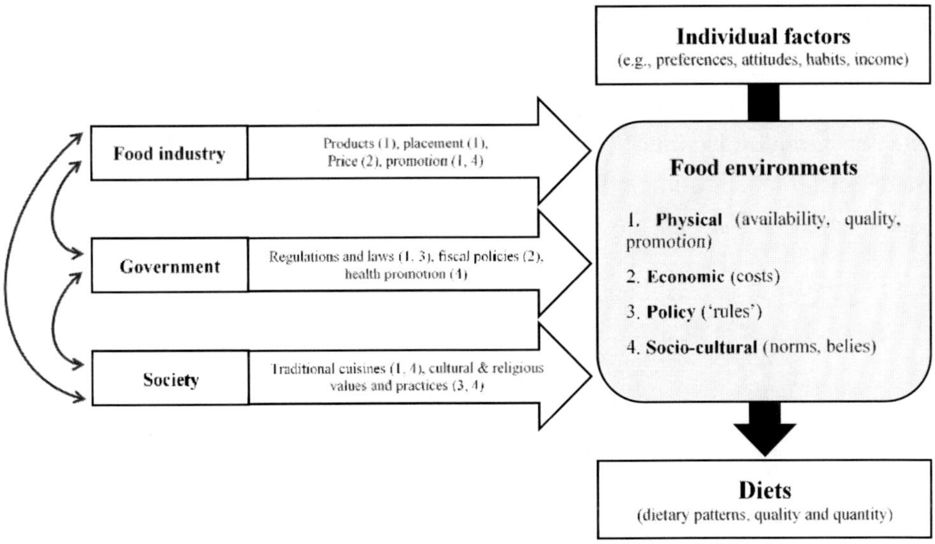

Figure 5. The major influences on food environments: the food industry, governments and society (and their interactions); and the interaction between individual factors and food environments to shape diets [9].

Multiple policies and programs have been implemented in efforts to improve the health of food environments. These efforts have been categorized into Micro and macro level approaches [23]:

Micro-Level Interventions

Several strategies have been used to improve children food environment through changing food availability, access and eating behaviors in different settings, including homes, child cares, schools, after schools, retail stores/supermarkets, restaurants and fast food outlets, as well as communities and clinics [103, 23]. Few studies have tried to reduce obesity and related chronic-disease risk factors in children and adolescents through modifying home food availability [104]. These efforts have been mainly implemented through providing parental social support for healthy eating and modeling of healthful dietary intake by parents and siblings.

School-based interventions aiming at dietary improvement and obesity prevention in children and youth have been started since 1990's. A recent review on school-based interventions in middle and high income countries have reported several strategies used to improve school food environment, including improving availability and intake of healthy foods, specifically fruits and vegetables and decreasing sweets and savory snacks, as well as marketing of healthy messages throughout the school [105]. In low to middle income countries limitations such as a lack of healthy food choices were found as a barrier to successful implementation of many interventions [106].

Some interventions were focused on increasing local availability and accessibility of healthy foods [107-112]. Opening a grocery store in a deprived area has been one of the interventions to increase fruit and vegetable accessibility that has led to increased fruit and vegetable consumption in some studies [112, 113]. Although similar efforts has not made a significant difference in some other studies [108]. Also, shelf labeling of healthy food is a successful intervention that has helped to increase purchasing of promoted foods [50, 111].

Macro Level Interventions

Policy approaches have been justified based on the idea that even if environmental influences on behavior are relatively weak, their daily influence on large segments of the population may help to facilitate improved diet quality at the population-level [114]. The main policy actions targeting at food environments to reduce obesity and non-communicable diseases have focused on fiscal food policy, restricting food advertising and product promotion, food transformation and processing, food labelling, providing high-quality foods in public institutions and incentives and rules to create a healthy retail and food service environment.

Fiscal Food Policy

One of the important factors in dietary choice is food price. Peoples' affordability of food has a direct impact on their purchasing and eating behaviors [115]. Application of fiscal tools as part of governments' efforts have been recommended by WHO global action plan on the prevention and control of NCDs, the WHO comprehensive implementation plan on maternal, infant and young child nutrition; and, more recently, by the WHO commission on ending childhood obesity [116]. However, few governments have used fiscal or price-control measures to influence food prices selectively to improve nutrition and health outcomes [117].

The fiscal food policy is mostly applied through food taxes and subsidies in order to improve nutrition and health by persuading people to buy and consume healthier foods [118, 119]. These policies have important role in discouraging the consumption of unhealthy foods, which containe harmful ingredients such as sugar, salt, and saturated fat and encouraging the consumption of healthy foods such as vegetables and fruits [120, 121].

An important consideration in this regard is optimal rate of tax for specific food items. A systematic review has shown that taxes on sugar-sweetened beverages (SSB) consistently decreased their consumption [122]. While some studies such as one by Waterlander et al. (2014) showed the link between existing soda sales taxes and weight outcomes is small [123]. Other natural experimental studies have generally shown that soda sale taxes (ranging from 1 to 8%) are too low to affect any population [124-126].

Experimental research suggests the tax level should be at least 20% [129] to 25% [130] to be effective.

Another example is junk food tax is in Hungary that was estimated to reduce purchases of processed foods by 3.4%, while purchased quantities of unprocessed foods increased by a statistically insignificant 1.1% at 16 months post-implementation [127]. An evidence gap that still needs to be addressed is quantifying the impact of taxes on a given food in improving body weight and other diet-related health risk factors.

Optimistic effects of fiscal policies can be augmented if a target food tax is joint to a subsidy on healthful foods such as fruits and vegetables [128], since reducing the price of healthy food may increase their intake. A 10% reduction in price of fruits and vegetables increases their consumption by 7.2% [129].

Food subsidies have also been applied to promote high-quality diets. Evidence on the implementation of vouchers, financial incentives and 'fruit and vegetable boxes' in high-income countries has shown that subsidies on more nutritious foods significantly increased the purchase and consumption of promoted foods within low-income groups [130, 131]. In South Africa, a 10% cash-back discount program for nutritious foods led to 5.7% increase in fruit and vegetables purchase, and a 5.6% decrease in the purchase of less nutritious foods, as a proportion of total food expenditure [132]. Other studies have shown modest impacts of subsidies on the purchase and consumption of more nutritious foods [133].

Overall, the goal of fiscal food policy must be encouraging higher-quality diets by enhancing supply and reducing the cost of high-quality food options. Policy coherence is essential to ensure optimal impact of fiscal policies on diets.

Restricting Food Advertising and Product Promotion

A powerful behavior change mechanism is the advertising and marketing in the food system which attracts good investment from governments, the private sector, charities and civil groups. Because children do not have the power of logical analysis of advertisements, most of the research and policy action on food marketing has focused on the advertising of foods to children [134]. Evidence from systematic reviews demonstrates that advertising and other forms of food marketing to children can directly influence their food preferences [135, 136]. In 2016, the WHO Commission on Ending Childhood Obesity established a set of recommended actions for its member states to effectively combat childhood obesity [137]. One of them was to reduce the exposure to, and the power of the marketing of foods and beverages high in saturated fatty acids, trans fatty acids, free sugars, or salt to children and adolescents.

Despite WHO recommendations [138], only 8% of countries regulate the marketing of foods and beverages to children and only 36% of countries have implemented provisions of the International Code of Marketing of Breast-milk Substitutes [139]. The complete effect of policy interventions to constrain the marketing and advertising of less nutritious foods to children on their dietary choices and later health indicators has not been completely assessed. However, some governments have well applied multi-sector legal marketing structures to encourage high-quality diets. In 2015, Chile adopted the most comprehensive marketing restriction law in the world to date (Law No. 20, 606) [140]. Since the law was implemented, food companies have been required to place front-of-package labels on foods and beverages that are high in sugar (≥10g/100g), sodium (≥ 400mg/100g), saturated fats (≥ 4g/100g) and energy (≥ 275kcal/100g). The law prohibits the advertising and marketing of these target foods to children aged 14 and younger. Further, these foods are not to be sold, marketed, promoted or advertised within establishments of preschool, primary or high school education [141]. Subsequent evaluation of this comprehensive strategy in terms of its impact on the quality of diets and health outcomes will be essential.

In South Korea, TV advertising of target food products to children under 18 years of age is prohibited during and after programs shown between 5-7 pm and during other children's programs. This law acquired good result in 2010 and has had a positive effect on the South Korean food environment by motivating around 50% of food companies to reformulate their products [142]. Part of the success in South Korea in maintaining nutritious traditional diets and keeping rates of obesity and NCDs at much lower levels than in other countries has been through the use of industry-developed social marketing techniques to promote the consumption of relatively nutritious traditional food [57].

The government in Mexico, Denmark and Latvia in collaboration with the food industry, have adopting codes for 'responsible' marketing to children. These law included restricting the commercial promotion of foods high in sugar, salt and fat, and prohibiting numerous forms of marketing through television, internet, videogames and product placements [143]. Despite these efforts, there is a high need for action to limit food marketing targeted at children to protect them from their negative impacts.

Food Transformation and Processing

The diversity of transformation and processing techniques can have mixed implications for diet quality. Yet processing can lead to lower nutritional quality of products [144]. From the perspective of generating policy impact in the food environment to explicitly improve diet quality, two key entry points in the food transformation subsystem are fortification and reformulation.

Food fortification has proven to be an effective strategy to address micronutrient deficiencies in many countries [145]. The mandatory fortification of wheat flour with folic acid and salt iodization illustrates what can be achieved. These fortified foods have helped reduce birth defects and brain damage, respectively, in many countries [146]. Fortifying widely-consumed foods involves public-private partnerships and can be an economically efficient way to treat micronutrient deficiencies. However, the public sector requires to match local nutrition priorities and rules to monitor the safety and coincidence of fortification. Fortification should not be taken as a substitute for a diverse diet and well-balanced, but as a supplement. The requisite for fortification should decrease in accordance with increasing of diet diversity, education levels and incomes [134].

On the other hand, the target of most reformulation policies to affect the obesity epidemic is ultra-processed products [147]. In this regard, Reformulation of food and beverages marketed directly to children to improve their nutritional quality, have been emphasized as a mean in improving the child-oriented food supply [147] The primary aim of these reformulation policies is to limit the set of negative nutrients, referred to as nutrients-to-limit reformulation. Over time the food industry has food product reformulation in format of added and removed ingredients to response to public health recommendations, regulatory actions and consumer demand [10]. Considering obesity and chronic disease epidemic, key nutrients of concern within product reformulation initiatives include Na, free sugars, SFA, trans-fatty acids and energy.

One policy that has been broadly implemented is reducing children's sugar intake through food reformulation. An example is the UK where since 2016, this policy has launched with the aim to reduce the amount of total sugar in foods commonly consumed by UK children, including breakfast cereals, yogurts, biscuits, morning goods, puddings, ice cream, and chocolate and sweet confectionery 20% by 2020 [148]. Sugar reformulation of packaged foods is one of the implementation steps of this policy. Manufacturers can achieve this goal by: 1) lowering sugar per 100 g of product, 2) decreasing the energy content or portion size of single-serving products, and/or 3) shifting consumer purchasing habits toward lower/no sugar products [149].

While the focus of reformulation strategies has been on reducing nutrients-to-limit, relatively little attention is given to the quality of the ingredients being substituted during reformulation [147]. A study on 120 child-oriented food products in Australia showed that reformulation is occurring in both directions - both towards and away from what is considered 'healthy' [150]. Such points need to be taken into account in monitoring food policies in the future. After all, trying to improve the nutrient profile of foods bring many opportunities to governments and the private sector collaboration to make food environment healthier.

Food Labelling

The main impact of food labelling on diet quality has been to stimulate the food industry to reformulate foods [128]. Food labels can help consumers make informed decisions either by providing lists of nutrient content, or by using interpretative labels (graphics, symbols or colors) related to the nutrient content. New forms of digital information for smartphones, computers and telephones, such as Smart Label [134], have also been developed to simplify the access to detailed information about food and beverage products. Systematic reviews have suggested that nutrition labelling, may be a valuable way to consumer awareness and empowerment to select more healthy and nutritious foods [151-153].

Mandatory disclosure of information about the nutritional content of packaged food can also effect the behaviour of food processors and retailers, encouraging reformulation. For example, mandatory labelling of trans-fats in the USA incentivised the food industry to remove this ingredient from their foods [154].

Another labeling approach is menu labeling in fast food restaurants. An experimental study on the effect of calorie labels on fast food choices of parents and adolescents in a low income community in New York City showed that adolescents noticed labels at similar rates to adults; however, those who did notice the information responded to it at a lower rates compared to adults. Overall, no significant effect on purchasing behavior was observed [155].

For better outcomes from labeling policy, it is necessary to provide more evidence on how consumers use the labels and how much their understanding of the scientific content of the labels is.

Providing High-Quality Foods in Schools

The shaping of the norms around foods via providing nutritious diets by public sector and schools has the potential to give priority to high-quality diets and incentivise providers and servicers to align their value chains accordingly [156]. The result of a review of interventions dedicated on changes in the schools food environment to avoid obesity and improve dietary intake showed that forbidding of sugary drinks in schools and increasing availability and accessibility of fruits and vegetables for children were positively effective in the prevention of childhood obesity and modifications in the environment according to the local needs [157].

The availability of food for pupils to purchase in schools is also an important issue. In many countries, there are requirements for foods allowed to be sold in the schools. In 2014, a United States Department of Agriculture (USDA) initiative, "Smart Snacks in Schools", required any snacks sold in schools to meet calorie, sugar, fat and sodium limits [158]. Also, in the UK, comprehensive food standards were introduced in 2015, with mandatory guidance for schools on the absence of drinks with added sugar, crisps, chocolate or sweets in school meals or vending machines, and provision of no more than two portions of deep fried, breaded or battered foods per week [159]. Another example is the Health Promoting Schools (IHPS) in public schools in Iran [160] where one of the components of the program is to promote haealthy food environment and healthy dietary behaviors among students. In this regard, schools are provided with a mandatory list of healthy snacks that could be sold and an unhealthy snacks list that their selling and consumption in schools is banned. A recent study found no significant difference between the school food environment and students' snacking behaviors in IHPS and non-IHPS schools ($P>0.05$) [161].

Incentives and Rules to Create a Healthy Retail and Food Service Environment

Retailers and food outlets are the means through which consumers access the food supply. These settings provide good entry points for policy interventions in food retailing. For example, in 2008, New York City provided 1,000 licenses for Green Carts, which were part of larger strategy to fight food deserts, the policy created a new vending permit class for the sale of fresh fruits and vegetables in neighborhoods with limited access to nutritious foods. However, only 7% of the green carts remained in the food deserts and the majority went where people and businesses congregate [162]. The investigators concluded that although most of the carts were not located in food deserts, their presence even in non–food desert areas may have effect on increasing overall fruit and vegetable accessibility by lowering prices through competition and increasing visibility of fresh produce. Effective approaches to implement such policies and the magnitude of their benefits deserves further evaluation. Other examples of policy attempts to manage food environment in urban neighborhoods include US approval of one-year moratorium on the opening of new fast food establishments in several neighborhoods with high fast-food density and high obesity in the Los Angeles City in 2008 [163]. Also, banning the establishment of fast-food restaurants within 500 feet of all types of preschools and schools in the US zoning code in Detroit is another good example [164]. In 2014, the US Congress developed the 'Healthy Food Financing Initiative', in which states use funds to incentivize retailers to sell healthy foods in deprived or unhealthy areas [165].

In Singapore, in 2006, Health Promotion Board initiated "Healthier Dining Program" which aimed to increase the availability of healthier dishes in restaurants [166]. The program, helped restaurants to modify their menu dishes to contain less oil, salt and sugar and to include more vegetables and fruits. The board promoted these restaurants in food magazines and national newspapers to encourage more patronage of healthy restaurants. This promotion was successful to increase the proportion of table orders with more than 1 healthier dish from 35% in 2004 to 63% in 2008 [167]. The Healthier Dining Program also worked with fast food chains to provide healthier options for customers. Fast food chains offered at least one of the following healthy food options in 2008 – salad (dressing served separately), pure fruit juices, potato fries with no salt (at the customer's request) and extra lettuce with burgers.

Planners, local government officials, food retailers and food policy councils can help ensure a healthy food environment at the city level. Overall, declarations of good practice in this domain contain the adaptation of zoning strategies to convince food venders to enlarge healthy food availability in low income neighborhoods (e.g., supporting farmers' markets and fresh fruit and vegetable outlets), and to control the availability of unhealthy food (e.g., fast-food outlets) around schools through zoning restrictions [168, 134].

Conclusion

Food environment, both internal and external environment, plays an important role in people's food acquisition and consumption. This effect is even higher when it comes to children and adolescents. Considering the rising prevalence of overweigh/obesity among these age groups, creating supportive food environments is known as the most promising strategies for creating population-wide improvements in eating, physical activity, and weight status. A number of environmental and policy interventions have been introduced, which their effectiveness has been very much dependent on the socio-economical context, as well as operational approaches taken. After all, ensuring a sustainable food environment for children and youth remains as a social responsibility of all stakeholders as well as societies.

References

[1] Kimm SY, Obarzanek E. "Childhood obesity: a new pandemic of the new millennium." *Pediatrics* 110, no. 5 (2002): 1003-7.

[2] Swinburn BA, Kraak VI, Allender S, Atkins VJ, Baker PI, Bogard JR, et al. "The global syndemic of obesity, undernutrition, and climate change: the Lancet Commission report." *The Lancet* 393, no. 10173 (2019): 791-846.

[3] Swinburn B, Egger G, Raza F. "Dissecting obesogenic environments: the development and application of a framework for identifying and prioritizing environmental interventions for obesity." *Preventive Medicine* 29, no. 6 (1999): 563-70.

[4] Bouchard C, Tremblay A, Després J-P, Nadeau A, Lupien PJ, Thériault G, et al. "The response to long-term overfeeding in identical twins." *New England Journal of Medicine* 322, no. 21 (1990): 1477-82.

[5] Swinburn BA, Sacks G, Hall KD, McPherson K, Finegood DT, Moodie ML, et al. "The global obesity pandemic: shaped by global drivers and local environments." *The Lancet* 378, no. 9793 (2011): 804-14.

[6] Penchansky R, Thomas JW. "The concept of access: definition and relationship to consumer satisfaction." *Medical Care* (1981): 127-40.

[7] Glanz K, Sallis JF, Saelens BE, Frank LD. "Healthy nutrition environments: concepts and measures." *American Journal of Health Promotion* 19, no. 5 (2005): 330-3.

[8] Townshend T, Lake AA. "Obesogenic urban form: theory, policy and practice." *Health & Place* 15, no. 4 (2009): 909-16.

[9] Swinburn B, Sacks G, Vandevijvere S, Kumanyika S, Lobstein T, Neal B, et al. "INFORMAS (I nternational N etwork for F ood and Obesity/non communicable diseases R esearch, M onitoring and A ction S upport): overview and key principles." *Obesity Reviews* 14 (2013): 1-12.

[10] FAO. "*Influencing food environments for healthy diets*." (2016): Food and Agriculture Organization of the United Nations, Rome.

[11] Tavares LF, Fonseca SC, Rosa MLG, Yokoo EM. "Relationship between ultra-processed foods and metabolic syndrome in adolescents from a Brazilian Family Doctor Program." *Public Health Nutrition* 15, no. 1 (2012): 82-7.

[12] Baker P, Hawkes C, Wingrove K, Demaio AR, Parkhurst J, Thow AM, et al. "What drives political commitment for nutrition? A review and framework synthesis to inform the United Nations Decade of Action on Nutrition." *BMJ Global Health* 3, no. 1 (2018): e000485.

[13] UNSCN. "Investments for Healthy Food Systems, Implementing the Framework for Action of the Second International Conference on Nutrition, Executive Summary." *United Nations System Standing Committee on Nutrition* (2016).

[14] Caspi CE, Sorensen G, Subramanian S, Kawachi I. "The local food environment and diet: a systematic review." *Health & place* 18, no. 5 (2012): 1172-87.

[15] Turner C, Aggarwal A, Walls H, Herforth A, Drewnowski A, Coates J, et al. "Concepts and critical perspectives for food environment research: A global framework with implications for action in low-and middle-income countries." *Global Food Security* 18 (2018): 93-101.

[16] UNICEF. "*The State of the World's Children 2019. Children, Food and Nutrition: Growing well in a changing world*." (2019): United Nations Children's Fund, New York.

[17] UNICEF. "*Food Systems for Children and Adolescents. Working Togetherto Secure Nutritious Diets*." (2018): Adolescents UNICEF Office of Research Innocent. Florence, Italy.

[18] Swinburn B, Kraak V, Rutter H, Vandevijvere S, Lobstein T, Sacks G, et al. "Strengthening of accountability systems to create healthy food environments and reduce global obesity." *The Lancet* 385, no. 9986 (2015): 2534-45.

[19] Heidari-Beni M, Kelishadi R. "Prevalence of Weight Disorders in Iranian Children and Adolescents." *Archives of Iranian Medicine (AIM)* 22, no. 9 (2019).

[20] Skinner AC, Ravanbakht SN, Skelton JA, Perrin EM, Armstrong SC. "Prevalence of obesity and severe obesity in US children, 1999–2016." *Pediatrics* 141, no. 3 (2018): e20173459.

[21] Storr R, Carins J, Rundle-Thiele S. "Assessing Support for Advantaged and Disadvantaged Groups: A Comparison of Urban Food Environments." *International Journal of Environmental Research and Public Health* 16, no. 7 (2019): 1135.

[22] Mackenbach JD, Nelissen KG, Dijkstra SC, Poelman MP, Daams JG, Leijssen JB, et al. "A systematic review on socioeconomic differences in the association between the food environment and dietary behaviors." *Nutrients* 11, no. 9 (2019): 2215.

[23] Story M, Kaphingst KM, Robinson-O'Brien R, Glanz K. "Creating healthy food and eating environments: policy and environmental approaches." *Annual Review of Public Health* 29 (2008): 253-72.

[24] Hawkes C, Harris J, Gillespie S. "Changing diets: Urbanization and the nutrition transition." *Global Food Policy Report.* Washington, DC: International Food Policy Research Institute. (2017): 34-41.

[25] Kearney J. "Food consumption trends and drivers." *Philosophical Transactions of the Royal Society B: Biological Sciences* 365, no. 1554 (2010): 2793-807.

[26] Van Der Horst K, Oenema A, Ferreira I, Wendel-Vos W, Giskes K, van Lenthe F, et al. "A systematic review of environmental correlates of obesity-related dietary behaviors in youth." *Health Education Research* 22, no. 2 (2007): 203-26.

[27] Blake CE, Wethington E, Farrell TJ, Bisogni CA, Devine CM. "Behavioral contexts, food-choice coping strategies, and dietary quality of a multiethnic sample of employed parents." *Journal of the American Dietetic Association* 111, no. 3 (2011): 401-7.

[28] Cairns G, Angus K, Hastings G, Caraher M. "Systematic reviews of the evidence on the nature, extent and effects of food marketing to children. A retrospective summary." *Appetite* 62 (2013): 209-15.

[29] Kelly B, Hattersley L, King L, Flood V. "Persuasive food marketing to children: use of cartoons and competitions in Australian commercial television advertisements." *Health Promotion International* 23, no. 4 (2008): 337-44.

[30] Li D, Wang T, Cheng Y, Zhang M, Yang X, Zhu Z, et al. "The extent and nature of television food advertising to children in Xi'an, China." *BMC Public Health* 16, no. 1 (2016): 770.

[31] Taveras EM, Sandora TJ, Shih MC, Ross-Degnan D, Goldmann DA, Gillman MW. "The association of television and video viewing with fast food intake by preschool-age children." *Obesity* 14, no. 11 (2006): 2034-41.

[32] *Cassar E. Food for thought: Understanding the role of food and food policy in low-income schools*: Temple University; 2017.

[33] Anderson PM, Butcher KF. "Reading, writing, and refreshments are school finances contributing to children's obesity?." *Journal of Human Resources* 41, no. 3 (2006): 467-94.

[34] Galvez MP, Hong L, Choi E, Liao L, Godbold J, Brenner B. "Childhood obesity and neighborhood food-store availability in an inner-city community." *Academic pediatrics* 9, no. 5 (2009): 339-43.

[35] Barrera LH, Rothenberg SJ, Barquera S, Cifuentes E. "The toxic food environment around elementary schools and childhood obesity in Mexican cities." *American journal of preventive medicine* 51, no. 2 (2016): 264-70.

[36] Howard PH, Fitzpatrick M, Fulfrost B. "Proximity of food retailers to schools and rates of overweight ninth grade students: an ecological study in California." *BMC Public Health* 11, no. 1 (2011): 68.

[37] Corrêa EN, Rossi CE, das Neves J, Silva DAS, de Vasconcelos FdAG. "Utilization and environmental availability of food outlets and overweight/obesity among schoolchildren in a city in the south of Brazil." *Journal of Public Health* 40, no. 1 (2018): 106-13.

[38] Elbel B, Tamura K, McDermott ZT, Wu E, Schwartz AE. "Childhood obesity and the food environment: A population-based sample of public school children in New York city." *Obesity* 28, no. 1 (2020): 65-72.

[39] Fiechtner L, Block J, Duncan DT, Gillman MW, Gortmaker SL, Melly SJ, et al. "Proximity to supermarkets associated with higher body mass index among overweight and obese preschool-age children." *Preventive Medicine* 56, no. 3-4 (2013): 218-21.

[40] Skidmore P, Welch A, van Sluijs E, Jones A, Harvey I, Harrison F, et al. "Impact of neighbourhood food environment on food consumption in children aged 9–10 years in the UK SPEEDY (Sport, Physical Activity and Eating behaviour: Environmental Determinants in Young people) study." *Public Health Nutrition* 13, no. 7 (2010): 1022-30.

[41] Timperio A, Ball K, Roberts R, Campbell K, Andrianopoulos N, Crawford D. "Children's fruit and vegetable intake: associations with the neighbourhood food environment." *Preventive Medicine* 46, no. 4 (2008): 331-5.

[42] Robinson TN, Banda JA, Hale L, Lu AS, Fleming-Milici F, Calvert SL, et al. "Screen media exposure and obesity in children and adolescents." *Pediatrics* 140, no. Supplement 2 (2017): S97-S101.

[43] Boulos R, Vikre EK, Oppenheimer S, Chang H, Kanarek RB. "ObesiTV: how television is influencing the obesity epidemic." *Physiology & Behavior* 107, no. 1 (2012): 146-53.

[44] Crespo CJ, Smit E, Troiano RP, Bartlett SJ, Macera CA, Andersen RE. "Television watching, energy intake, and obesity in US children: results from the third National Health and Nutrition Examination Survey, 1988-1994." *Archives of Pediatrics & Adolescent Medicine* 155, no. 3 (2001): 360-5.

[45] Wiecha JL, Peterson KE, Ludwig DS, Kim J, Sobol A, Gortmaker SL. "When children eat what they watch: Impact of television viewing on dietary intake in youth." *Archives of Pediatrics & Adolescent Medicine* 160, no. 4 (2006): 436-42.

[46] Falciglia GA, Gussow JD. "Television commercials and eating behavior of obese and normal-weight women." *Journal of Nutrition Education* 12, no. 4 (1980): 196-9.

[47] Halford JC, Boyland EJ, Hughes G, Oliveira LP, Dovey TM. "Beyond-brand effect of television (TV) food advertisements/commercials on caloric intake and food choice of 5–7-year-old children." *Appetite* 49, no. 1 (2007): 263-7.

[48] Aktas Arnas Y. "The effects of television food advertisement on children's food purchasing requests." *Pediatrics International* 48, no. 2 (2006): 138-45.

[49] Amini M, Omidvar N, Yeatman H, Shariat-Jafari S, Eslami-Amirabadi M, Zahedirad M. "Content analysis of food advertising in Iranian children's television programs." *International Journal of Preventive Medicine* 5, no. 10 (2014): 1337.

[50] Chamberlain LJ, Wang Y, Robinson TN. "Does children's screen time predict requests for advertised products?: Cross-sectional and prospective analyses." *Archives of Pediatrics & Adolescent Medicine* 160, no. 4 (2006): 363-8.

[51] Kaiser HJ. "The role of media in childhood obesity." *The Henry J Kaiser Family Foundation* (2004).

[52] Boynton-Jarrett R, Thomas TN, Peterson KE, Wiecha J, Sobol AM, Gortmaker SL. "Impact of television viewing patterns on fruit and vegetable consumption among adolescents." *Pediatrics* 112, no. 6 (2003): 1321-6.

[53] Coon KA, Goldberg J, Rogers BL, Tucker KL. "Relationships between use of television during meals and children's food consumption patterns." *Pediatrics* 107, no. 1 (2001): e7.

[54] Halford JC, Boyland EJ, Cooper GD, Dovey TM, Smith CJ, Williams N, et al. "Children's food preferences: Effects of weight status, food type, branding and television food advertisements (commercials)." *International Journal of Pediatric Obesity* 3, no. 1 (2008): 31-8.

[55] Boyland EJ, Halford JC. "Television advertising and branding. Effects on eating behaviour and food preferences in children." *Appetite* 62 (2013): 236-41.

[56] Robinson TN, Borzekowski DL, Matheson DM, Kraemer HC. "Effects of fast food branding on young children's taste preferences." *Archives of Pediatrics & Adolescent Medicine* 161, no. 8 (2007): 792-7.

[57] Herforth A, Ahmed S. "The food environment, its effects on dietary consumption, and potential for measurement within agriculture-nutrition interventions." *Food Security* 7, no. 3 (2015): 505-20.

[58] Minaker L, Fisher P, Raine K, Frank L. "Measuring the food environment: From theory to planning practice." *Journal of Agriculture, Food Systems, and Community Development* 2, no. 1 (2011): 65-82.

[59] Moore LV, Diez Roux AV, Nettleton JA, Jacobs Jr DR. "Associations of the local food environment with diet quality—a comparison of assessments based on surveys

and geographic information systems: The multi-ethnic study of atherosclerosis." *American Journal of Epidemiology* 167, no. 8 (2008): 917-24.

[60] Befort C, Kaur H, Nollen N, Sullivan DK, Nazir N, Choi WS, et al. "Fruit, vegetable, and fat intake among non-Hispanic black and non-Hispanic white adolescents: Associations with home availability and food consumption settings." *Journal of the American Dietetic Association* 106, no. 3 (2006): 367-73.

[61] Cullen KW, Baranowski T, Owens E, Marsh T, Rittenberry L, De Moor C. "Availability, accessibility, and preferences for fruit, 100% fruit juice, and vegetables influence children's dietary behavior." *Health Education & Behavior* 30, no. 5 (2003): 615-26.

[62] Watts AW, Barr SI, Hanning RM, Lovato CY, Mâsse LC. "The home food environment and associations with dietary intake among adolescents presenting for a lifestyle modification intervention." *BMC Nutrition* 4, no. 1 (2018): 3.

[63] Couch SC, Glanz K, Zhou C, Sallis JF, Saelens BE. "Home food environment in relation to children's diet quality and weight status." *Journal of the Academy of Nutrition and Dietetics* 114, no. 10 (2014): 1569-79.

[64] Neumark-Sztainer D, Wall M, Perry C, Story M. "Correlates of fruit and vegetable intake among adolescents: Findings from project EAT." *Preventive Medicine* 37, no. 3 (2003): 198-208.

[65] Pearson N, Biddle SJ, Gorely T. "Family correlates of fruit and vegetable consumption in children and adolescents: A systematic review." *Public Health Nutrition* 12, no. 2 (2009): 267-83.

[66] Bryant M, Stevens J. "Measurement of food availability in the home." *Nutrition Reviews* 64, no. 2 (2006): 67-76.

[67] Gattshall ML, Shoup JA, Marshall JA, Crane LA, Estabrooks PA. "Validation of a survey instrument to assess home environments for physical activity and healthy eating in overweight children." *International Journal of Behavioral Nutrition and Physical Activity* 5, no. 1 (2008): 3.

[68] Hanson NI, Neumark-Sztainer D, Eisenberg ME, Story M, Wall M. "Associations between parental report of the home food environment and adolescent intakes of fruits, vegetables and dairy foods." *Public Health Nutrition* 8, no. 1 (2005): 77-85.

[69] Stevens J, Bryant M, Wang L, Borja J, Bentley ME. "Exhaustive measurement of food items in the home using a universal product code scanner." *Public Health Nutrition* 14, no. 2 (2011): 314-8.

[70] Nepper M, Ludemann M, Chai W. "Validation of instruments to assess home food environment of pre-adolescents: A pilot study." *Journal of Nutritional Health & Food Science* 2, no. 4 (2014): 1-9.

[71] Boles RE, Scharf C, Filigno SS, Saelens BE, Stark LJ. "Differences in home food and activity environments between obese and healthy weight families of preschool children." *Journal of Nutrition Education and Behavior* 45, no. 3 (2013): 222-31.

[72] Boles RE, Burdell A, Johnson SL, Gavin WJ, Davies PL, Bellows LL. "Home food and activity assessment. Development and validation of an instrument for diverse families of young children." *Appetite* 80 (2014): 23-7.

[73] Block G, Hartman AM, Naughton D. "A reduced dietary questionnaire: Development and validation." *Epidemiology* 1, no. 1 (1990): 58-64.

[74] Willett WC, Stampfer MJ, Underwood BA, Speizer FE, Rosner B, Hennekens CH. "Validation of a dietary questionnaire with plasma carotenoid and α-tocopherol levels." *The American Journal of Clinical Nutrition* 38, no. 4 (1983): 631-9.

[75] Kennedy ET, Ohls J, Carlson S, Fleming K. "The healthy eating index: Design and applications." *Journal of the American Dietetic Association* 95, no. 10 (1995): 1103-8.

[76] Krebs-Smith SM, Reedy J, Bosire C. "Healthfulness of the US food supply: Little improvement despite decades of dietary guidance." *American Journal of Preventive Medicine* 38, no. 5 (2010): 472-7.

[77] Reedy J, Krebs-Smith SM, Bosire C. "Evaluating the food environment: Application of the Healthy Eating Index-2005." *American Journal of Preventive Medicine* 38, no. 5 (2010): 465-71.

[78] Allison KR, Adlaf EM. "Structured opportunities for student physical activity in Ontario elementary and secondary schools." *Canadian Journal of Public Health* 91, no. 5 (2000): 371-5.

[79] Kyle TM, Brener ND, Kann L, Ross JG, Roberts AM, Iachan R, et al. "Methods: School health policies and programs study 2006." *Journal of School Health* 77, no. 8 (2007): 398-407.

[80] Kubik MY, Lytle LA, Hannan PJ, Perry CL, Story M. "The association of the school food environment with dietary behaviors of young adolescents." *American Journal of Public Health* 93, no. 7 (2003): 1168-73.

[81] Krukowski RA, Philyaw Perez AG, Bursac Z, Goodell M, Raczynski JM, Smith West D, et al. "Development and evaluation of the school cafeteria nutrition assessment measures." *Journal of School Health* 81, no. 8 (2011): 431-6.

[82] Nathan N, Wolfenden L, Morgan PJ, Bell AC, Barker D, Wiggers J. "Validity of a self-report survey tool measuring the nutrition and physical activity environment of primary schools." *International Journal of Behavioral Nutrition and Physical Activity* 10, no. 1 (2013): 75.

[83] Anderson AS, Dewar J, Marshall D, Cummins S, Taylor M, Dawson J, et al. "The development of a healthy eating indicator shopping basket tool (HEISB) for use in food access studies—identification of key food items." *Public Health Nutrition* 10, no. 12 (2007): 1440-7.

[84] Farley TA, Rice J, Bodor JN, Cohen DA, Bluthenthal RN, Rose D. "Measuring the food environment: Shelf space of fruits, vegetables, and snack foods in stores." *Journal of Urban Health* 86, no. 5 (2009): 672-82.

[85] Rose D, Hutchinson PL, Bodor JN, Swalm CM, Farley TA, Cohen DA, et al. "Neighborhood food environments and body mass index: The importance of in-store contents." *American Journal of Preventive Medicine* 37, no. 3 (2009): 214-9.

[86] Glanz K, Sallis JF, Saelens BE, Frank LD. "Nutrition Environment Measures Survey in stores (NEMS-S): Development and evaluation." *American Journal of Preventive Medicine* 32, no. 4 (2007): 282-9.

[87] Ghirardelli A, Quinn V, Sugerman S. "Reliability of a retail food store survey and development of an accompanying retail scoring system to communicate survey findings and identify vendors for healthful food and marketing initiatives." *Journal of Nutrition Education and Behavior* 43, no. 4 (2011): S104-S12.

[88] Kerr J, Sallis JF, Bromby E, Glanz K. "Assessing reliability and validity of the GroPromo audit tool for evaluation of grocery store marketing and promotional environments." *Journal of Nutrition Education and Behavior* 44, no. 6 (2012): 597-603.

[89] Black C, Ntani G, Inskip H, Cooper C, Cummins S, Moon G, et al. "Measuring the healthfulness of food retail stores: Variations by store type and neighbourhood deprivation." *International Journal of Behavioral Nutrition and Physical Activity* 11, no. 1 (2014): 69.

[90] Andreyeva T, Blumenthal DM, Schwartz MB, Long MW, Brownell KD. "Availability and prices of foods across stores and neighborhoods: The case of New Haven, Connecticut." *Health Affairs* 27, no. 5 (2008): 1381-8.

[91] Kanter R, Alvey J, Fuentes D. "Creation of a mobile-phone application for assessing supermarket offerings for a Guatemalan-based exploration of the Nutrient Environment Measurement Survey-Stores (255.1)." *The FASEB Journal* 28, no. 1_supplement (2014): 255.1.

[92] Saelens BE, Glanz K, Sallis JF, Frank LD. "Nutrition Environment Measures Study in restaurants (NEMS-R): Development and evaluation." *American Journal of Preventive Medicine* 32, no. 4 (2007): 273-81.

[93] Babey SH, Diamant AL, Hastert TA, Harvey S. "*Designed for disease: The link between local food environments and obesity and diabetes*." California: UCLA Center for Health Policy Research (2008).

[94] Spence JC, Cutumisu N, Edwards J, Raine KD, Smoyer-Tomic K. "Relation between local food environments and obesity among adults." *BMC Public Health* 9, no. 1 (2009): 192.

[95] Caldwell EM, Kobayashi MM, DuBow W, Wytinck S. "Perceived access to fruits and vegetables associated with increased consumption." *Public Health Nutrition* 12, no. 10 (2009): 1743-50.

[96] Freedman DA, Bell BA. "Access to healthful foods among an urban food insecure population: perceptions versus reality." *Journal of Urban Health* 86, no. 6 (2009): 825-38.

[97] Moore LV, Diez Roux AV, Nettleton JA, Jacobs DR, Franco M. "Fast-food consumption, diet quality, and neighborhood exposure to fast food: the multi-ethnic study of atherosclerosis." *American Journal of Epidemiology* 170, no. 1 (2009): 29-36.

[98] Williams LK, Thornton L, Ball K, Crawford D. "Is the objective food environment associated with perceptions of the food environment?." *Public Health Nutrition* 15, no. 2 (2012): 291-8.

[99] Winkler E, Turrell G, Patterson C. "Does living in a disadvantaged area mean fewer opportunities to purchase fresh fruit and vegetables in the area? Findings from the Brisbane food study." *Health & Place* 12, no. 3 (2006): 306-19.

[100] Cummins S. "Neighbourhood food environment and diet: Time for improved conceptual models?." *Preventive Medicine* 44, no. 3 (2007): 196.

[101] Penney TL, Brown HE, Maguire ER, Kuhn I, Monsivais P. "Local food environment interventions to improve healthy food choice in adults: A systematic review and realist synthesis protocol." *BMJ Open* 5, no. 4 (2015).

[102] Carducci B, Oh C, Keats EC, Gaffey MF, Roth DE, Bhutta ZA. "PROTOCOL: Impact of the food environment on diet-related health outcomes in school-age children and adolescents in low-and middle-income countries: A systematic review." *Campbell Systematic Reviews* 14, no. 1 (2018): 1-55.

[103] Flynn M, McNeil D, Maloff B, Mutasingwa D, Wu M, Ford C, et al. "Reducing obesity and related chronic disease risk in children and youth: A synthesis of evidence with 'best practice'recommendations." *Obesity Reviews* 7 (2006): 7-66.

[104] Harvey-Berino J, Rourke J. "Obesity prevention in preschool native-american children: a pilot study using home visiting." *Obesity Research* 11, no. 5 (2003): 606-11.

[105] Evans CE, Albar SA, Vargas-Garcia EJ, Xu F. "School-based interventions to reduce obesity risk in children in high-and middle-income countries." *Advances in Food and Nutrition Research*: Elsevier; 2015. p. 29-77.

[106] Skar M, Kirstein E, Kapur A. "Lessons learnt from school-based health promotion projects in low-and middle-income countries." *Child: Care, Health and Development* 41, no. 6 (2015): 1114-23.

[107] Cummins S, Findlay A, Higgins C, Petticrew M, Sparks L, Thomson H. "Reducing inequalities in health and diet: Findings from a study on the impact of a food retail development." *Environment and Planning A* 40, no. 2 (2008): 402-22.

[108] Cummins S, Findlay A, Petticrew M, Sparks L. "Retail-led regeneration and store-switching behaviour." *Journal of Retailing and Consumer Services* 15, no. 4 (2008): 288-95.

[109] Gittelsohn J, Song H-J, Suratkar S, Kumar MB, Henry EG, Sharma S, et al. "An urban food store intervention positively affects food-related psychosocial variables and food behaviors." *Health Education & Behavior* 37, no. 3 (2010): 390-402.

[110] Gittelsohn J, Vijayadeva V, Davison N, Ramirez V, Cheung LW, Murphy S, et al. "A food store intervention trial improves caregiver psychosocial factors and children's dietary intake in Hawaii." *Obesity* 18, no. S1 (2010): S84-S90.

[111] Song H-J, Gittelsohn J, Kim M, Suratkar S, Sharma S, Anliker J. "A corner store intervention in a low-income urban community is associated with increased availability and sales of some healthy foods." *Public Health Nutrition* 12, no. 11 (2009): 2060-7.

[112] Wrigley N, Warm D, Margetts B. "Deprivation, diet, and food-retail access: Findings from the Leeds 'food deserts' study." *Environment and Planning A* 35, no. 1 (2003): 151-88.

[113] Wrigley N, Warm D, Margetts B, Whelan A. "Assessing the impact of improved retail access on diet in a'food desert': A preliminary report." *Urban Studies* 39, no. 11 (2002): 2061-82.

[114] Booth SL, Sallis JF, Ritenbaugh C, Hill JO, Birch LL, Frank LD, et al. "Environmental and societal factors affect food choice and physical activity: Rationale, influences, and leverage points." *Nutrition Reviews* 59, no. 3 (2001): S21-S36.

[115] WHO. "*Using price policies to promote healthier diets*." (2015): Europe: World Health Organization.

[116] WHO. "*Commission on ending childhood obesity 2016. 2017*." [last accessed 5th December 2016]. Available at http://www.who.int/end-childhood-obesity/en.

[117] WHO. "*Assessing national capacity for the prevention and control of noncommunicable diseases: report of the 2015 global survey*." (2016): World Health Organization, Geneva.

[118] Hyseni L, Atkinson M, Bromley H, Orton L, Lloyd-Williams F, McGill R, et al. "The effects of policy actions to improve population dietary patterns and prevent diet-related non-communicable diseases: Scoping review." *European Journal of Clinical Nutrition* 71, no. 6 (2017): 694-711.

[119] WHO. "*Fiscal policies for diet and prevention of non-communicable diseases: Technical meeting report*." (2016): World Health Organization, Geneva.

[120] Eyles H, Mhurchu CN, Nghiem N, Blakely T. "Food pricing strategies, population diets, and non-communicable disease: A systematic review of simulation studies." *PLoS Medicine* 9, no. 12 (2012).

[121] Thow AM, Jan S, Leeder S, Swinburn B. "The effect of fiscal policy on diet, obesity and chronic disease: A systematic review." *Bulletin of the World Health Organization* 88 (2010): 609-14.

[122] Colchero MA, Popkin BM, Rivera JA, Ng SW. "Beverage purchases from stores in Mexico under the excise tax on sugar sweetened beverages: Observational study." *BMJ* 352 (2016).

[123] Silver LD, Ng SW, Ryan-Ibarra S, Taillie LS, Induni M, Miles DR, et al. "Changes in prices, sales, consumer spending, and beverage consumption one year after a tax on sugar-sweetened beverages in Berkeley, California, US: A before-and-after study." *PLoS Medicine* 14, no. 4 (2017).

[124] Fletcher JM, Frisvold D, Tefft N. "Can soft drink taxes reduce population weight?." *Contemporary Economic Policy* 28, no. 1 (2010): 23-35.

[125] Kim D, Kawachi I. "Food taxation and pricing strategies to "thin out" the obesity epidemic." *American Journal of Preventive Medicine* 30, no. 5 (2006): 430-7.

[126] Thow AM, Downs S, Jan S. "A systematic review of the effectiveness of food taxes and subsidies to improve diets: Understanding the recent evidence." *Nutrition Reviews* 72, no. 9 (2014): 551-65.

[127] Bíró A. "Did the junk food tax make the Hungarians eat healthier?." *Food Policy* 54 (2015): 107-15.

[128] Hawkes C, Smith TG, Jewell J, Wardle J, Hammond RA, Friel S, et al. "Smart food policies for obesity prevention." *The Lancet* 385, no. 9985 (2015): 2410-21.

[129] Huang KS, Lin B-H. *Estimation of food demand and nutrient elasticities from household survey data*. 2000.

[130] Black AP, Brimblecombe J, Eyles H, Morris P, Vally H, Kerin O. "Food subsidy programs and the health and nutritional status of disadvantaged families in high income countries: A systematic review." *BMC Public Health* 12, no. 1 (2012): 1099.

[131] McFadden A, Green JM, Williams V, McLeish J, McCormick F, Fox-Rushby J, et al. "Can food vouchers improve nutrition and reduce health inequalities in low-income mothers and young children: A multi-method evaluation of the experiences of beneficiaries and practitioners of the Healthy Start programme in England." *BMC Public Health* 14, no. 1 (2014): 148.

[132] Sturm R, An R, Segal D, Patel D. "A cash-back rebate program for healthy food purchases in South Africa: Results from scanner data." *American Journal of Preventive Medicine* 44, no. 6 (2013): 567-72.

[133] An R. "Effectiveness of subsidies in promoting healthy food purchases and consumption: A review of field experiments." *Public Health Nutrition* 16, no. 7 (2013): 1215-28.

[134] Global Panel. "Improving nutrition through enhanced food environments." *Global Panel on Agriculture and Food Systems for Nutrition:* London, UK (2017).

[135] Cairns G, Angus K, Hastings G. The extent, nature and effects of food promotion to children: a review of the evidence to December 2008: *World Health Organization*, WHO Press; 2009.

[136] Hastings G, McDermott L, Angus K, Stead M, Thomson S. "*The extent, nature and effects of food promotion to children: a review of the evidence*." Geneva: World Health Organization 20 (2006).

[137] WHO. "*Report of the commission on ending childhood obesity: World Health Organization*." (2016) World Health Organization; Geneva.

[138] WHO. "*Set of recommendations on the marketing of foods and non-alcoholic beverages to children*." (2010) World Health Organization; Geneva.

[139] Turner C, Kadiyala S, Aggarwal A, Coates J, Drewnowski A, Hawkes C, et al. "*Concepts and methods for food environment research in low and middle income countries. Agriculture*." (2017) Nutrition, and Health Academy.

[140] WIPO. "*Chile – Ley NO 20.606 sobre Composición Nutricional de los Alimentosy su Publicidad (modificada por la Ley NO 20.869 sobre Publicidad de los Alimentos) [Chile - Law NO 20.606 on Nutritional Composition of Food and its Advertising (as amended by Law NO 20.869 on Food Advertising)]*." (2016): World Intellectual Property Organization.

[141] Ramirez N, Katial A. "*Chile New Nutrition Labelling Regulation (GAIN Report No. CI1506)*." (2015) United States Department of Agriculture Foreign Agricultural Service, Washington, DC.

[142] Lee Y, Yoon J, Chung S-J, Lee S-K, Kim H, Kim S. "Effect of TV food advertising restriction on food environment for children in South Korea." *Health Promotion International* 32, no. 1 (2017): 25-34.

[143] World Bank Group. "*The World Bank Group A to Z 2016*." (2016) World Bank Publications.

[144] Monteiro CA, Moubarac JC, Cannon G, Ng SW, Popkin B. "Ultra-processed products are becoming dominant in the global food system." *Obesity Reviews* 14 (2013): 21-8.

[145] Bailey RL, West Jr KP, Black RE. "The epidemiology of global micronutrient deficiencies." *Annals of Nutrition and Metabolism* 66, no. Suppl. 2 (2015): 22-33.

[146] Global Panel. "Biofortification: An agricultural investment for nutrition." *Policy Brief*, no. 1 (2015): 1-8.

[147] Scrinis G, Monteiro CA. "Ultra-processed foods and the limits of product reformulation." *Public Health Nutrition* 21, no. 1 (2018): 247-52.

[148] Public Health England. *Sugar reduction programme Progress made by industry in the first year*: Accessed 26/09/18. [Internet]. Available from: https://publichealthengland.exposure.co/sugar reduction-programme. 2018.

[149] Public Health England. "*Sugar reduction: achieving the 20%*." Accessed 23/02/2018. [Internet]. Available from: https://www.gov.uk/government/ publications/sugar-reduction-achieving-the-20. 7.

[150] Savio S, Mehta K, Udell T, Coveney J. "A survey of the reformulation of Australian child-oriented food products." *BMC Public Health* 13, no. 1 (2013): 836.

[151] Campos S, Doxey J, Hammond D. "Nutrition labels on pre-packaged foods: A systematic review." *Public Health Nutrition* 14, no. 8 (2011): 1496-506.

[152] Cecchini M, Warin L. "Impact of food labelling systems on food choices and eating behaviours: a systematic review and meta-analysis of randomized studies." *Obesity Reviews* 17, no. 3 (2016): 201-10.
[153] Cowburn G, Stockley L. "Consumer understanding and use of nutrition labelling: a systematic review." *Public Health Nutrition* 8, no. 1 (2005): 21-8.
[154] Martinez SW. "Introduction of new food products with voluntary health-and Nutrition-Related Claims, 1989-2010." *USDA-ERS Economic Information Bulletin*, no. 108 (2013).
[155] Elbel B, Gyamfi J, Kersh R. "Child and adolescent fast-food choice and the influence of calorie labeling: A natural experiment." *International Journal of Obesity* 35, no. 4 (2011): 493-500.
[156] Haddad L, Hawkes C, Waage J, Webb P, Godfray C, Toulmin C. "*Food systems and diets: Facing the challenges of the 21st century*." (2016).
[157] Pineda E, Swinburn B, Sassi F. "Effective school food environment interventions for the prevention of childhood obesity: systematic review and meta-analysis." *The Lancet* 394 (2019): S77.
[158] USDA. "*Help make the healthy choice the easy choice for kids at school. A Guide to Smart Snacks in School*." 2016. United States Department of Agriculture.
[159] Dimbleby H, Vincent J. "*The school food plan*." (2013).
[160] Motlagh M, Chinian M, Dashti M. "*A national guideline for implementation health promoting schools in Islamic Republic of Iran*." Iran, 2011.
[161] Yazdi-Feyzabadi V, Omidvar N, Keshavarz Mohammadi N, Nedjat S, Karimi-Shahanjarini A, Rashidian A. "Is an Iranian Health Promoting School Status Associated with Improving School Food Environment and Snacking Behaviors in Adolescents?" *Health Promotion International* 33, no. 6 (2018): 1010-21.
[162] Li KY, Cromley EK, Fox AM, Horowitz CR. "Peer reviewed: Evaluation of the placement of mobile fruit and vegetable vendors to alleviate food deserts in New York city." *Preventing Chronic Disease* 11, (2014): E158.
[163] Sturm R, Cohen DA. "Zoning for health? The year-old ban on new fast-food restaurants in south LA: The ordinance isn't a promising approach to attacking obesity." *Health Affairs* 28, no. Suppl1 (2009): w1088-w97.
[164] Hopkins J, Universities G, Pierce MW. "*The use of zoning to restrict fast food outlets: A potential strategy to combat obesity*." (2005).
[165] WCRFI. "*NOURISHING framework*." (2017): World Cancer Research Fund International.
[166] Henderson JC. "Foodservice in Singapore: Retaining a place for hawkers?." *Journal of Foodservice Business Research* 19, no. 3 (2016): 272-86.
[167] Soon G, Koh Y, Wong M, Lam P. "*Obesity prevention and control efforts in Singapore*." (2008) Seattle: The National Bureau of Asian Research.

[168] Ni Mhurchu C, Vandevijvere S, Waterlander W, Thornton LE, Kelly B, Cameron AJ, et al. "Monitoring the availability of healthy and unhealthy foods and non-alcoholic beverages in community and consumer retail food environments globally." *Obesity Reviews* 14 (2013): 108-19.

In: Childhood Obesity
Editor: Roya Kelishadi

ISBN: 978-1-53618-158-6
© 2020 Nova Science Publishers, Inc.

Chapter 4

THE ASSOCIATION OF ENDOCRINE DISRUPTING CHEMICALS AND CHILDHOOD OBESITY

Karim Ebrahimpour[1], PhD, Mohammad Mehdi. Amin[1], PhD, Bahareh Shoshtari-Yeganeh[1,*], PhD and Roya Kelishadi[2], MD

[1]Environment Research Center,
Research Institute for Primordial Prevention of Non-Communicable Disease,
Isfahan University of Medical Sciences, Isfahan, Iran
[2]Child Growth and Development Research Center,
Research Institute for Primordial Prevention of Non-Communicable Disease,
Isfahan University of Medical Sciences, Isfahan, Iran

ABSTRACT

Obesity, as a specific disease, is rapidly becoming significant public health problems, and its prevalence has increased dramatically around the world. Epidemiological and toxicological studies suggest that environmental chemicals might have a crucial role in the development of obesity. By increase in exposure to environmental pollutants, including chemicals that disrupt the hormonal functions, the prevalence of obesity has increased as well. Among these toxins, endocrine-disrupting chemicals (EDCs) may increase the risk of obesity by disrupting hormonally mediated processes. Many of these compounds are human-made chemicals that are released into the environment and have a negative impact on the health of animals and humans. EDCs consist of various chemical compounds with widespread use. Some EDCs, including organochlorine and polychlorinated biphenyl, are stable and would persist in the environment. Although their use is prohibited, their use in food constituents, packaging industry, and pesticides still continues, and their concentrations have increased over time. Recent *in-vitro*, *in-vivo*, and epidemiological studies documented the link of EDCs exposure with obesity. Several recent studies have

* Corresponding Author's Email: baharshoshtary@gmail.com.

revealed the association between early-life exposure to EDCs, including bisphenol A, phthalates, and childhood obesity; however, the results of these studies are inconsistent.

In this chapter, we provide an overview of the role of EDCs in the development of obesity from early life in order to underscore the importance of preventing production and reducing exposure to EDCs as one of the important strategies for preventing childhood obesity and its health consequences.

Keywords: endocrine disruptors, obesity, childhood

1. Introduction

In modern society, obesity has been recognized as a social problem, and the World Health Organization (WHO) has called obesity a worldwide epidemic and has warned that it is a chronic disease that needs treatment (James 2008). Over the last 2 to 3 decades, the prevalence of childhood overweight and obesity has increased rapidly (De Onis, Blössner et al. 2010). The global prevalence of overweight and obesity in preschool children has increased from 4.2% to 6.7% in the years 1990 to 2012 (De Onis, Blössner et al. 2010). It has more than tripled in the United States, with a 17% prevalence in preschoolers and children (Ogden, Carroll et al. 2014). In South Korea, the prevalence of obesity among children and adolescents increased from 6.8% in 1998 to 10.0% in 2013 (Ha and Kim 2016). Likewise, 15% of children in southern Europe, including Greece, Italy, and Spain, are overweight and obese (Fat 2012). The trend is expected to continue, and the World Health Organization (WHO) suggests that by 2020 60 million preschoolers (9.1%) will become overweight or obese worldwide (De Onis, Blössner et al. 2010). Obesity is a problem for all ages, but it is particularly important for children because most obese and overweight children have obesity in the adolescent. The number of overweight and obese children has risen in parallel with the increase in obesity in adults, (Ogden, Flegal et al. 2002). Although various studies have examined the effects of obesity, there is no evidence of a decrease in prevalence.

Childhood obesity is a risk factor for several chronic diseases such as Type 2 diabetes, insulin resistance, cardiovascular disease, high blood pressure, and some forms of cancer (Mokdad, Serdula et al. 1999, Mokdad, Ford et al. 2003, Collins 2005, Park, Falconer et al. 2012). The effects of diet, genetics/epigenetics, the use of certain pharmaceuticals, and a sedentary lifestyle can be attributed to the rise in obesity and overweight. However, the exact etiology of obesity is unknown (Baillie-Hamilton 2002, McAllister, Dhurandhar et al. 2009). Obesity is most likely due to the complex interaction between genetic, behavioral, and environmental factors. Although genetic factors, high-calorie fatty diets, and decreased physical activity are the most common causes of obesity, this alone cannot justify an increase in obesity prevalence. Recent evidence suggests that environmental factors play a decisive role as well (Baillie-Hamilton 2002, Grün and Blumberg 2006,

Hatch, Nelson et al. 2010). Interestingly, as obesity grows, the production and use of synthetic chemicals have increased dramatically. One of the environmental factors that have recently been attention is the contribution of endocrine disrupters (EDCs) to the high prevalence of obesity (Baillie-Hamilton 2002, Elobeid and Allison 2008, Newbold, Padilla-Banks et al. 2008). EDCs can alter endogenous hormone signaling and metabolism, which regulate vital body functions, including growth, sex development, gender behavior, and production and utilization of insulin (Newbold 2010). Recent evidence suggests that EDCs can act as obesity and interfere with standard bodyweight control mechanisms (Baillie-Hamilton 2002, Grün and Blumberg 2006). Biological mechanisms that may underlie this relationship include changes in thyroid function and steroid hormone and activation of peroxisome proliferative activating receptors, which have an essential effect in fat differentiation and energy storage (Hatch, Nelson et al. 2008). Exposure to EDCs in early life stages can lead to interfering with the pathways of the endocrine-signaling programs established during vulnerable periods of life (Newbold, Padilla-Banks et al. 2007). Besides, exposure to EDCs is associated with increased triglycerides and cholesterol, impaired fasting glucose, and diabetes in humans, all of which are related to obesity (Steinberg, Freni-Titulaer et al. 1986, Vasiliu, Cameron et al. 2006, Codru, Schymura et al. 2007, Langer, Kočan et al. 2007, Everett, Mainous III et al. 2008, Goncharov, Haase et al. 2008).

There is a general concern that fetuses, infants, and children, due to different diets, behavior, physiology, and anatomy, may have higher exposure to EDCs than adults (Miller, Marty et al. 2002). For instance, more consumption of water and more enormous quantities of specific foods, and also a higher intestinal absorption, surface area to volume ratios, and hand-to-mouth activity can cause more exposure to some EDCs in infants and children (Selevan, Kimmel et al. 2000). Thus, endocrine disruptive compounds, compared to adults, adversely affect a sensitive group of fetuses, infants, and children and may increase the risk of disease in children (Braun 2017). Recent epidemiological studies have evaluated the potential effects of exposure to EDCs and indicated that exposure to EDCs during development is associated with overweight and obesity in children (Newbold 2010). For example, urinary BPA concentration has been associated with increased BMI z-score, waist circumference, and the sum of skinfold thickness in a RHEA pregnancy cohort in Crete, Greece (Vafeiadi, Roumeliotaki et al. 2016). Likewise, a study on US children aged 6-18 years revealed that there is a positive association between increasing levels of BPA in urine and obesity (Bhandari, Xiao et al. 2013). Likewise, the cross-sectional studies on 2836 children aged 6-18 years found a significant association between increasing BPA and the weight-to-height ratio (Wells, Jackson et al. 2014). Other studies reported the association between endocrine disruptive compounds, including phthalates, organochlorine, and obesity in children. A cross-sectional study on Iranian children found a significant association between phthalate metabolites and obesity (Amin, Ebrahimpour et al. 2018); another study reported similar findings in the Center for the Health Assessment of Mothers and Children of Salinas (CHAMACOS) participants (Harley, Berger et al. 2017). Likewise, in a study by Hatch et al., urinary mono-ethyl phthalate (MEP) levels of girls in the United States are associated with increased BMI and WC (Knudsen, Laurberg et al. 2005). On the evaluation of organochlorine, the longitudinal study based on CHAMACOS cohort data in 9-year-old children found a positive association between DDT and DDE with BMI and waist circumference only in boys (Warner, Wesselink et al. 2014). Furthermore, polychlorinated (PCB) 153 was shown to be directly associated with the overweight/obesity of Swedish children (Lauritzen, Larose et al. 2018).

Overall, an increasing number of birth or pregnancy cohort studies indicate that exposure to endocrine-disrupting compounds very early in life plays an important role in childhood obesity (Botton, Kadawathagedara et al. 2017, Zarean and Poursafa 2019). In contrast, obesity is a severe concern for children and a risk to adult health. (Xue, Wu et al. 2015, Helaleh, Diboun et al. 2018).

2. EDCs Overview

Endocrine disrupters are chemicals that interfere with the hormone system and cause adverse effects on growth, reproduction, serology, and immunity in mammals. These compounds are found in many products, including plastic bottles, metal cans, detergents, flame retardants, foodstuffs, toys, cosmetics, and pesticides (Yang, Kim et al. 2015). Scientific information shows that even very low levels of EDCs have adverse effects. Some pollutants that interfere with the endocrine system have received more attention due to the specific chemical properties. Preliminary results from clinical and epidemiological studies have also shown that these substances also have an adverse affecting human health and lead to increased obesity, diabetes, and some cancers (Yang, Kim et al. 2015). Hence, it has become a global health challenge (Kester, Bulduk et al. 2000). Recently, numerous studies examining the association between EDCs and measures like Body mass index (BMI), Waist circumference (WC), have revealed a notable positive association between weight gain and obesity and increased endocrine disruptors level (Braun, Chen et al. 2016, Amin, Ebrahimpour et al. 2018, Amin, Parastar et al. 2018, Kalloo, Calafat et al. 2018, Lauritzen, Larose et al. 2018, Amin, Ebrahim et al. 2019).

2.1. Sources and Exposure Routs of Endocrine Disruptive

Some Endocrine disruptive compounds are present in nature (e.g., plant phytoestrogens); however, most of these compounds are synthetic chemicals released by human activities in the environment. Using EDCs in pesticides, herbicides, plastics, industrial and household products, flame retardants, detergents, and as ingredients of personal care products can be considered as the primary agents of human exposure to these compounds in daily life (Darbre 2015). Food is the major route of intake of EDCs to the human body. According to the report by the U.S. FDA in 1971, concentrations of PCBs as high as 35 ppm in fish, 28 ppm in milk, 3.7 ppm in eggs, and one ppm in cheese were measured (Sawhney and Hankin 1985). Likewise, BPA exposure also occurs due to contaminated food and water (Cichna-Markl 2012). Consumers may be exposed to bisphenol A that are transported from cans to beverages and foods, or products resulting from polymer hydrolysis (Almeida, Raposo et al. 2018). Increasing household products containing pollutants and decreasing indoor conditioning has become a significant source of EDCs exposure (Weschler 2009). Besides, EDCS can also intake to the human body by inhalation or dermal adsorption (Darbre 2015). In summary, some of the most important EDCs that are likely to contribute to the obesogenic processes are shown in Figure 1.

The origins and activities of the mentioned EDCs are outlined below, and the mechanism of EDCs actions and obesogenic properties of them will also be discussed.

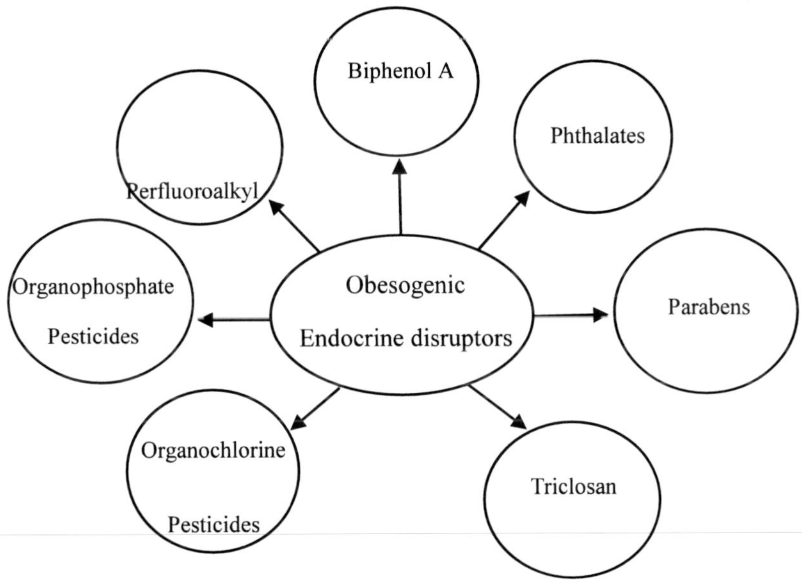

Figure 1. The most important environmental endocrine-disruptive compounds which have an obesogenic properties.

2.1.1. Bisphenol A (BPA)

Bisphenol A is one of the important EDCs that used as the monomer or additive in the manufacture of polycarbonate (PC), epoxy resins and other polymeric materials (Almeida, Raposo et al. 2018), which are now used in consumer products such as beverage bottles, linings of water pipes, thermal paper, toys children, and coating of canned food (Darbre 2017). Global consumption of BPA was estimated at 8 million metric tons in 2016 and is expected to reach 10.6 million metric tons in 2020 (Almeida, Raposo et al. 2018). Although some countries, such as the United States, Canada, and the European Union, have banned the use of BPA, 36% of BPA's market share is in Western Europe and the United States. Therefore, these data indicate that BPA consumption has been increasing in recent years (LI, HAN et al. 2011). Oral ingestion, inhalation, and dermal absorption are the main routs of BPA exposure (Carwile, Ye et al. 2011). BPA has a biological half-life of 6 hours, so it does not persist in the body. Once absorption, BPA is conjugated in the liver and excreted through the bile and also urine (Thayer, Doerge et al. 2015). In blood, BPA comes in a nonconjugated form, so BPA exposure assessed by measuring the urinary concentration of BPA, including free and conjugated form (Calafat 2016). BPA can also accumulate in adipose tissue due to the lipophilic properties (Almeida, Raposo et al. 2018). Some other factors, including gender, age, liver function, and physiological status, are influence in BPA metabolism (Bertoli, Leone et al. 2015).

2.1.2. Phthalates

One of the most important classes of EDCs is phthalates, which are used in personal care products, medication coatings, fragrances, and plastics (Harley, Berger et al. 2017). Many of the phthalates are also listed by the Organisation for Economic Cooperation and Development (OECD) as high production volume chemicals in 2004 that have endocrine-disrupting properties (Co-operation and Development 2002, Kamrin 2009, Huang, Liou et al. 2012). Biomonitoring studies indicate that exposure to phthalates among pregnant women, infants, and children is almost ubiquitous (Braun 2017). Phthalates categorized into two groups, including high-molecular-weight (HMW) and low-molecular-weight (LMW). High-molecular-weight of phthalates, including di-isononyl phthalate (DiNP), butyl benzyl phthalates (BBzP), di-isodecyl phthalate (DiDP), and di(2-ethylhexyl) phthalate (DEHP), are widely used as plasticizers in food packages, PVC building material, medical devices, and vinyl flooring (Braun 2017, Harley, Berger et al. 2017). Phthalates with low-molecular-weight, including di-ethyl phthalate (DEP), di-n-butyl phthalate (DBP), di-iso butyl phthalate (DiBP), and di-n- octyl phthalate (DOP), are mainly used in personal care products such as shampoo, lotions, and cosmetics (Amin, Ebrahimpour et al. 2018). Phthalates exposure the same as BPA occurs through ingestion, inhalation, and dermal absorption (Bornehag, Lundgren et al. 2005, Rudel, Gray et al. 2011, Braun, Just et al. 2014, Langer, Bekö et al. 2014). Within 24-48 h after adsorption, phthalates can break down into monoester metabolites by hydrolysis mechanism, then excreted in the urine as glucuronides (Amin, Ebrahimpour et al. 2018). Phthalate exposure is assessed using urine, blood, breast milk, and feces samples. However, the urinary concentration of phthalate metabolites is used as the most useful biomarker since phthalates are mainly excreted in the urine (Teitelbaum, Britton et al. 2008, Wittassek and Angerer 2008).

2.1.3. Paraben

Parabens are the alkyl or aryl ester of para-hydroxybenzoic acid, which are used as antimicrobial agents for the preservation of pharmaceutical, personal care products, foods, and paper products (Darbre 2017). Methylparaben (MP), ethylparaben (EtP), propylparaben (PrP), butylparaben (BuP), and benzyl paraben (BEP) are the available commercial metabolites (Guo, Wu et al. 2017). Parabens exposure occurs through ingestion or topical contact (Liao, Chen et al. 2013, Guo, Wang et al. 2014). Human exposure to parabens is evaluated using urine, serum, breast milk, amniotic fluid, and placenta tissue (Philippat, Wolff et al. 2013, Hines, Mendola et al. 2015, Valle-Sistac, Molins-Delgado et al. 2016). Besides, parabens are also found in the fat components of human body tissue (Wang, Asimakopoulos et al. 2015). Parabens are not persistent and, after absorption, rapidly metabolized and excreted in the urine (Moos, Angerer et al. 2016). Therefore, the Urinary concentration of parabens used as a valid biomarker of exposure (Ye, Bishop et al. 2006).

2.1.4. Triclosan

Triclosan, also known as 5-chloro-2-(2,4-dichloro phenoxy) phenolic is an antibacterial chemical compound which widely used in household and care products such as mouthwash, soaps, toothpaste, textiles, toys, and medical devices (Koeppe, Ferguson et al. 2013, Ginsberg and Balk 2016). Exposure to triclosan is mainly through the oral and dermal routes (Rodricks, Swenberg et al. 2010). Various studies indicated that levels of triclosan are detectable in urine, fat tissue, blood, nails, and human milk (Li, Zhao et al. 2015). The biological half-life of triclosan is less than 24 hours, so it is not persistent and is mainly excreted in the urine as glucuronide or sulfate conjugate (Braun 2017). Like BPA, phthalates, and parabens, exposure to triclosan is assessed by measuring the urine concentration of triclosan (Calafat 2016). Although triclosan has a short biological half-life, urinary triclosan concentrations are relatively stable than BPA and phthalates over time (Braun 2017). Biomonitoring studies indicated that about 75% of the U.S and Belgian population and 85% of the pregnant women in the U.S have a detectable concentration of triclosan in their urine samples (Calafat, Ye et al. 2008, Woodruff, Zota et al. 2011, Li, Zhao et al. 2015).

2.1.5. Organochlorine Pesticide

Organochlorines (OC) are a class of EDCs which widely used as pesticides. These compounds belong to the group of high persistent organic pollutants (POPs). The major organochlorine pesticides are including Dichlorodiphenyltrichloroethane (DDT), 1,1-dichloro-2,2bis (p-chlorophenyl)ethane (DDD), Dichloro diphenyl dichloroethane (DDE), Dicofol, Endrin, Dieldrin, Heptachlor, Lindane, Endosulfan, Chloropropylate, Aldrin, and Pentachlorophenol (Jayaraj, Megha et al. 2016). Organochlorine compounds have stability against degradation process in the environment and also have a low vapor pressure.

Additionally, these compounds have very low solubility in water and high solubility in the lipid and fatty tissue. Their properties made them desirable for industrial usage (Kleanthi, Katerina et al. 2008). In contrast, these properties cause bioaccumulation of organochlorines through absorption in the human body and subsequent deposition in adipose tissue (Genuis, Lane et al. 2016). Although, the use of organochlorine pesticides is presently banned or restricted in some countries, statistical studies show that 40% of all pesticides used to belong to the organochlorine compounds (Jayaraj, Megha et al. 2016). Exposure to pesticides occurs via the ingestion of food and water, inhalation of air, and skin absorption (Nicolopoulou-Stamati and Pitsos 2001). However, due to the bioaccumulation of pesticides in fish and the other animal that humans consume, food is the primary route of exposure to pesticides (Hall 1992). Solubility in lipid and slow degradation of the organochlorine compounds causes bioaccumulation of them in the human body, thus being found in adipose tissue, blood, and breast milk (Kleanthi, Katerina et al. 2008). Human hair is also used to measure the biological level of organochlorine pesticides (Althuis, Dozier et al. 2005). Long-term exposure to small amounts of pesticides can lead to the accumulation of these substances in human tissues. Thus, the level of organochlorines in human tissues has a positive relationship with age (Cocco 2002) and the rate of consumption of contaminated products (Pagni 2006).

2.1.6. Organophosphates Pesticides

Organophosphates (OP) are esters of phosphoric acid, and they are one of the most common pesticides (Ranjbar, Rotondi et al. 2015). According to world statistics, 1 million accidental severe poisonings and 3 million suicides worldwide each year are attributed to organophosphate compounds (Adhikari, Ghosh et al. 2011). Organophosphate exposure occurs through the consumption of contaminated vegetables and fruits, contacting residential pest control programs, or through occupation (Ranjbar, Rotondi et al. 2015). Organophosphate pesticides can enter the body through intake and inhalation as well as through dermal absorption (Reigart and Roberts 1999, Kavvalakis and Tsatsakis 2012). Once absorbance, organophosphate pesticides via hydrolyzes or oxidative desulfuration were metabolized to non-specific metabolites, including dimethyl phosphate (DMP), dimethyl thiophosphate (DMTP), dimethyl dithiophosphate (DMDTP), diethyl phosphate (DEP), diethyl thiophosphate (DETP), and diethyl dithiophosphate (DEDTP) (Richardson 1995, Whyatt and Barr 2001, Tsatsakis, Tzatzarakis et al. 2009). Exposure to OPs is assessed using biological samples such as urine, blood, hair, post-mortem tissue, and amniotic fluid (Koutroulakis, Sifakis et al. 2014). However, most biomonitoring studies used the urinary concentration of OPs as the valid biomarkers of exposure.

2.1.7. Perfluoroalkyl Substances

Perfluoroalkyl substances (PFAs) are a class of synthetic fluorinated compounds used in food packaging, non-stick cookware, insecticides, floor polish, firefighting foams, and industrial surfactants (Lau, Anitole et al. 2007). Ingestion of contaminated food, drinking water, ingestion, or inhalation of contaminated dust and soil are considered as major routes of human exposure to PFAs (Mora, Oken et al. 2017). Due to the strong carbon-fluorine bond, PFAs are stable in the environment, leading to biological accumulation and persistence in human tissues for years (Buck, Franklin et al. 2011). Perfluorooctanoic acid (PFOA) and perfluorooctanesulfonic acid (PFOS), perfluorononanoic acid (PFNA), perfluorohexane sulfonate (PFHxS) have been identified as important endocrine disruptors with the potential to impair weight regulation (Hofmann, Ardelt-Gattinger et al. 2015). Detectable levels of these compounds were founded in the serum of pregnant women, neonates, and children, which indicated that exposure to PFAs is ubiquitous (Braun 2017). As mentioned above, PFAs are persistent in the environment, and they have a long half-life in humans, ranging from 3 to 5 years (Mora, Oken et al. 2017). Therefore, epidemiological studies used serum and plasma concentration of PFAs to characterize exposure (Braun 2017).

3. Mechanism of EDCs Function

One of the most commonly proposed mechanisms of EDC function is the alteration of endocrine function by acting as an agonist or antagonist of nuclear receptors, particularly androgen receptors (ARs), estrogen receptors (ER), thyroid receptors (TRs), and also nonnuclear receptors, including aryl hydrocarbon receptors (AhR) (Newbold 2010). Additionally, endocrine disruptors are thought to affect in regulating the pregnane X receptor, and the peroxisome proliferator-activated receptors (PPARα, β, and γ) and the constitutive androstane receptor (Vasiliu, Cameron et al. 2006). The above mentioned nuclear receptors, such as ER, AhR, and PPAR, are also present in the mitochondria, and many EDCs can disrupt mitochondria function by moving to the mitochondria (Park, Jun et al. 2013, Hwang, Dornbos et al. 2016).

3.1. Plausible Mechanisms of Action of Obesogenic EDCs

Endocrine-disrupting chemicals are likely to exert their effects through various mechanisms. However, investigation of the mechanisms related to the effect of EDC on weight homeostasis is at the early stages. Regarding possible mechanisms, the most common mechanism involves direct bindings of EDC to PPARs, which play a key role in adipogenesis and lipid metabolism (Grün and Blumberg 2006). PPAR-gamma has been defined as a master regulator of fat cell development, with activation required for fat differentiation and maturation (Tontonoz, Hu et al. 1994). In animal studies, exposure to some organotins (Grün and Blumberg 2006) and phthalates as PPARgamma agonists show weight gain. Activation of PPAR-γ and retinoic X receptor (RXR) heterodimer favors the differentiation of preadipocytes and adipocytes progenitors and acts as a regulator of lipid biosynthesis and storage (Grun, Watanabe et al. 2006). EDCs can directly stimulate adipogenesis by targeting the RXR-PRAP γ, which cause to increase adipocyte differentiation and adipose tissue amounts following the exposure (Kim and Lee 2017). BPA, nonylphenol, and some metabolites of phthalate have been shown to promote adipogenesis (Maloney and Waxman 1999, Masuno, Kidani et al. 2002, Masuno, Okamoto et al. 2003, Feige, Gelman et al. 2007, Li, Pham et al. 2012).

Another obesogens mechanism is through interference with steroid receptors. Steroid hormones can affect fat storage and fat deposition and, therefore, can influence adipose tissue development (Law, Bloor et al. 2014). Some EDCs may act directly through cellular steroid receptors, while others may act by stimulating less estrogen synthesis. The cytochrome P450 enzyme aromatase from the adipocyte's cytoplasm converts testosterone to estrogen. Some studies indicated that several EDCs can affect intracellular aromatase activity and can, therefore, act indirectly to increase intracellular estrogen levels in adipocytes, which lead to increased obesity in humans (Whitehead and Rice 2006, Williams 2012).

Another plausible mechanism may be thyroid dysfunction, which plays a key role in the maintenance of basal metabolism. The cross-sectional study by Knudsen et al. revealed that after the dysfunction of thyroid, reduced thyroid hormone is associated with an increase in BMI of the individuals (Knudsen, Laurberg et al. 2005). Several endocrine disruptors compounds with anti-thyroid activities are including Polychlorinated biphenyls (PCB), polychlorinated dibenzodioxins (PCDD), PFASs, phthalates, and BPA (Ghassabian and Trasande 2018). Based on the proposed mechanism, biological activity and epidemiological studies on children related to the obesogenic EDCs are as follow:

3.1.1. BPA and Obesity

BPA may interact with various receptors, including genomic estrogen receptors 1 and 2, membrane-bound estrogen receptors, androgen receptor, PPAR γ, and thyroid hormone receptor (Vafeiadi, Roumeliotaki et al. 2016). In-vitro studies have shown that prenatal exposure to BPA is associated with the level of T4 in offspring (Zoeller, Bansal et al. 2005) and also thyroid-specific gene expression (Gentilcore, Porreca et al. 2013). Similarly, some studies on rodents indicated that prenatal exposure to BPA could lead to increased body weight and adiposity (Vafeiadi, Roumeliotaki et al. 2016). A small number of studies have examined the association between BPA exposure and childhood obesity. Thirteen publications from cross-sectional, prospective cohort and case-control studies have examined this relationship. The cross-sectional study by Bhandari et al. shows a positive association between BPA exposure and obesity among U.S. children aged 6-18 years old (Bhandari, Xiao et al. 2013). Three cross-sectional studies linked the levels of BPA with an increased risk of obesity (Trasande, Attina et al. 2012, Li, Miao et al. 2013, McGuinn,

Ghazarian et al. 2015). Likewise, the cross-sectional studies in the US on children and adolescents found that higher BPA level was associated with increased fat mass in girls, not in boys (Li, Lai et al. 2017). Likewise, a case-control study of 54 participants aged 5-16 years in Italy found free and total BPA levels were associated with the increase in BMI (D'Aniello, Troisi et al. 2015). Up to now, three prospective cohort studies examined BPA exposure in association with childhood obesity (Valvi, Casas et al. 2013, Braun, Lanphear et al. 2014, Harley, Berger et al. 2017). However, the results are inconsistent. One of them found that BPA exposure is weakly associated with obesity (Valvi, Casas et al. 2013). Another case reported that the urinary BPA concentrations were not associated with BMI at age 5, but BPA levels were associated with BMI at age nine (Harley, Schall et al. 2013). The other cohort study reported a lower BMI with higher childhood exposure (Braun, Lanphear et al. 2014). In contrast, some cross-sectional studies reported that there is no association between BPA exposure and obesity (Choi, Eom et al. 2014, Wang, Wang et al. 2014, Pornkunwilai, Nosoongnoen et al. 2015). For instance, the cross-sectional study of Wang et al. was found that there is no significant association between BPA level and obesity (Wang, Wang et al. 2014). Two other cross-sectional studies reported the same results (Choi, Eom et al. 2014, Pornkunwilai, Nosoongnoen et al. 2015). The available epidemiological studies show the inconsistent results related to the association between early-life BPA exposure and obesity. So a systematic review and meta-analyses by Kim et al. in 2019 investigated the association between BPA exposure and obesity in children (Kim, Lee et al. 2019). This study elucidated that BPA exposure itself increased the risk of obesity in children. However, more investigation is needed for a plausible association between BPA exposure and obesity on each developmental stage and sex.

3.1.2. Phthalates and Obesity

Phthalates may interfere with the mechanism of androgen. They cannot interact with the androgen receptor directly; rather, the anti-androgenic effect of these substances is mediated through PPARα (Foster, Mylchreest et al. 2001, Corton and Lapinskas 2005). The anti-androgenic effect of phthalates results in decreased androgen activity and, consequently, obesity. The anti-androgenic effect of various metabolites of phthalate has been demonstrated in infants and adults (Main, Mortensen et al. 2006, Pan, Hanaoka et al. 2006). Also, phthalates action as PPARγ agonists leads to the differentiation and accumulation of lipids in 3T3-L1 cells (Hurst and Waxman 2003, Bility, Thompson et al. 2004). Thus, phthalates are likely to have an adipogenic effect through the activation of PPARγ. The disruption of thyroid function is considered as another effect of phthalates exposure. Recent human studies demonstrated the effect of phthalate exposure on thyroid function in children and adults (Kim and Park 2014). For instance, a cohort study of Boas et al. observed the inverse association between urinary phthalate metabolites, such as di(2-ethylhexyl) phthalate and diisononyl phthalate and thyroid hormone serum levels in children (Boas, Frederiksen et al. 2010). Several epidemiological studies have examined the association of phthalate metabolites exposure and obesity or body size measurements in children. In a study of Teitelbaum et al. (Teitelbaum, Mervish et al. 2012), a positive relationship was observed between urinary concentrations of monoethyl phthalate (MEP) and the sum of low molecular-weight phthalates and body size measures in overweight children. Likewise, a cross-sectional study by Wang et al. investigated the association of phthalate metabolites exposure with body mass index (BMI) and waist circumference (WC). The results revealed the positive association between some metabolites and BMI and WC (Wang, Zhou et al. 2013). A cross-sectional study on 493 Chinese children found that urinary concentrations of monobutyl phthalate (MBP) and the sum of LMW metabolites were positively associated with obesity in boys. In contrast, MEHP, MEHHP, and the sum of DEHP metabolites were negatively associated with girl's obesity (Zhang, Meng et al. 2014). A cohort study in France that examined only boys, the significant association was found between prenatal urinary concentrations of DEP and increased BMI at the age of 5 years (Botton, Philippat et al. 2016). However, three other studies have found the inverse association between the prenatal levels of phthalate and BMI in boys (Buckley, Engel et al. 2016, Buckley, Engel et al. 2016, Maresca, Hoepner et al. 2016). A cohort study in Spain found that urinary concentration of high molecular weight of phthalate metabolites was positively (although non-significantly) with BMI z-score in girls but was negatively in boys aged in the range of 4 to 7 years (Valvi, Casas et al. 2015). Likewise, in a cohort study in American children, a positive association was found between levels of diethyl phthalate (DEP), di-n-butyl phthalate (DBP), butyl benzyl phthalate, and di(2-ethylhexyl) phthalate (DEHP) with BMI z-score, and waist circumference a-score at multiple age (Harley, Berger et al. 2017). Likewise, a cross-sectional study in Iranian children and adolescents was found that except for MEOHP, all other metabolites were significantly associated with obesity (Amin, Ebrahimpour et al. 2018). Besides, a study examined in both overweight/obese children and normal-weight children found that higher levels of phthalate metabolites detected in urinary samples of overweight/obese children, though a positive association was found between phthalate levels and increased prevalence of obesity (Xia, Zhu et al. 2018). In contrast, a cohort study of 180 children aged 4 to 9 years in the US, found no association between prenatal phthalate exposure and childhood adiposity (Buckley, Engel et al. 2016). In summary, the associations between phthalate exposure and childhood obesity or adiposity have been inconsistent, and it does not support that phthalates are chemical obesogenic.

3.1.3. Parabens and Obesity

Similar to the two previous compounds, parabens may also interfere with thyroid hormones and activate the peroxisome proliferator-activated receptors (PPARg) (Pereira-Fernandes, Demaegdt et al. 2013). Besides, a study by Hu et al. reported that parabens could promote the development and differentiation of multipotent cells into mature adipocyte cells, which leads to obesity (Hu, Chen et al. 2013). In addition to estrogenic properties, some parabens also exhibit anti-androgenic activity by binding to androgen receptors and inducing testosterone-induced transcriptional inhibition (Błędzka, Gromadzińska et al. 2014).

Epidemiological researches related to the association between paraben exposure and body growth is scarce. The cross-sectional study of Xue et al. that investigated methylparaben (MeP), ethylparaben (EtP), propylparaben (PrP), 4-hydroxybenzoic acid (4-HB), 3,4-dihydroxybenzoic acid (3,4-DHB), the positive association with obesity was shown only for 3,4-DHB. However, other metabolites did not have any association (Xue, Wu et al. 2015). A cohort study on 436 children in China, found a positive association between five parabens and weigh z-score only in boys (Guo, Wu et al. 2017). This study suggested that exposure to parabens may be affected the physical growth in 3-year-old boy children. In contrast, a cross-sectional study in American adults and children observed the significant inverse associations between adiposity measures and urinary concentrations of paraben among adults (BP, EP, MP, PP) and children (MP) (Quirós-Alcalá, Buckley et al. 2018). Because of the inconsistent results, further researches are needed regarding the underlying mechanism of interfering with paraben with body growth in the children.

3.1.4. Triclosan and Obesity

Triclosan can impair the glands and the thyroid hormone's homeostasis. Animal studies indicated that triclosan disrupts the cholesterol biosynthesis in Leydig cell, which causes to reduce testosterone production (Kumar, Balomajumder et al. 2008, Adam and Kumari 2009). Besides, a systematic review and meta-analyses on rodents indicated that thyroxine concentrations in the fetus, dam, neonate, and juvenile reduced due to the triclosan exposure (Johnson, Koustas et al. 2016). Epidemiological studies related to triclosan exposure and thyroid function have inconsistent results (Cullinan, Palmer et al. 2012, Koeppe, Ferguson et al. 2013). However, there are no prospective epidemiological studies to investigate the relationship between triclosan exposure and thyroid hormone during pregnancy, infant, and childhood. Additionally, in vitro studies show that triclosan reduces the global methylation in HepG2 cells (Ma, Zheng et al. 2013), increases estradiol (E2), and progesterone secretion (Gee, Charles et al. 2008, Honkisz, Zieba-Przybylska et al. 2012), and inhibits lipid differentiation and inflammation (Barros, Wirojchanasak et al. 2010, Udoji, Martin et al. 2010, Guo, Wu et al. 2012).

Several human studies investigated the association between triclosan exposure and obesity in childhood. For instance, Buser and colleagues reported that there is no association between triclosan and BMI z-score, waist circumference (Buser, Murray et al. 2014). Likewise, a prospective cohort study confirms that triclosan exposure has not an association with child adiposity at 4 to 9 years of age (Buckley, Herring et al. 2016). In contrast, the cross-sectional study of Li et al. was found an inverse association between urinary concentration of triclosan and BMI and waist circumference among American children in the range age of 6-19 years old (Li, Zhao et al. 2015). So far, publishing data related to the association between triclosan exposure and child obesity is limited. In summary, the published data on EDC and child obesity is limited, and evidence to determine the effect of triclosan exposure on childhood obesity is insufficient.

3.1.5. Organochlorine Pesticides and Obesity

Due to the four-ring steroid structure similar to the Endogenous hormones (estradiol), Organochlorine chemicals have shown the weak estrogenic effects in both in-vitro and in-vivo studies (Kortenkamp 2006). These compounds altered the structure and metabolism of hormones and change the number of hormone receptors and lead to the estrogenic or anti-estrogenic effects (Kleanthi, Katerina et al. 2008). Besides, organochlorines have been shown to affect thyroid hormones (Kleanthi, Katerina et al. 2008). Nevertheless, compared with relatively extensive animal studies, epidemiological studies that investigated the association of organochlorine exposure with children's obesity is limited. Several longitudinal birth cohort studies investigated the association between prenatal exposure to organochlorine, including DDT and DDE and child growth (Verhulst, Nelen et al. 2009, Cupul-Uicab, Hernández-Ávila et al. 2010, Mendez, Garcia-Esteban et al. 2011, Garced, Torres-Sánchez et al. 2012, Valvi, Mendez et al. 2012). Birth cohort studies conducted in European children reported a positive association between prenatal exposure to DDE and DDT and BMI z-score from 1 to 7 years of age (Verhulst, Nelen et al. 2009, Mendez, Garcia-Esteban et al. 2011, Valvi, Mendez et al. 2012). Likewise, using data from the Center for the Health Assessment of Mothers and Children of Salinas (CHAMACOS) Study, a longitudinal birth cohort study was found an association between prenatal exposure to DDT and DDE several measures of obesity at nine years of age in boys but not in girls (Warner, Wesselink et al. 2014). However, conducted studies in the United States (Cupul-Uicab, Klebanoff et al. 2013, Warner, Schall et al. 2013) and Mexico (Cupul-Uicab, Hernández-Ávila et al. 2010, Garced, Torres-Sánchez et al. 2012) did not confirm the relationship between organochlorine exposure and obesity. Likewise, two prospective studies found no significant association between prenatal exposure to DDE or DDT and growth in the first year of Dutch children (De Cock, De Boer et al. 2014) or BMI in Greenland, Polish, and Ukrainian children from 5 to 9 years (Høyer, Ramlau-Hansen et al. 2014). In summary, there is insufficient evidence to determine the possible association between organochlorine exposure and obesity. Therefore, further research is needed to determine how these compounds effect.

3.1.6. Organophosphate Pesticides and Obesity

Organophosphates maybe act as metabolism-disrupting compounds and interfere with energy homeostasis, satiety, lipid metabolism, sensitivity to insulin, which leads to metabolic dysregulation or increased body fat (Boyle, Buckley et al. 2019). The findings of animal and human studies showed that OPs might interfere with sex steroid and thyroid hormones (Meeker and Stapleton 2010, Liu, Ji et al. 2012, Farhat, Crump et al. 2013, Kim,

Jung et al. 2015, Wang, Lam et al. 2015, Krivoshiev, Dardenne et al. 2016, Zhang, Ji et al. 2016) peroxisome proliferator-activated receptors (PPARs) (Kojima, Takeuchi et al. 2013, Belcher, Cookman et al. 2014, Hu, Gao et al. 2017). These biological pathways have a well-known role in adipose tissue growth and the risk of obesity. Two independent studies on rodents indicated that prenatal exposure to organophosphates increases body mass, fat mass, leptin, fasting glucose, and also total energy intake (Patisaul, Roberts et al. 2013, Green, Graham et al. 2017). Despite sufficient laboratory evidence, epidemiological studies evaluating the association between OPs exposure and obesity are extremely limited. Two cross-sectional studies reported the positive association between OPs biomarker concentrations and BMI among pregnant women (Hoffman, Lorenzo et al. 2017, Romano, Hawley et al. 2017). Besides, several studies investigated the association between parental exposure to OPs and birth outcomes, including birth weight, birth length, and head circumference (Rauch, Braun et al. 2012, Wang, Tian et al. 2012, Koutroulakis, Sifakis et al. 2014, Huang, Pan et al. 2017, Dalsager, Christensen et al. 2018). However, these studies did not include children, but Boyle et al. examined the association between urinary organophosphate ester metabolites and adiposity among US children (Boyle, Buckley et al. 2019). This cross-sectional study showed that dibutyl phosphate (DBUP) significantly associated with lower BMI z-scores (β: -0.08, 95% CI: -0.17, 0.01), and waist circumference (β: -0.71, 95% CI: -1.49,0.07). Also, bis (1-chloro-2-propyl) phosphate (BCPP) concentrations were associated with increased prevalence odds of being overweight vs. normal weight (aPOR: 1.15, 95% CI: 1.01, 1.32) (Boyle, Buckley et al. 2019). Given the paucity of studies investigating the association between exposure to organophosphates and obesity, especially in children, further studies are needed to understand the role of organophosphates in obesity.

3.1.7. Perfluoroalkyl Substances

Perfluoroalkyl substances (PFASs), especially PFOA and PFOS as an endocrine disruptor, may affect on weight regulation (Liu, Dhana et al. 2018). Animal researches suggested that PFAs can alter energy metabolism and thyroid hormone homeostasis (Chang, Thibodeaux et al. 2008, Yu, Liu et al. 2009, Kirkley and Sargis 2014). PFASs can activate the peroxisome proliferator-activated receptor (PPARs), which leads to an increase in adipocyte differentiation and increase body fat (Vanden Heuvel, Thompson et al. 2006, Sales, Kamstra et al. 2013). Also, PFAS s may alter the estrogen and androgen receptor function and inhibit the enzyme 11-β-hydroxysteroid dehydrogenase (Mora, Oken et al. 2017). However, the number of animal and human studies that examined the association between PFASs exposure and adiposity or obesity is limited. Additionally, observed results in human studies are somewhat contradictory. Two studies reported that prenatal PFAS serum concentrations were associated with higher body mass index, waist circumference, and body fat in 8-year-old boys and girls (Braun, Chen et al. 2016). Likewise, the cohort study Greenlandic and Ukrainian children determined that prenatal serum concentrations of PFOA and PFOS were associated with increased waist-to-height ratio in girls ages 5–9 years (Høyer, Ramlau-Hansen et al. 2015). Likewise, the findings of a cohort study in the US pregnant women and their offspring in early childhood (median 3.2 years) and mid-childhood (median 7.7 years) showed that exposure to PFASs (PFAO, PFSO, PFHxS, PFNA) during pregnancy are associated with a small increase in mid-childhood adiposity measurements, but only among girls (Mora, Oken et al. 2017). In contrast, a Danish cohort study revealed that prenatal plasma PFOS and PFOA concentrations have an inverse association with BMI and waist circumference in 7-year-old boys and girls (Andersen, Fei et al. 2013). Given the scarce available human study and also inconsistent reported results related to the association between PFAS exposure and obesity in childhood, further researches are needed.

CONCLUSION

Exposure to obesogenic EDCs, including BPA, phthalates, paraben, triclosan, organochlorine pesticides, organophosphate pesticides, and PFAS, is ubiquitous and can occur during potentially sensitive periods of development that are important in obesity of children. Therefore, serious measures should be taken to reduce production and use as well as exposure to these compounds. In the past decades, EDC studies have increased, and increasing knowledge and information are provided in the areas of environmental contamination and the risk of obesity. Although it is difficult to establish causality between EDC and obesity, there is sufficient evidence to support measures to control human exposure to obesity in the community. Until then, it may be the most useful way is to provide enough information to people in the community to reduce exposure of themselves and their children ahead of EDCs.

REFERENCES

Adam, E. K. and Kumari, M. (2009). Assessing salivary cortisol in large-scale, epidemiological research. *Psychoneuroendocrinology*, 34 (10): 1423-1436.

Adhikari, K., Ghosh, A., Alauddin, M., Moitra, A. and Datta, A. (2011). Organophosphate poisoning in pregnancy. *Journal of Obstetrics and Gynaecology*, 31 (4): 290-292.

Almeida, S., Raposo, A., Almeida-González, M. and Carrascosa, C. (2018). Bisphenol A: food exposure and impact on human health. *Comprehensive Reviews in Food Science and Food Safety*, 17 (6): 1503-1517.

Althuis, M. D., Dozier, J. M., Anderson, W. F., Devesa, S. S. and Brinton, L. A. (2005). Global trends in breast cancer incidence and mortality 1973–1997. *International journal of epidemiology*, 34 (2): 405-412.

Amin, M. M., Ebrahim, K., Hashemi, M., Shoshtari-Yeganeh, B., Rafiei, N., Mansourian, M. and Kelishadi, R. (2019). Association of exposure to Bisphenol A with obesity and cardiometabolic risk factors in children and adolescents. *International journal of environmental health research*, 29 (1): 94-106.

Amin, M. M., Ebrahimpour, K., Parastar, S., Shoshtari-Yeganeh, B., Hashemi, M., Mansourian, M., Poursafa, P., Fallah, Z., Rafiei, N. and Kelishadi, R. (2018). Association of urinary concentrations of phthalate metabolites with cardiometabolic risk factors and obesity in children and adolescents. *Chemosphere*, 211: 547-556.

Amin, M. M., Parastar, S., Ebrahimpour, K., Shoshtari-Yeganeh, B., Hashemi, M., Mansourian, M. and Kelishadi, R. (2018). Association of urinary phthalate metabolites concentrations with body mass index and waist circumference. *Environmental Science and Pollution Research*, 25 (11): 11143-11151.

Andersen, C. S., Fei, C., Gamborg, M., Nohr, E. A., Sørensen, T. I. and Olsen, J. (2013). Prenatal exposures to perfluorinated chemicals and anthropometry at 7 years of age. *American journal of epidemiology*, 178 (6): 921-927.

Baillie-Hamilton, P. F. (2002). Chemical toxins: a hypothesis to explain the global obesity epidemic. *The Journal of Alternative & Complementary Medicine*, 8 (2): 185-192.

Barros, S. P., Wirojchanasak, S., Barrow, D. A., Panagakos, F. S., DeVizio, W. and Offenbacher, S. (2010). Triclosan inhibition of acute and chronic inflammatory gene pathways. *Journal of clinical periodontology*, 37 (5): 412-418.

Belcher, S. M., Cookman, C. J., Patisaul, H. B. and Stapleton, H. M. (2014). In vitro assessment of human nuclear hormone receptor activity and cytotoxicity of the flame retardant mixture FM 550 and its triarylphosphate and brominated components. *Toxicology letters*, 228 (2): 93-102.

Bertoli, S., Leone, A. and Battezzati, A. (2015). Human bisphenol A exposure and the "diabesity phenotype". *Dose-Response*, 13 (3): 1559325815599173.

Bhandari, R., Xiao, J. and Shankar, A. (2013). Urinary bisphenol A and obesity in US children. *American journal of epidemiology*, 177 (11): 1263-1270.

Bility, M. T., Thompson, J. T., McKee, R. H., David, R. M., Butala, J. H., Vanden Heuvel, J. P. and Peters, J. M. (2004). Activation of mouse and human peroxisome proliferator-activated receptors (PPARs) by phthalate monoesters. *Toxicological sciences*, 82 (1): 170-182.

Błędzka, D., Gromadzińska, J. and Wąsowicz, W. (2014). Parabens. From environmental studies to human health. *Environment international*, 67: 27-42.

Boas, M., Frederiksen, H., Feldt-Rasmussen, U., Skakkebæk, N. E., Hegedüs, L., Hilsted, L., Juul, A. and Main, K. M. (2010). Childhood exposure to phthalates: associations with thyroid function, insulin-like growth factor I, and growth. *Environmental health perspectives*, 118 (10): 1458-1464.

Bornehag, C.-G., Lundgren, B., Weschler, C. J., Sigsgaard, T., Hagerhed-Engman, L. and Sundell, J. (2005). Phthalates in indoor dust and their association with building characteristics. *Environmental health perspectives*, 113 (10): 1399-1404.

Botton, J., Kadawathagedara, M. and de Lauzon-Guillain, B. (2017). *Endocrine disrupting chemicals and growth of children*. Annales d'endocrinologie, Elsevier.

Botton, J., Philippat, C., Calafat, A. M., Carles, S., Charles, M.-A., Slama, R. and Group, E. M. C. C. S. (2016). Phthalate pregnancy exposure and male offspring growth from the intra-uterine period to five years of age. *Environmental research*, 151: 601-609.

Boyle, M., Buckley, J. P. and Quirós-Alcalá, L. (2019). Associations between urinary organophosphate ester metabolites and measures of adiposity among US children and adults: NHANES 2013–2014. *Environment international*, 127: 754-763.

Braun, J. M. (2017). Early-life exposure to EDCs: role in childhood obesity and neurodevelopment. *Nature Reviews Endocrinology*, 13 (3): 161.

Braun, J. M., Chen, A., Romano, M. E., Calafat, A. M., Webster, G. M., Yolton, K. and Lanphear, B. P. (2016). Prenatal perfluoroalkyl substance exposure and child adiposity at 8 years of age: The HOME study. *Obesity*, 24 (1): 231-237.

Braun, J. M., Just, A. C., Williams, P. L., Smith, K. W., Calafat, A. M. and Hauser, R. (2014). Personal care product use and urinary phthalate metabolite and paraben concentrations during pregnancy among women from a fertility clinic. *Journal of exposure science & environmental epidemiology*, 24 (5): 459-466.

Braun, J. M., Lanphear, B. P., Calafat, A. M., Deria, S., Khoury, J., Howe, C. J. and Venners, S. A. (2014). Early-life bisphenol a exposure and child body mass index: a prospective cohort study. *Environmental health perspectives*, 122 (11): 1239-1245.

Buck, R. C., Franklin, J., Berger, U., Conder, J. M., Cousins, I. T., De Voogt, P., Jensen, A. A., Kannan, K., Mabury, S. A. and van Leeuwen, S. P. (2011). Perfluoroalkyl and polyfluoroalkyl substances in the environment: terminology, classification, and origins. *Integrated environmental assessment and management*, 7 (4): 513-541.

Buckley, J. P., Engel, S. M., Braun, J. M., Whyatt, R. M., Daniels, J. L., Mendez, M. A., Richardson, D. B., Xu, Y., Calafat, A. M. and Wolff, M. S. (2016). Prenatal phthalate exposures and body mass index among 4 to 7 year old children: A pooled analysis. *Epidemiology (Cambridge, Mass.)*, 27 (3): 449.

Buckley, J. P., Engel, S. M., Mendez, M. A., Richardson, D. B., Daniels, J. L., Calafat, A. M., Wolff, M. S. and Herring, A. H. (2016). Prenatal phthalate exposures and childhood fat mass in a New York City cohort. *Environmental health perspectives*, 124 (4): 507-513.

Buckley, J. P., Herring, A. H., Wolff, M. S., Calafat, A. M. and Engel, S. M. (2016). Prenatal exposure to environmental phenols and childhood fat mass in the Mount Sinai Children's Environmental Health Study. *Environment international*, 91: 350-356.

Buser, M. C., Murray, H. E. and Scinicariello, F. (2014). Association of urinary phenols with increased body weight measures and obesity in children and adolescents. *The Journal of pediatrics*, 165 (4): 744-749.

Calafat, A. M. (2016). Contemporary issues in exposure assessment using biomonitoring. *Current epidemiology reports*, 3 (2): 145-153.

Calafat, A. M., Ye, X., Wong, L. Y., Reidy, J. A. and Needham, L. L. (2008). Urinary concentrations of triclosan in the US population: 2003–2004. *Environmental health perspectives*, 116 (3): 303-307.

Carwile, J. L., Ye, X., Zhou, X., Calafat, A. M. and Michels, K. B. (2011). Canned soup consumption and urinary bisphenol A: a randomized crossover trial. *Jama*, 306 (20): 2218-2220.

Chang, S.-C., Thibodeaux, J. R., Eastvold, M. L., Ehresman, D. J., Bjork, J. A., Froehlich, J. W., Lau, C., Singh, R. J., Wallace, K. B. and Butenhoff, J. L. (2008). Thyroid hormone status and pituitary function in adult rats given oral doses of perfluorooctanesulfonate (PFOS). *Toxicology*, 243 (3): 330-339.

Choi, J., Eom, J., Kim, J., Lee, S. and Kim, Y. (2014). Association between some endocrine-disrupting chemicals and childhood obesity in biological samples of young girls: a cross-sectional study. *Environmental toxicology and pharmacology*, 38 (1): 51-57.

Cichna-Markl, M. (2012). Sample clean-up by sol–gel immunoaffinity chromatography for the determination of bisphenol A in food and urine. *Methods*, 56 (2): 186-191.

Co-operation, O. f. E. and Development (2002). *Education at a glance: OECD indicators* 2002, OECD Paris.

Cocco, P. (2002). On the rumors about the silent spring: review of the scientific evidence linking occupational and environmental pesticide exposure to endocrine disruption health effects. *Cadernos de Saúde pública*, 18 (2): 379-402.

Codru, N., Schymura, M. J., Negoita, S., Rej, R., Carpenter, D. O. and Environment, A. T. F. o. t. (2007). Diabetes in relation to serum levels of polychlorinated biphenyls and chlorinated pesticides in adult Native Americans. *Environmental health perspectives*, 115 (10): 1442-1447.

Collins, S. (2005). Overview of clinical perspectives and mechanisms of obesity. *Birth Defects Research Part A: Clinical and Molecular Teratology*, 73 (7): 470-471.

Corton, J. C. and Lapinskas, P. J. (2005). Peroxisome proliferator-activated receptors: mediators of phthalate ester-induced effects in the male reproductive tract? *Toxicological sciences*, 83 (1): 4-17.

Cullinan, M. P., Palmer, J. E., Carle, A. D., West, M. J. and Seymour, G. J. (2012). Long term use of triclosan toothpaste and thyroid function. *Science of the Total Environment*, 416: 75-79.

Cupul-Uicab, L. A., Hernández-Ávila, M., Terrazas-Medina, E. A., Pennell, M. L. and Longnecker, M. P. (2010). Prenatal exposure to the major DDT metabolite 1, 1-

dichloro-2, 2-bis (p-chlorophenyl) ethylene (DDE) and growth in boys from Mexico. *Environmental research*, 110 (6): 595-603.

Cupul-Uicab, L. A., Klebanoff, M. A., Brock, J. W. and Longnecker, M. P. (2013). Prenatal exposure to persistent organochlorines and childhood obesity in the US collaborative perinatal project. *Environmental health perspectives*, 121 (9): 1103-1109.

D'Aniello, R., Troisi, J., D'Amico, O., Sangermano, M., Massa, G., Moccaldo, A., Pierri, L., Poeta, M. and Vajro, P. (2015). Emerging pathomechanisms involved in obesity. *Journal of pediatric gastroenterology and nutrition*, 60 (1): 113-119.

Dalsager, L., Christensen, L. E., Kongsholm, M. G., Kyhl, H. B., Nielsen, F., Schoeters, G., Jensen, T. K. and Andersen, H. R. (2018). Associations of maternal exposure to organophosphate and pyrethroid insecticides and the herbicide 2, 4-D with birth outcomes and anogenital distance at 3 months in the Odense Child Cohort. *Reproductive toxicology*, 76: 53-62.

Darbre, P. D. (2015). *Endocrine disruption and human health*, Academic Press.

Darbre, P. D. (2017). Endocrine disruptors and obesity. *Current obesity reports*, 6 (1): 18-27.

De Cock, M., De Boer, M. R., Lamoree, M., Legler, J. and Van de Bor, M. (2014). First year growth in relation to prenatal exposure to endocrine disruptors—a Dutch prospective cohort study. *International journal of environmental research and public health*, 11 (7): 7001-7021.

De Onis, M., Blössner, M. and Borghi, E. (2010). Global prevalence and trends of overweight and obesity among preschool children. *The American journal of clinical nutrition*, 92 (5): 1257-1264.

Elobeid, M. A. and Allison, D. B. (2008). Putative environmental-endocrine disruptors and obesity: a review. *Current opinion in endocrinology, diabetes, and obesity*, 15 (5): 403.

Everett, C. J., Mainous III, A. G., Frithsen, I. L., Player, M. S. and Matheson, E. M. (2008). Association of polychlorinated biphenyls with hypertension in the 1999–2002 National Health and Nutrition Examination Survey. *Environmental research*, 108 (1): 94-97.

Farhat, A., Crump, D., Chiu, S., Williams, K. L., Letcher, R. J., Gauthier, L. T. and Kennedy, S. W. (2013). In ovo effects of two organophosphate flame retardants—TCPP and TDCPP—on pipping success, development, mRNA expression, and thyroid hormone levels in chicken embryos. *Toxicological sciences*, 134 (1): 92-102.

Fat, O. (2012). Overweight and Obesity. *Centers for Disease Control and Prevention:* http://www.cdc.gov.

Feige, J. N., Gelman, L., Rossi, D., Zoete, V., Métivier, R., Tudor, C., Anghel, S. I., Grosdidier, A., Lathion, C. and Engelborghs, Y. (2007). The endocrine disruptor monoethyl-hexyl-phthalate is a selective peroxisome proliferator-activated receptor γ modulator that promotes adipogenesis. *Journal of Biological Chemistry*, 282 (26): 19152-19166.

Foster, P., Mylchreest, E., Gaido, K. and Sar, M. (2001). Effects of phthalate esters on the developing reproductive tract of male rats. *Apmis*, 109 (S103): S272-S277.

Garced, S., Torres-Sánchez, L., Cebrián, M. E., Claudio, L. and López-Carrillo, L. (2012). Prenatal dichlorodiphenyldichloroethylene (DDE) exposure and child growth during the first year of life. *Environmental research*, 113: 58-62.

Gee, R., Charles, A., Taylor, N. and Darbre, P. (2008). Oestrogenic and androgenic activity of triclosan in breast cancer cells. *Journal of Applied Toxicology: An International Journal*, 28 (1): 78-91.

Gentilcore, D., Porreca, I., Rizzo, F., Ganbaatar, E., Carchia, E., Mallardo, M., De Felice, M. and Ambrosino, C. (2013). Bisphenol A interferes with thyroid specific gene expression. *Toxicology*, 304: 21-31.

Genuis, S. J., Lane, K. and Birkholz, D. (2016). Human elimination of organochlorine pesticides: blood, urine, and sweat study. *BioMed research international*, 2016.

Ghassabian, A. and Trasande, L. (2018). Disruption in thyroid signaling pathway: a mechanism for the effect of endocrine-disrupting chemicals on child neurodevelopment. *Frontiers in endocrinology*, 9: 204.

Ginsberg, G. L. and Balk, S. J. (2016). Consumer products as sources of chemical exposures to children: case study of triclosan. *Current opinion in pediatrics*, 28 (2): 235-242.

Goncharov, A., Haase, R. F., Santiago-Rivera, A., Morse, G., McCaffrey, R. J., Rej, R., Carpenter, D. O. and Environment, A. T. F. o. t. (2008). High serum PCBs are associated with elevation of serum lipids and cardiovascular disease in a Native American population. *Environmental research*, 106 (2): 226-239.

Green, A. J., Graham, J. L., Gonzalez, E. A., La Frano, M. R., Petropoulou, S.-S. E., Park, J.-S., Newman, J. W., Stanhope, K. L., Havel, P. J. and La Merrill, M. A. (2017). Perinatal triphenyl phosphate exposure accelerates type 2 diabetes onset and increases adipose accumulation in UCD-type 2 diabetes mellitus rats. *Reproductive toxicology*, 68: 119-129.

Grün, F. and Blumberg, B. (2006). Environmental obesogens: organotins and endocrine disruption via nuclear receptor signaling. *Endocrinology*, 147 (6): s50-s55.

Grun, F., Watanabe, H., Zamanian, Z., Maeda, L., Arima, K., Cubacha, R., Gardiner, D. M., Kanno, J., Iguchi, T. and Blumberg, B. (2006). Endocrine-disrupting organotin compounds are potent inducers of adipogenesis in vertebrates. *Molecular Endocrinology*, 20 (9): 2141-2155.

Guo, J., Wu, C., Lu, D., Jiang, S., Liang, W., Chang, X., Xu, H., Wang, G. and Zhou, Z. (2017). Urinary paraben concentrations and their associations with anthropometric measures of children aged 3 years. *Environmental Pollution*, 222: 307-314.

Guo, L.-W., Wu, Q., Green, B., Nolen, G., Shi, L., LoSurdo, J., Deng, H., Bauer, S., Fang, J. L. and Ning, B. (2012). Cytotoxicity and inhibitory effects of low-concentration triclosan on adipogenic differentiation of human mesenchymal stem cells. *Toxicology and applied pharmacology*, 262 (2): 117-123.

Guo, Y., Wang, L. and Kannan, K. (2014). Phthalates and parabens in personal care products from China: concentrations and human exposure. *Archives of environmental contamination and toxicology*, 66 (1): 113-119.

Ha, K. H. and Kim, D. J. (2016). Epidemiology of childhood obesity in Korea. *Endocrinology and Metabolism*, 31 (4): 510-518.

Hall, R. H. (1992). A new threat to public health: organochlorines and food. *Nutrition and health*, 8 (1): 33-43.

Harley, K. G., Berger, K., Rauch, S., Kogut, K., Henn, B. C., Calafat, A. M., Huen, K., Eskenazi, B. and Holland, N. (2017). Association of prenatal urinary phthalate metabolite concentrations and childhood BMI and obesity. *Pediatric research*, 82 (3): 405-415.

Harley, K. G., Schall, R. A., Chevrier, J., Tyler, K., Aguirre, H., Bradman, A., Holland, N. T., Lustig, R. H., Calafat, A. M. and Eskenazi, B. (2013). Prenatal and postnatal bisphenol A exposure and body mass index in childhood in the CHAMACOS cohort. *Environmental health perspectives*, 121 (4): 514-520.

Hatch, E. E., Nelson, J. W., Qureshi, M. M., Weinberg, J., Moore, L. L., Singer, M. and Webster, T. F. (2008). Association of urinary phthalate metabolite concentrations with body mass index and waist circumference: a cross-sectional study of NHANES data, 1999–2002. *Environmental Health*, **7** (1): 27.

Hatch, E. E., Nelson, J. W., Stahlhut, R. W. and Webster, T. F. (2010). Association of endocrine disruptors and obesity: perspectives from epidemiological studies. *International journal of andrology*, 33 (2): 324-332.

Helaleh, M., Diboun, I., Al-Tamimi, N., Al-Sulaiti, H., Al-Emadi, M., Madani, A., Mazloum, N. A., Latiff, A. and Elrayess, M. A. (2018). Association of polybrominated diphenyl ethers in two fat compartments with increased risk of insulin resistance in obese individuals. *Chemosphere*, 209: 268-276.

Hines, E. P., Mendola, P., von Ehrenstein, O. S., Ye, X., Calafat, A. M. and Fenton, S. E. (2015). Concentrations of environmental phenols and parabens in milk, urine and serum of lactating North Carolina women. *Reproductive toxicology*, 54: 120-128.

Hoffman, K., Lorenzo, A., Butt, C. M., Adair, L., Herring, A. H., Stapleton, H. M. and Daniels, J. L. (2017). Predictors of urinary flame retardant concentration among pregnant women. *Environment international*, 98: 96-101.

Hofmann, J., Ardelt-Gattinger, E., Paulmichl, K., Weghuber, D. and Blechert, J. (2015). Dietary restraint and impulsivity modulate neural responses to food in adolescents with obesity and healthy adolescents. *Obesity*, 23 (11): 2183-2189.

Honkisz, E., Zieba-Przybylska, D. and Wojtowicz, A. K. (2012). The effect of triclosan on hormone secretion and viability of human choriocarcinoma JEG-3 cells. *Reproductive toxicology*, 34 (3): 385-392.

Høyer, B., Ramlau-Hansen, C., Henriksen, T., Pedersen, H., Góralczyk, K., Zviezdai, V., Jönsson, B., Heederik, D., Lenters, V. and Vermeulen, R. (2014). Body mass index in young school-age children in relation to organochlorine compounds in early life: a prospective study. *International journal of obesity*, 38 (7): 919-925.

Høyer, B. B., Ramlau-Hansen, C. H., Vrijheid, M., Valvi, D., Pedersen, H. S., Zviezdai, V., Jönsson, B. A., Lindh, C. H., Bonde, J. P. and Toft, G. (2015). Anthropometry in 5-to 9-year-old Greenlandic and Ukrainian children in relation to prenatal exposure to perfluorinated alkyl substances. *Environmental health perspectives*, 123 (8): 841-846.

Hu, P., Chen, X., Whitener, R. J., Boder, E. T., Jones, J. O., Porollo, A., Chen, J. and Zhao, L. (2013). Effects of parabens on adipocyte differentiation. *Toxicological sciences*, 131 (1): 56-70.

Hu, W., Gao, F., Zhang, H., Hiromori, Y., Arakawa, S., Nagase, H., Nakanishi, T. and Hu, J. (2017). Activation of peroxisome proliferator-activated receptor gamma and disruption of progesterone synthesis of 2-ethylhexyl diphenyl phosphate in human placental choriocarcinoma cells: comparison with triphenyl phosphate. *Environmental science & technology*, 51 (7): 4061-4068.

Huang, P. C., Liou, S. H., Ho, I. K. and Chiang, H. C. (2012). Phthalates exposure and endocrinal effects: an epidemiological review. *Journal of Food and Drug Analysis*, 20 (4).

Huang, Y. F., Pan, W. C., Tsai, Y. A., Chang, C. H., Chen, P. J., Shao, Y. S., Tsai, M. S., Hou, J. W., Lu, C. A. and Chen, M. L. (2017). Concurrent exposures to nonylphenol, bisphenol A, phthalates, and organophosphate pesticides on birth outcomes: A cohort study in Taipei, Taiwan. *Science of the Total Environment*, 607: 1126-1135.

Hurst, C. H. and Waxman, D. J. (2003). Activation of PPARα and PPARγ by environmental phthalate monoesters. *Toxicological sciences*, 74 (2): 297-308.

Hwang, H. J., Dornbos, P., Steidemann, M., Dunivin, T. K., Rizzo, M. and LaPres, J. J. (2016). Mitochondrial-targeted aryl hydrocarbon receptor and the impact of 2, 3, 7, 8-tetrachlorodibenzo-p-dioxin on cellular respiration and the mitochondrial proteome. *Toxicology and applied pharmacology*, 304: 121-132.

James, W. P. T. (2008). WHO recognition of the global obesity epidemic. *International journal of obesity*, 32 (7): S120-S126.

Jayaraj, R., Megha, P. and Sreedev, P. (2016). Organochlorine pesticides, their toxic effects on living organisms and their fate in the environment. *Interdisciplinary toxicology*, 9 (3-4): 90-100.

Johnson, P. I., Koustas, E., Vesterinen, H. M., Sutton, P., Atchley, D. S., Kim, A. N., Campbell, M., Donald, J. M., Sen, S. and Bero, L. (2016). Application of the Navigation Guide systematic review methodology to the evidence for developmental and reproductive toxicity of triclosan. *Environment international*, 92: 716-728.

Kalloo, G., Calafat, A. M., Chen, A., Yolton, K., Lanphear, B. P. and Braun, J. M. (2018). Early life Triclosan exposure and child adiposity at 8 Years of age: a prospective cohort study. *Environmental Health*, 17 (1): 24.

Kamrin, M. A. (2009). Phthalate risks, phthalate regulation, and public health: a review. *Journal of Toxicology and Environmental Health, Part B*, 12 (2): 157-174.

Kavvalakis, M. P. and Tsatsakis, A. M. (2012). The atlas of dialkylphosphates; assessment of cumulative human organophosphorus pesticides' exposure. *Forensic science international*, 218 (1-3): 111-122.

Kester, M. H., Bulduk, S., Tibboel, D., Meinl, W., Glatt, H., Falany, C. N., Coughtrie, M. W., Bergman, A., Safe, S. H. and Kuiper, G. G. (2000). Potent inhibition of estrogen sulfotransferase by hydroxylated PCB metabolites: a novel pathway explaining the estrogenic activity of PCBs. *Endocrinology*, 141 (5): 1897-1900.

Kim, J. T. and Lee, H. K. (2017). Childhood obesity and endocrine disrupting chemicals. *Annals of pediatric endocrinology & metabolism*, 22 (4): 219.

Kim, K. Y., Lee, E. and Kim, Y. (2019). The Association between Bisphenol A Exposure and Obesity in Children—A Systematic Review with Meta-Analysis. *International journal of environmental research and public health*, 16 (14): 2521.

Kim, S., Jung, J., Lee, I., Jung, D., Youn, H. and Choi, K. (2015). Thyroid disruption by triphenyl phosphate, an organophosphate flame retardant, in zebrafish (Danio rerio) embryos/larvae, and in GH3 and FRTL-5 cell lines. *Aquatic Toxicology*, 160: 188-196.

Kim, S. H. and Park, M. J. (2014). Phthalate exposure and childhood obesity. *Annals of pediatric endocrinology & metabolism*, 19 (2): 69.

Kirkley, A. G. and Sargis, R. M. (2014). Environmental endocrine disruption of energy metabolism and cardiovascular risk. *Current diabetes reports*, 14 (6): 494.

Kleanthi, G., Katerina, L., Evaggelia, P. and Andreas, L. (2008). Mechanisms of Actions and Health Effects of Organochlorine Substances: A Review. *Health Science Journal*, 2 (2).

Knudsen, N., Laurberg, P., Rasmussen, L. B., Bülow, I., Perrild, H., Ovesen, L. and Jørgensen, T. (2005). Small differences in thyroid function may be important for body mass index and the occurrence of obesity in the population. *The Journal of Clinical Endocrinology & Metabolism*, 90 (7): 4019-4024.

Koeppe, E. S., Ferguson, K. K., Colacino, J. A. and Meeker, J. D. (2013). Relationship between urinary triclosan and paraben concentrations and serum thyroid measures in NHANES 2007–2008. *Science of the Total Environment*, 445: 299-305.

Kojima, H., Takeuchi, S., Itoh, T., Iida, M., Kobayashi, S. and Yoshida, T. (2013). In vitro endocrine disruption potential of organophosphate flame retardants via human nuclear receptors. *Toxicology*, 314 (1): 76-83.

Kortenkamp, A. (2006). Breast cancer, oestrogens and environmental pollutants: A re-evaluation from a mixture perspective. *International journal of andrology*, 29 (1): 193-198.

Koutroulakis, D., Sifakis, S., Tzatzarakis, M., Alegakis, A., Theodoropoulou, E., Kavvalakis, M., Kappou, D. and Tsatsakis, A. (2014). Dialkyl phosphates in amniotic fluid as a biomarker of fetal exposure to organophosphates in Crete, Greece; association with fetal growth. *Reproductive toxicology*, 46: 98-105.

Krivoshiev, B. V., Dardenne, F., Covaci, A., Blust, R. and Husson, S. J. (2016). Assessing in-vitro estrogenic effects of currently-used flame retardants. *Toxicology in Vitro*, 33: 153-162.

Kumar, V., Balomajumder, C. and Roy, P. (2008). Disruption of LH-induced testosterone biosynthesis in testicular Leydig cells by triclosan: probable mechanism of action. *Toxicology*, 250 (2-3): 124-131.

Langer, P., Kočan, A., Tajtaková, M., Petrík, J., Chovancová, J., Drobná, B., Jursa, S., Rádiková, Ž., Koška, J. and Kšinantová, L. (2007). Fish from industrially polluted freshwater as the main source of organochlorinated pollutants and increased frequency of thyroid disorders and dysglycemia. *Chemosphere*, 67 (9): S379-S385.

Langer, S., Bekö, G., Weschler, C. J., Brive, L. M., Toftum, J., Callesen, M. and Clausen, G. (2014). Phthalate metabolites in urine samples from Danish children and correlations with phthalates in dust samples from their homes and daycare centers. *International journal of hygiene and environmental health*, 217 (1): 78-87.

Lau, C., Anitole, K., Hodes, C., Lai, D., Pfahles-Hutchens, A. and Seed, J. (2007). Perfluoroalkyl acids: a review of monitoring and toxicological findings. *Toxicological sciences*, 99 (2): 366-394.

Lauritzen, H. B., Larose, T. L., Øien, T., Sandanger, T. M., Odland, J. Ø., Van De Bor, M. and Jacobsen, G. W. (2018). Prenatal exposure to persistent organic pollutants and child overweight/obesity at 5-year follow-up: a prospective cohort study. *Environmental Health*, 17 (1): 9.

Law, J., Bloor, I., Budge, H. and Symonds, M. E. (2014). The influence of sex steroids on adipose tissue growth and function. *Hormone molecular biology and clinical investigation*, 19 (1): 13-24.

Li, D.-K., Miao, M., Zhou, Z., Wu, C., Shi, H., Liu, X., Wang, S. and Yuan, W. (2013). Urine bisphenol-A level in relation to obesity and overweight in school-age children. *PloS one*, 8 (6).

Li, J., Lai, H., Chen, S., Zhu, H. and Lai, S. (2017). Gender differences in the associations between urinary bisphenol A and body composition among American children: The National Health and Nutrition Examination Survey, 2003–2006. *Journal of epidemiology*, 27 (5): 228-234.

Li, S., Zhao, J., Wang, G., Zhu, Y., Rabito, F., Krousel-Wood, M., Chen, W. and Whelton, P. K. (2015). Urinary triclosan concentrations are inversely associated with body mass index and waist circumference in the US general population: experience in NHANES 2003–2010. *International journal of hygiene and environmental health*, 218 (4): 401-406.

Li, X., Pham, H. T., Janesick, A. S. and Blumberg, B. (2012). Triflumizole is an obesogen in mice that acts through peroxisome proliferator activated receptor gamma (PPAR γ). *Environmental health perspectives*, 120 (12): 1720-1726.

LI, Z. D., HAN, Z. Y. and Guo, G. R. (2011). Bisphenol A market trend [J]. *Thermosetting Resin*, 4.

Liao, C., Chen, L. and Kannan, K. (2013). Occurrence of parabens in foodstuffs from China and its implications for human dietary exposure. *Environment international*, 57: 68-74.

Liu, G., Dhana, K., Furtado, J. D., Rood, J., Zong, G., Liang, L., Qi, L., Bray, G. A., DeJonge, L. and Coull, B. (2018). Perfluoroalkyl substances and changes in body weight and resting metabolic rate in response to weight-loss diets: A prospective study. *PLoS medicine*, 15 (2).

Liu, X., Ji, K. and Choi, K. (2012). Endocrine disruption potentials of organophosphate flame retardants and related mechanisms in H295R and MVLN cell lines and in zebrafish. *Aquatic Toxicology*, 114: 173-181.

Ma, H., Zheng, L., Li, Y., Pan, S., Hu, J., Yu, Z., Zhang, G., Sheng, G. and Fu, J. (2013). Triclosan reduces the levels of global DNA methylation in HepG2 cells. *Chemosphere*, 90 (3): 1023-1029.

Main, K. M., Mortensen, G. K., Kaleva, M. M., Boisen, K. A., Damgaard, I. N., Chellakooty, M., Schmidt, I. M., Suomi, A. M., Virtanen, H. E. and Petersen, J. H. (2006). Human breast milk contamination with phthalates and alterations of endogenous reproductive hormones in infants three months of age. *Environmental health perspectives*, 114 (2): 270-276.

Maloney, E. K. and Waxman, D. J. (1999). Trans-Activation of PPARα and PPARγ by structurally diverse environmental chemicals. *Toxicology and applied pharmacology*, 161 (2): 209-218.

Maresca, M. M., Hoepner, L. A., Hassoun, A., Oberfield, S. E., Mooney, S. J., Calafat, A. M., Ramirez, J., Freyer, G., Perera, F. P. and Whyatt, R. M. (2016). Prenatal exposure to phthalates and childhood body size in an urban cohort. *Environmental health perspectives*, 124 (4): 514-520.

Masuno, H., Kidani, T., Sekiya, K., Sakayama, K., Shiosaka, T., Yamamoto, H. and Honda, K. (2002). Bisphenol A in combination with insulin can accelerate the conversion of 3T3-L1 fibroblasts to adipocytes. *Journal of lipid research*, 43 (5): 676-684.

Masuno, H., Okamoto, S., Iwanami, J., Honda, K., Shiosaka, T., Kidani, T., Sakayama, K. and Yamamoto, H. (2003). Effect of 4-nonylphenol on cell proliferation and adipocyte formation in cultures of fully differentiated 3T3-L1 cells. *Toxicological sciences*, 75 (2): 314-320.

McAllister, E. J., Dhurandhar, N. V., Keith, S. W., Aronne, L. J., Barger, J., Baskin, M., Benca, R. M., Biggio, J., Boggiano, M. M. and Eisenmann, J. C. (2009). Ten putative contributors to the obesity epidemic. *Critical reviews in food science and nutrition*, 49 (10): 868-913.

McGuinn, L. A., Ghazarian, A. A., Su, L. J. and Ellison, G. L. (2015). Urinary bisphenol A and age at menarche among adolescent girls: evidence from NHANES 2003–2010. *Environmental research*, 136: 381-386.

Meeker, J. D. and Stapleton, H. M. (2010). House dust concentrations of organophosphate flame retardants in relation to hormone levels and semen quality parameters. *Environmental health perspectives*, 118 (3): 318-323.

Mendez, M. A., Garcia-Esteban, R., Guxens, M., Vrijheid, M., Kogevinas, M., Goñi, F., Fochs, S. and Sunyer, J. (2011). Prenatal organochlorine compound exposure, rapid weight gain, and overweight in infancy. *Environmental health perspectives*, 119 (2): 272-278.

Miller, M. D., Marty, M. A., Arcus, A., Brown, J., Morry, D. and Sandy, M. (2002). Differences between children and adults: implications for risk assessment at California EPA. *International journal of toxicology*, 21 (5): 403-418.

Mokdad, A. H., Ford, E. S., Bowman, B. A., Dietz, W. H., Vinicor, F., Bales, V. S. and Marks, J. S. (2003). Prevalence of obesity, diabetes, and obesity-related health risk factors, 2001. *Jama*, 289 (1): 76-79.

Mokdad, A. H., Serdula, M. K., Dietz, W. H., Bowman, B. A., Marks, J. S. and Koplan, J. P. (1999). The spread of the obesity epidemic in the United States, 1991-1998. *Jama*, 282 (16): 1519-1522.

Moos, R. K., Angerer, J., Dierkes, G., Brüning, T. and Koch, H. M. (2016). Metabolism and elimination of methyl, iso-and n-butyl paraben in human urine after single oral dosage. *Archives of toxicology*, 90 (11): 2699-2709.

Mora, A. M., Oken, E., Rifas-Shiman, S. L., Webster, T. F., Gillman, M. W., Calafat, A. M., Ye, X. and Sagiv, S. K. (2017). Prenatal exposure to perfluoroalkyl substances and adiposity in early and mid-childhood. *Environmental health perspectives*, 125 (3): 467-473.

Newbold, R. R. (2010). Impact of environmental endocrine disrupting chemicals on the development of obesity. *Hormones*, 9 (3): 206-217.

Newbold, R. R., Padilla-Banks, E., Jefferson, W. N. and Heindel, J. J. (2008). Effects of endocrine disruptors on obesity. *International journal of andrology*, 31 (2): 201-208.

Newbold, R. R., Padilla-Banks, E., Snyder, R. J. and Jefferson, W. N. (2007). Perinatal exposure to environmental estrogens and the development of obesity. *Molecular nutrition & food research*, 51 (7): 912-917.

Nicolopoulou-Stamati, P. and Pitsos, M. (2001). The impact of endocrine disrupters on the female reproductive system. *Human Reproduction Update*, 7 (3): 323-330.

Ogden, C. L., Carroll, M. D., Kit, B. K. and Flegal, K. M. (2014). Prevalence of childhood and adult obesity in the United States, 2011-2012. *Jama*, 311 (8): 806-814.

Ogden, C. L., Flegal, K. M., Carroll, M. D. and Johnson, C. L. (2002). Prevalence and trends in overweight among US children and adolescents, 1999-2000. *Jama*, 288 (14): 1728-1732.

Pagni, R. (2006). *Environmental Chemistry*, (Baird, Colin; Cann, Michael), ACS Publications.

Pan, G., Hanaoka, T., Yoshimura, M., Zhang, S., Wang, P., Tsukino, H., Inoue, K., Nakazawa, H., Tsugane, S. and Takahashi, K. (2006). Decreased serum free testosterone in workers exposed to high levels of di-n-butyl phthalate (DBP) and di-2-ethylhexyl phthalate (DEHP): a cross-sectional study in China. *Environmental health perspectives*, 114 (11): 1643-1648.

Park, M. H., Falconer, C., Viner, R. a. and Kinra, S. (2012). The impact of childhood obesity on morbidity and mortality in adulthood: a systematic review. *Obesity reviews*, 13 (11): 985-1000.

Park, W. H., Jun, D. W., Kim, J. T., Jeong, J. H., Park, H., Chang, Y. S., Park, K. S., Lee, H. K. and Pak, Y. K. (2013). Novel cell-based assay reveals associations of circulating serum AhR-ligands with metabolic syndrome and mitochondrial dysfunction. *Biofactors*, 39 (4): 494-504.

Patisaul, H. B., Roberts, S. C., Mabrey, N., McCaffrey, K. A., Gear, R. B., Braun, J., Belcher, S. M. and Stapleton, H. M. (2013). Accumulation and endocrine disrupting effects of the flame retardant mixture Firemaster® 550 in rats: an exploratory assessment. *Journal of biochemical and molecular toxicology*, 27 (2): 124-136.

Pereira-Fernandes, A., Demaegdt, H., Vandermeiren, K., Hectors, T. L., Jorens, P. G., Blust, R. and Vanparys, C. (2013). Evaluation of a screening system for obesogenic compounds: screening of endocrine disrupting compounds and evaluation of the PPAR dependency of the effect. *PloS one*, 8 (10).

Philippat, C., Wolff, M. S., Calafat, A. M., Ye, X., Bausell, R., Meadows, M., Stone, J., Slama, R. and Engel, S. M. (2013). Prenatal exposure to environmental phenols: concentrations in amniotic fluid and variability in urinary concentrations during pregnancy. *Environmental health perspectives*, 121 (10): 1225-1231.

Pornkunwilai, S., Nosoongnoen, W., Jantarat, C., Wachrasindhu, S. and Supornsilchai, V. (2015). Urinary bisphenol A detection is significantly associated with young and obese Thai children. *Asian Biomedicine*, 9 (3): 363-372.

Quirós-Alcalá, L., Buckley, J. P. and Boyle, M. (2018). Parabens and measures of adiposity among adults and children from the US general population: NHANES 2007–2014. *International journal of hygiene and environmental health*, 221 (4): 652-660.

Ranjbar, M., Rotondi, M. A., Ardern, C. I. and Kuk, J. L. (2015). The influence of urinary concentrations of organophosphate metabolites on the relationship between BMI and Cardiometabolic health risk. *Journal of obesity*, 2015.

Rauch, S. A., Braun, J. M., Barr, D. B., Calafat, A. M., Khoury, J., Montesano, M. A., Yolton, K. and Lanphear, B. P. (2012). Associations of prenatal exposure to organophosphate pesticide metabolites with gestational age and birth weight. *Environmental health perspectives*, 120 (7): 1055-1060.

Reigart, J. R. and Roberts, J. R. (1999). *Recognition and management of pesticide poisonings,* US Environmental Protection Agency.

Richardson, R. J. (1995). Assessment of the neurotoxic potential of chlorpyrifos relative to other organophosphorus compounds: a critical review of the literature. *Journal of Toxicology and Environmental Health, Part A Current Issues*, 44 (2): 135-165.

Rodricks, J. V., Swenberg, J. A., Borzelleca, J. F., Maronpot, R. R. and Shipp, A. M. (2010). Triclosan: a critical review of the experimental data and development of margins of safety for consumer products. *Critical reviews in toxicology*, 40 (5): 422-484.

Romano, M. E., Hawley, N. L., Eliot, M., Calafat, A. M., Jayatilaka, N. K., Kelsey, K., McGarvey, S., Phipps, M. G., Savitz, D. A. and Werner, E. F. (2017). Variability and predictors of urinary concentrations of organophosphate flame retardant metabolites among pregnant women in Rhode Island. *Environmental Health*, 16 (1): 40.

Rudel, R. A., Gray, J. M., Engel, C. L., Rawsthorne, T. W., Dodson, R. E., Ackerman, J. M., Rizzo, J., Nudelman, J. L. and Brody, J. G. (2011). Food packaging and bisphenol A and bis (2-ethyhexyl) phthalate exposure: findings from a dietary intervention. *Environmental health perspectives*, 119 (7): 914-920.

Sales, L. B., Kamstra, J., Cenijn, P., Van Rijt, L., Hamers, T. and Legler, J. (2013). Effects of endocrine disrupting chemicals on in vitro global DNA methylation and adipocyte differentiation. *Toxicology in Vitro*, 27 (6): 1634-1643.

Sawhney, B. L. and Hankin, L. (1985). Polychlorinated biphenyls in food: A review. *Journal of food protection*, 48 (5): 442-448.

Selevan, S. G., Kimmel, C. A. and Mendola, P. (2000). Identifying critical windows of exposure for children's health. *Environmental health perspectives*, 108 (suppl 3): 451-455.

Steinberg, K., Freni-Titulaer, L., Rogers, T., Burse, V., Mueller, P., Stehr, P., Miller, D. and Steele, G. (1986). Effects of polychlorinated biphenyls and lipemia on serum analytes. *Journal of Toxicology and Environmental Health, Part A Current Issues*, 19 (3): 369-381.

Teitelbaum, S., Britton, J., Calafat, A., Ye, X., Silva, M., Reidy, J., Galvez, M., Brenner, B. and Wolff, M. (2008). Temporal variability in urinary concentrations of phthalate metabolites, phytoestrogens and phenols among minority children in the United States. *Environmental research*, 106 (2): 257-269.

Teitelbaum, S. L., Mervish, N., Moshier, E. L., Vangeepuram, N., Galvez, M. P., Calafat, A. M., Silva, M. J., Brenner, B. L. and Wolff, M. S. (2012). Associations between phthalate metabolite urinary concentrations and body size measures in New York City children. *Environmental research*, 112: 186-193.

Thayer, K. A., Doerge, D. R., Hunt, D., Schurman, S. H., Twaddle, N. C., Churchwell, M. I., Garantziotis, S., Kissling, G. E., Easterling, M. R. and Bucher, J. R. (2015). Pharmacokinetics of bisphenol A in humans following a single oral administration. *Environment international*, 83: 107-115.

Tontonoz, P., Hu, E. and Spiegelman, B. M. (1994). Stimulation of adipogenesis in fibroblasts by PPARγ2, a lipid-activated transcription factor. *Cell*, 79 (7): 1147-1156.

Trasande, L., Attina, T. M. and Blustein, J. (2012). Association between urinary bisphenol A concentration and obesity prevalence in children and adolescents. *Jama*, 308 (11): 1113-1121.

Tsatsakis, A., Tzatzarakis, M., Koutroulakis, D., Toutoudaki, M. and Sifakis, S. (2009). Dialkyl phosphates in meconium as a biomarker of prenatal exposure to organophosphate pesticides: a study on pregnant women of rural areas in Crete, Greece. *Xenobiotica*, 39 (5): 364-373.

Udoji, F., Martin, T., Etherton, R. and Whalen, M. M. (2010). Immunosuppressive effects of triclosan, nonylphenol, and DDT on human natural killer cells in vitro. *Journal of immunotoxicology*, 7 (3): 205-212.

Vafeiadi, M., Roumeliotaki, T., Myridakis, A., Chalkiadaki, G., Fthenou, E., Dermitzaki, E., Karachaliou, M., Sarri, K., Vassilaki, M. and Stephanou, E. G. (2016). Association of early life exposure to bisphenol A with obesity and cardiometabolic traits in childhood. *Environmental research*, 146: 379-387.

Valle-Sistac, J., Molins-Delgado, D., Díaz, M., Ibáñez, L., Barceló, D. and Díaz-Cruz, M. S. (2016). Determination of parabens and benzophenone-type UV filters in human placenta. First description of the existence of benzyl paraben and benzophenone-4. *Environment international*, 88: 243-249.

Valvi, D., Casas, M., Mendez, M. A., Ballesteros-Gómez, A., Luque, N., Rubio, S., Sunyer, J. and Vrijheid, M. (2013). Prenatal bisphenol a urine concentrations and early rapid growth and overweight risk in the offspring. *Epidemiology*: 791-799.

Valvi, D., Casas, M., Romaguera, D., Monfort, N., Ventura, R., Martinez, D., Sunyer, J. and Vrijheid, M. (2015). Prenatal phthalate exposure and childhood growth and blood pressure: evidence from the Spanish INMA-Sabadell Birth Cohort Study. *Environmental health perspectives*, 123 (10): 1022-1029.

Valvi, D., Mendez, M. A., Martinez, D., Grimalt, J. O., Torrent, M., Sunyer, J. and Vrijheid, M. (2012). Prenatal concentrations of polychlorinated biphenyls, DDE, and DDT and overweight in children: a prospective birth cohort study. *Environmental health perspectives*, 120 (3): 451-457.

Vanden Heuvel, J. P., Thompson, J. T., Frame, S. R. and Gillies, P. J. (2006). Differential activation of nuclear receptors by perfluorinated fatty acid analogs and natural fatty acids: a comparison of human, mouse, and rat peroxisome proliferator-activated receptor-α,-β, and-γ, liver X receptor-β, and retinoid X receptor-α. *Toxicological sciences*, 92 (2): 476-489.

Vasiliu, O., Cameron, L., Gardiner, J., DeGuire, P. and Karmaus, W. (2006). Polybrominated biphenyls, polychlorinated biphenyls, body weight, and incidence of adult-onset diabetes mellitus. *Epidemiology*: 352-359.

Verhulst, S. L., Nelen, V., Hond, E. D., Koppen, G., Beunckens, C., Vael, C., Schoeters, G. and Desager, K. (2009). Intrauterine exposure to environmental pollutants and body mass index during the first 3 years of life. *Environmental health perspectives*, 117 (1): 122-126.

Wang, B., Wang, H., Zhou, W., He, Y., Zhou, Y., Chen, Y. and Jiang, Q. (2014). Exposure to bisphenol A among school children in eastern China: a multicenter cross-sectional study. *Journal of exposure science & environmental epidemiology*, 24 (6): 657-664.

Wang, H., Zhou, Y., Tang, C., He, Y., Wu, J., Chen, Y. and Jiang, Q. (2013). Urinary phthalate metabolites are associated with body mass index and waist circumference in Chinese school children. *PloS one*, 8 (2).

Wang, L., Asimakopoulos, A. G. and Kannan, K. (2015). Accumulation of 19 environmental phenolic and xenobiotic heterocyclic aromatic compounds in human adipose tissue. *Environment international*, 78: 45-50.

Wang, P., Tian, Y., Wang, X. J., Gao, Y., Shi, R., Wang, G. Q., Hu, G. H. and Shen, X. M. (2012). Organophosphate pesticide exposure and perinatal outcomes in Shanghai, China. *Environment international*, 42: 100-104.

Wang, Q., Lam, J. C., Han, J., Wang, X., Guo, Y., Lam, P. K. and Zhou, B. (2015). Developmental exposure to the organophosphorus flame retardant tris (1, 3-dichloro-2-propyl) phosphate: estrogenic activity, endocrine disruption and reproductive effects on zebrafish. *Aquatic Toxicology*, 160: 163-171.

Warner, M., Schall, R. A., Harley, K. G., Bradman, A., Barr, D. and Eskenazi, B. (2013). In utero DDT and DDE exposure and obesity status of 7-year-old Mexican-American children in the CHAMACOS cohort. *Environmental health perspectives*, 121 (5): 631-636.

Warner, M., Wesselink, A., Harley, K. G., Bradman, A., Kogut, K. and Eskenazi, B. (2014). Prenatal exposure to dichlorodiphenyltrichloroethane and obesity at 9 years of age in the CHAMACOS study cohort. *American journal of epidemiology*, 179 (11): 1312-1322.

Wells, E. M., Jackson, L. W. and Koontz, M. B. (2014). Association between bisphenol A and waist-to-height ratio among children: National Health and Nutrition Examination Survey, 2003–2010. *Annals of epidemiology*, 2 (24): 165-167.

Weschler, C. J. (2009). Changes in indoor pollutants since the 1950s. *Atmospheric Environment*, 43 (1): 153-169.

Whitehead, S. A. and Rice, S. (2006). Endocrine-disrupting chemicals as modulators of sex steroid synthesis. *Best practice & research Clinical endocrinology & metabolism*, 20 (1): 45-61.

Whyatt, R. M. and Barr, D. B. (2001). Measurement of organophosphate metabolites in postpartum meconium as a potential biomarker of prenatal exposure: a validation study. *Environmental health perspectives*, 109 (4): 417-420.

Williams, G. (2012). Aromatase up-regulation, insulin and raised intracellular oestrogens in men, induce adiposity, metabolic syndrome and prostate disease, via aberrant ER-α and GPER signalling. *Molecular and cellular endocrinology*, 351 (2): 269-278.

Wittassek, M. and Angerer, J. (2008). Phthalates: metabolism and exposure. *International journal of andrology*, 31 (2): 131-138.

Woodruff, T. J., Zota, A. R. and Schwartz, J. M. (2011). Environmental chemicals in pregnant women in the United States: NHANES 2003–2004. *Environmental health perspectives*, 119 (6): 878-885.

Xia, B., Zhu, Q., Zhao, Y., Ge, W., Zhao, Y., Song, Q., Zhou, Y., Shi, H. and Zhang, Y. (2018). Phthalate exposure and childhood overweight and obesity: urinary metabolomic evidence. *Environment international*, 121: 159-168.

Xue, J., Wu, Q., Sakthivel, S., Pavithran, P. V., Vasukutty, J. R. and Kannan, K. (2015). Urinary levels of endocrine-disrupting chemicals, including bisphenols, bisphenol A diglycidyl ethers, benzophenones, parabens, and triclosan in obese and non-obese Indian children. *Environmental research*, 137: 120-128.

Yang, O., Kim, H. L., Weon, J. I. and Seo, Y. R. (2015). Endocrine-disrupting chemicals: review of toxicological mechanisms using molecular pathway analysis. *Journal of cancer prevention*, 20 (1): 12.

Ye, X., Bishop, A. M., Reidy, J. A., Needham, L. L. and Calafat, A. M. (2006). Parabens as urinary biomarkers of exposure in humans. *Environmental health perspectives*, 114 (12): 1843-1846.

Yu, W. G., Liu, W. and Jin, Y. H. (2009). Effects of perfluorooctane sulfonate on rat thyroid hormone biosynthesis and metabolism. *Environmental Toxicology and Chemistry: An International Journal*, 28 (5): 990-996.

Zarean, M. and Poursafa, P. (2019). The Role of Environmental Disruptor Chemicals in the Development of Non Communicable Disease. *Primordial Prevention of Non Communicable Disease,* Springer**:** 21-31.

Zhang, Q., Ji, C., Yin, X., Yan, L., Lu, M. and Zhao, M. (2016). Thyroid hormone-disrupting activity and ecological risk assessment of phosphorus-containing flame retardants by in vitro, in vivo and in silico approaches. *Environmental Pollution*, 210: 27-33.

Zhang, Y., Meng, X., Chen, L., Li, D., Zhao, L., Zhao, Y., Li, L. and Shi, H. (2014). Age and sex-specific relationships between phthalate exposures and obesity in Chinese children at puberty. *PloS one*, 9 (8).

Zoeller, R. T., Bansal, R. and Parris, C. (2005). Bisphenol-A, an environmental contaminant that acts as a thyroid hormone receptor antagonist in vitro, increases serum thyroxine, and alters RC3/neurogranin expression in the developing rat brain. *Endocrinology*, 146 (2): 607-612.

In: Childhood Obesity
Editor: Roya Kelishadi

ISBN: 978-1-53618-158-6
© 2020 Nova Science Publishers, Inc.

Chapter 5

FAMILY-RELATED RISK FACTORS OF CHILDHOOD OBESITY

Xin'nan Zong[1] and Bo Xi[2,*]
[1]Department of Growth and Development,
Capital Institute of Pediatrics, Beijing, China
[2]Department of Epidemiology, School of Public Health,
Shandong University, Jinan, China

INTRODUCTION

Obesity has become a major global health challenge in the 21 century because of its substantial increases in prevalence and established health risks. To date, no national success stories to combat obesity epidemic have been reported over the three decades [1]. It is estimated that obese children exceeded 120 million in 2016 [2].

Childhood obesity is not a disease in itself but rather a complex symptom. An important consequence of childhood obesity is the increasing number of children experiencing obesity-related morbidity, such as hypertension, diabetes mellitus, metabolic syndrome, stroke, ischemic heart disease, and several cancers in childhood or adulthood [3-4]. Obesity persists from childhood to adolescence and even adulthood which is not only a leading cause of health problems, but also the rise in obesity-related health conditions that contributes to great economic costs [5].

* Corresponding Author's Email: xibo2007@126.com.

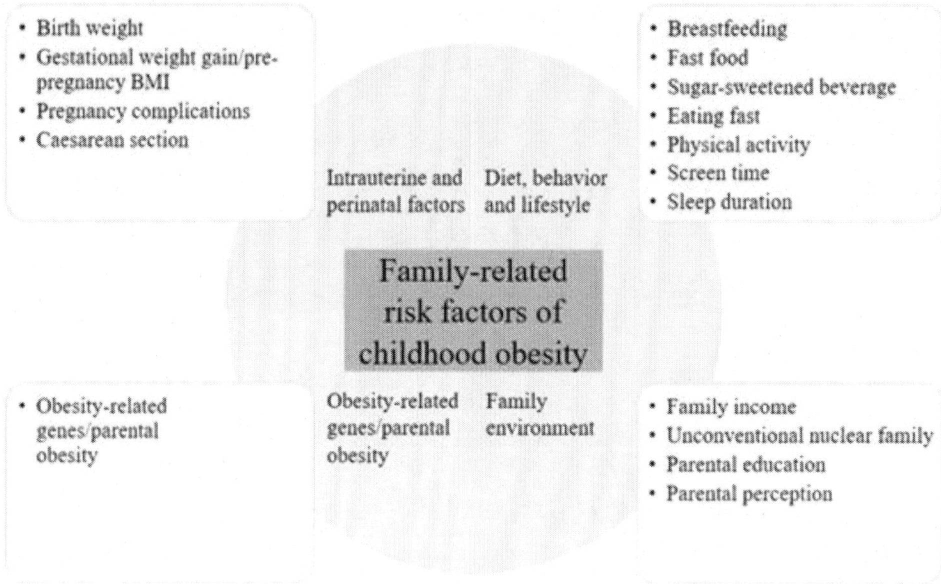

Figure 1. Structural outline of family-related risk factors of childhood obesity.

Rapid increase in obesity prevalence and associated disease burden highlights the need for continued focus on surveillance of obesity and identification, implementation, and evaluation of evidence-based interventions to address this problem. Alarming increase in childhood obesity appears to be connected to living in an obesogenic society with increasing social, cultural, and technological changes that lead to unhealthy lifestyles [6]. Current evidence indicates that modifiable environmental influences and learned unhealthy behaviors significantly contribute to obesity and its rising rate [7]. Recognition and consideration of these environmental, social, cultural, and family factors are critical to develop prevention and intervention strategies of childhood obesity.

Childhood obesity is an ongoing concern all over the world. The development of obesity may be already in early childhood, suggesting a timely intervention targeted at young children was very necessary [8]. Obesity prevention and control in early childhood was paid less attention comparing with school-aged children and adults, to some extent, which may be due to the lack of systematic integration of some highly suspected risk factors of childhood obesity. Childhood obesity epidemic driven by complex forces requires system thinking to conceptualize the causes and to develop evidence needed for action [9]. Family-related risk factors of childhood obesity shown in Figure 1, as an integrated concept would evidence science and the feasibility of the development of family-based prevention and control strategies of childhood obesity. Parents and families should participate in learning how to prevent their children from overweight or obesity and what to do if their children are already overweight or obese.

COMPONENTS OF FAMILY-RELATED RISK FACTORS OF CHILDHOOD OBESITY

Intrauterine and Perinatal Factors

Birth Weight

Several cohort studies have indicated that high birth weight is associated with an increased risk of obesity in childhood or adolescence [10-12]. A meta-analysis of 66 studies from 26 countries demonstrated that high birth weight (>4000 g) was significantly associated with increased odds of childhood overweight (odds ratio (OR), 1.66; 95% confidence interval (CI), 1.55-1.77) compared with normal birth weight (2500-4000 g) [13]. A 12-country study of 5141 children aged 9-11 years found that obesity risk was significantly higher among children whose birth weight were 3500-4000 g (OR, 1.45; 95% CI, 1.10-1.92), and >4000 g (OR, 2.08; 95% CI, 1.47-2.93) compared with the reference group (2500-3000 g) [14]. Furthermore, high birth weight is also associated with risk of type 2 diabetes mellitus and cardiovascular disease in adulthood [15].

A prospective birth cohort study in China also showed that higher birth weight was associated with an increased risk of childhood overweight, and lower birth weight with an increased risk of childhood underweight [16]. A meta-analysis of 8 studies reported that low birth weight (<2500 g) was associated with an increased risk of diabetes mellitus (OR, 1.55; 95% CI, 1.39-1.73) compared with normal birth weight (2500-4000 g) [17]. Another meta-analysis of 21 studies also reported that low birth weight (<2500 g) increased the risk of diabetes mellitus (OR, 1.41; 95% CI, 1.26-1.58) compared with normal birth weight (2500-4000 g) [18]. Thus, normal birth weight should be informed by health counselling to women of childbearing age before and during pregnancy in order to guide weight control for the women.

Gestational Weight Gain/Pre-Pregnancy BMI

Excessive weight gain during pregnancy increases the risk for having heavy babies, and studies suggest these babies are programmed to be overweight or obese later in life [19-20]. A meta-analysis of 15 studies concluded that gestational weight gain greater than or less than the Institute of Medicine guideline recommendations (gain of 12.5-18 kg for underweight women [body mass index (BMI) <18.5], 11.5-16 kg for normal-weight women [BMI 18.5-24.9], 7-11 kg for overweight women [BMI 25-29.9], and 5-9 kg for obese women [BMI ≥30]) was associated with higher risk of adverse maternal and infant outcomes [21].

Pre-pregnancy BMI is significantly associated with pregnancy complications and offspring obesity and also is associated with gestational weight gain [22-23]. A meta-analysis of 25 cohort studies suggests that maternal pre-pregnancy BMI was more strongly associated with adverse maternal and infant outcomes than gestational weight gain [24]. Furthermore, an individual participant data meta-analysis including 160757 mother-offspring pairs from 34 European or North American cohorts confirmed that preventive strategies for reducing childhood obesity should focus on maternal BMI rather than on pregnancy complications [25].

Higher maternal pre-pregnancy BMI and gestational weight gain are also associated with higher risks of gestational hypertensive disorders, gestational diabetes, and large for gestational age at birth [26]. Therefore, women with overweight and obesity need support to lose weight before they conceive and to minimize their weight gain in pregnancy. Risk assessment and hazard analysis of gestational weight gain and pre-pregnancy BMI may be very necessary for preconception counseling.

Pregnancy Complications

A meta-analysis of over 24000 infants showed that infants of diabetic mothers had greater fat mass than infants of mothers without diabetes (mean difference (95% CI)): 83 g (49 to 117), and fat mass is greater in infants of mothers with gestational diabetes: 62 g (29 to 94) and type 1 diabetes: 268 g (139 to 397) [27]. Another meta-analysis of 20 observational studies also reported that intrauterine exposure to hyperglycemia was associated with offspring obesity and abnormal glucose tolerance especially in offspring of mothers with type 1 diabetes mellitus [28]. Pregnancy-induced hypertension raises the risk of childhood obesity by 50% [29]. A birth cohort suggested that hypertension during pregnancy, independent of maternal body size before pregnancy, was a risk factor for offspring childhood obesity [30]. Maternal gestational diabetes mellitus alone or joint gestational diabetes mellitus and hypertensive disorder during pregnancy were associated with increased ratios of offspring's overweight [31]. Thus, lowering maternal risk of pregnancy complications, such as gestational diabetes mellitus and gestational hypertension, may be necessary and effective to prevent the risk of overweight and obesity of the offspring.

Caesarean Section

Children born by caesarean section are at higher risk of developing overweight and obesity compared with vaginal birth [32-33]. A prospective cohort study showed that cesarean birth was associated with offspring obesity after accounting for major confounding factors [34]. Children delivered by both elective and non-elective caesarean section are at increased risk of overweight and obesity [35]. Caesarean section with or without medical indications is associated with increased risks of overweight and obesity in school-aged children [36]. Although additional research is needed to clarify the mechanisms underlying the association between caesarean section and obesity, health care professionals and childbearing women should weigh this risk when considering cesarean delivery in the absence of a clear medical indication.

Diet, Behavior and Lifestyle

Breastfeeding

Breast milk is rich in effective ingredients with higher nutritional value. Based on the known benefits of breastfeeding for women and children, the WHO recommended in 2002 that infants should be exclusively breastfed for the first 6 months, and breastfeeding should be supplemented with additional foods for the first 2 years. A longitudinal birth cohort study of 918 children showed that bottle feeding from birth or breast-fed for less than 3 months was a risk factor for overweight and adiposity at 6 year of age, and early bottle-feeding brings forward the obesity rebound and predicts obesity later in life [37]. A longitudinal data of 1234 children showed breastfeeding within 1 month and beyond 6 months reduced the risk of childhood obesity [38]. A retrospective cohort study showed that exclusive breastfeeding in the first 6 months was a significant protective factor against overweight/obesity in children with high birth weight [39]. A meta-analysis of 28 studies showed breastfeeding was associated with a reduced risk of obesity compared with formula feeding (OR, 0.87; 95% CI, 0.85-0.89) [40]. A meta-analysis of 17 studies also supported a dose-dependent association between longer duration of breastfeeding and decrease in overweight risk [41]. In addition, promoting exclusive breastfeeding was also reported to be important in preventing both stunting and overweight among children [42].

Fast Food

Most studies reported that a diet with a lower percentage of obesogenic foods (including fatty cheeses, sugary drinks, processed foods, fast food, candies, snacks, cakes, animal products, whole milk, and refined grains) should be effective in reducing the obesity risk in childhood [43]. Fast food intake was associated with overweight and measures of adiposity (BMI, waist circumference, and body fat mass percentage) in children [44]. Fast food consumption was also associated with the incidence of metabolic syndrome, abdominal obesity, and hypertriglyceridemia in children and adolescents [45]. Researches have shown that TV/video viewing was correlated with fast food consumption among children, which raised the possibility that greater exposure to TV/video may influence children's consumption of unhealthful foods [46-47]. Thus, limiting fast food consumption and reducing TV/video viewing time should be considered together as means of improving dietary patterns and reducing childhood obesity risk.

Sugar-Sweetened Beverage

Most studies reported that there was a direct association between sugar-sweetened beverage consumption and weight gain, overweight, and obesity in children and adolescents [48]. Recent evidence further showed that sugar-sweetened beverage consumption was positively associated with or has an effect on obesity inices (weight/BMI/BMI z-score) in children and adults [49]. A meta-analysis reported that sweet nutriments preference (OR, 2.78; 95% CI, 1.97-3.93) was associated with overweight/obesity in children and adolescents [50]. A significant association between sugar-sweetened beverage and general and central adiposity was also observed among children under 12 years [51]. Because sugar-sweetened beverage consumption is associated with obesity and other adverse health outcomes, the consumption of sugar-sweetened beverage by children and adolescents should be limited, and the consumption of water and other non-sweetened beverages should be advised.

Eating Fast

Fast eating speed is significantly associated with risk of childhood general and abdominal obesity in China [52-53]. Research has shown a synergistic interaction between late bedtime and fast eating speed in increasing overweight and obesity risk in preschool children [54]. Fast eating speed was associated with overweight among adolescents, and furthermore, the combination of both fast eating speed and eating too much may have a joint effect on overweight [55]. A meta-analysis further showed the pooled OR for eating quickly on the development of obesity was 2.15 (95% CI, 1.84-2.51) compared with eating slowly [56]. Eating fast may be related to more energy intake, therefore, the modification of eating fast could help prevent overweight and obesity in children.

Physical Activity

World Health Organization recommended that children and youth aged 5-17 should accumulate at least 60 minutes of moderate- to vigorous-intensity physical activity daily [57]. Early childhood period is important for the establishment of healthy behavioral patterns, especially limitation of screen time and encouragement of physical activity. Strong evidence has showed an inverse association between total physical activity and overweight in preschool children, and a positive association between television viewing and overweight [58]. A meta-analysis of more than 6000 children and adolescents showed physical activity of moderate-to-vigorous intensity but limited sedentary time was independently inversely associated with the metabolic syndrome [59]. Physical activity interventions in a school-based setting in combination with healthy diets, and participation of home and community may have the most effectiveness [60].

Screen Time

Screen-media use among young children is highly prevalent in today's society. Current evidence showed that higher duration or frequency of screen time such as TV viewing was associated with unfavourable body composition and higher cardio-metabolic risk [61]. Total screen time was closely related to obesity in preschool children, with 1-2 hr/day (OR, 1.37; 95% CI, 1.17-1.61) and ≥2 hr/day (OR, 2.00; 95% CI, 1.60-2.49) both having obesity risk compared with <half hr/day [52]. A meta-analysis showed an increased risk of overweight/obesity among children with screen time ≥2 hr/day (OR, 1.67; 95% CI, 1.48-

1.88) compared with those with screen time <2 hr/day [62]. In addition, the encouragement and support from parents can increase children's physical activity, and the reduce of parents' own screen time was correlated with decrease of children's screen time [63]. Interventions for reducing screen time in children might be effective in preventing excess weight gain [64]. Thus, limiting total screen time, such as TV, mobile phone and ipad, should be taken as a necessary means to decrease obesity risk in children and adolescents.

The American Academy of Pediatrics recommended New Guidelines for Screen Time for Children in 2016 [65]. For children younger than 18 months, avoid use of screen media other than video-chatting. Parents of children 18 to 24 months of age who want to introduce digital media should choose high-quality programming, and watch it with their children to help them understand what they're seeing. For children ages 2 to 5 years, limit screen use to 1 hour per day of high-quality programs. Parents should co-view media with children to help them understand what they are seeing and apply it to the world around them. For children ages 6 and older, place consistent limits on the time spent using media, and the types of media, and make sure media does not take the place of adequate sleep, physical activity and other behaviors essential to health. Designate media-free times together, such as dinner or driving, as well as media-free locations at home, such as bedrooms. Have ongoing communication about online citizenship and safety, including treating others with respect online and offline.

Sleep Duration

A meta-analysis of prospective studies demonstrated that short sleep duration was associated with a greater risk of developing overweight or obesity in infancy (relative risk (RR), 1.40; 95% CI, 1.19-1.65), early childhood (RR, 1.57; 95% CI, 1.40-1.76), middle childhood (RR, 2.23; 95% CI, 2.18-2.27), and adolescence (RR, 1.30; 95% CI, 1.11-1.53) [66]. Short sleep duration may be linked to the development of insulin resistance, increased sedentary behavior and unhealthy dietary patterns from the underlying explanatory mechanisms [67]. A systematic review of 67 studies found that screen time is adversely associated with sleep outcomes (primarily shortened duration and delayed timing) in 90% of studies [68]. Short sleep duration increases childhood obesity risk, and public health efforts that encourage children to have sufficient sleep duration may be important in combating against overweight and obesity risk. Sleep promotion should be therefore included in family-based or school-based interventions to prevent childhood overweight and obesity by educating parents or teachers on age-appropriate sleep duration.

The American Academy of Sleep Medicine developed a set of consensus recommendations for amounts of sleep for children of different ages based on evidence review and expert discussion [69]. The recommendations state that to promote optimal health, children should regularly sleep the following amounts per 24 hours: infants aged 4 to 12 months: 12 to 16 hours, children aged 1 to 2 years: 11 to 14 hours, children aged 3 to

5 years: 10 to 13 hours, children aged 6 to 12 years: 9 to 12 hours, teenagers aged 13 to 18 years: 8 to 10 hours.

Obesity-Related Genes/Parental Obesity

Obesity has genetic basis, and inter-generational obesity link exists. A GWAS-identified single-nucleotide polymorphisms (SNPs) study of 69775 participants demonstrated the association between several SNPs and BMI and obesity in an ethnically diverse population [70]. Further, coding-altering variants associated with BMI implicate pathways that control energy intake and expenditure [71]. In a Mendelian randomization study, genetically elevated maternal BMI and blood glucose levels were potentially causally associated with higher offspring birth weight, which may have implications for counseling and managing pregnancy to avoid maternal complications and high birth weight of the offspring [72]. A meta-analysis of 27 studies showed a strong parent-child obesity association (OR, 2.22; 95% CI, 2.09-2.36), suggesting that families and parents should be a key target for obesity intervention efforts [73]. A national epidemiological study in China also showed that parental obesity and maternal/paternal obesity affected the weight status of the offsprings [52]. There are modest genetic/epigenetic influences on environmental factors behind adverse adiposity [74]. Individuals with family history of obesity should be targeted from an early age to prevent childhood obesity.

Family Environment

Family Income

Family level risk factors such as higher socioeconomic status may increase overweight/obesity risk among children and adolescents [75]. Childhood obesity appears to be predominantly a problem of the rich in low- and middle-income countries [76]. A meta-analysis showed a positive association between high family incomes and overweight/obesity risk among children and adolescents (OR, 3.16; 95% CI, 1.87-5.34) [50]. In contrast, a cross-sectional study in California from 2010 through 2012 reported children with lower family incomes tend to have higher risk of obesity than children with higher family incomes [77]. A systematic review showed that over half the studies indicated increasing obesity prevalence among low socioeconomic position children and adolescents compared to a third of studies showing a positive association among high socioeconomic position children and adolescents in economically advanced countries [78]. Children in high income families in developing countries and low income families in developed countries with greater access to energy-dense diets are both at increased risk of being obese than their counterparts [79].

Unconventional Nuclear Family

A systematic review showed that children from single-parent households were at a higher risk of obesity [80]. A cohort study reported that parental separation before child birth was associated with higher BMI and increased risk of overweight and obesity in children [81]. Children living in single-mother households may have an increased risk of overweight/obesity (OR, 3.67; 95% CI, 1.27-10.62) as a result of single-mothers with high level of psychological stress [82]. Future interventions should increase resources for single-parents to lower obesity risk in children.

Grandparents are increasingly providing care to grandchildren and therefore have an important role in children's eating and activity behaviors. Evidence from China showed that grandparents' co-residence affected grandchildren's weight outcome through changes in dietary patterns and physical activity [83]. A national epidemiological study in China showed that those children mainly raised by their grandparents might be more susceptible to the occurrence and development of obesity than those brought up by parents [52]. A national cohort study in Japan also showed that children living with grandparents may increase the likelihood of overweight and obesity [84]. The findings can help provide clinicians and public health professionals with a better understanding of the role of grandparents in prevention of obesity-related behaviors in children.

Parental Education

Parents with low educational level may result in unhealthy diets of their children. Children from less educated families had a three times higher risk of obesity at 8 year of age, independent of parental income [85]. A prospective cohort in 11 European countries demonstrated that low maternal education yielded a substantial risk of early childhood overweight (OR, 1.58; 95% CI, 1.34-1.85) [86]. Both family income and parental educational attainment were negatively associated with the prevalence of overweight and obesity, the population groups with low income and/or lower education level had the highest prevalence of obesity in children under 10 years [87]. The UK Millennium Cohort Study reported that children of mothers with no academic qualifications were more likely to be overweight (RR, 1.72; 95% CI, 1.48-2.01) compared with children of mothers with degrees and higher degrees at 11 years of age [88].

Parental Perception

Maternal perception of the child's health status seems to influence both overestimation and underestimation of the child's actual weight status [89]. If parents and families fail to recognize that their children with overweight are overweight, then it is unlikely that they will recognize that interventions targeting obesity are relevant to their families [90]. Therefore, parents and other members from families need to be educated on how to identify if their children are overweight or obese.

Many Chinese adults have traditionally viewed plumpness as a sign of prosperity and healthy development, and thinness as a sign of poverty or ill-health [91]. A national epidemiological study in China reported that 18.7% of parents believed that obesity was a good thing for boys in the obese group and the proportion was 14.7% in the normal weight group [52]. Such attitudes are found in many societies that have recently experienced food insecurity, where a degree of adiposity reflects the ability to survive episodes of ill-health from infectious disease. Therefore, efforts to prevent overweight and obesity in childhood should address parents' and grandparents' attitudes and practices in those developing countries.

CHARACTERISTICS OF FAMILY-RELATED RISK FACTORS OF CHILDHOOD OBESITY

First, mother plays a key role of the build-up of adipose tissue of the offspring, and the early growth and development and the formation of good behavior habits of their children. A synthesis of existing empirical evidence posits obesity is the consequence of the competitive dominance of adipocytes over other cell types in the acquisition and sequestering of nutrient energy, and childhood obesity epidemic is the result of nongenetic evolutionary processes altering the interplay between maternal energy resources (eg, body mass and adiposity), maternal patterns of physical activity, and the ensuing metabolic sequelae of pregnancy that affect subsequent fetal outcomes [92]. Intrauterine exposures can raise or lower disease risk, but so too can a plethora of other intertwined genetic, lifestyle, socio-economic and environmental factors which are poorly understood [93]. Hence, society should help mothers to improve their health without constraining women's freedom, instead of blaming the mothers.

Second, family sharing environment is the theoretical basis for developing family-based prevention and control strategies of childhood obesity. Childhood is a critical period for a person to develop behaviors, habits and lifestyles which mostly originate from their parents and other members from families. Except for similar genetic background, sharing dietary patterns, behaviors, lifestyles and perception for parents and their children in the same family may produce a similar effect on health conditions [94-96]. Efforts are warranted to correct parents' and families' wrong attitudes and perceptions on childhood obesity and to modify unhealthy behaviors and lifestyles of parents and other members from families.

Third, the majority of risk factors of childhood obesity are modifiable at parental, child and environmental levels. Although the cause of obesity is complex and multi-factorial, most identified non-genetic risk factors are modifiable, such as pre-pregnancy obesity, gestational weight gain, gestational diabetes, sugar sweetened beverage, fast food, low frequency of physical activity, excessive screen time, short sleep duration, which suggests intervening childhood obesity should firstly modify these unhealthy environmental risk factors to a relative healthy level based on current cumulative evidence.

Fourth, developing family-based prevention and control strategies of childhood obesity is feasible, but should be differentiated according to the social and cultural background of different countries. An umbrella review reported that family-based interventions targeting parents, alone or with their children, are effective for children weight management [97]. Nevertheless, the designs of family-based interventions also reveal numerous inconsistencies and a significant void between research results and health care practice [98]. In addition, because obesity is a chronic condition in need of ongoing management, long-term interventions, the differentiated family-based strategies should be implemented sustainably in practice.

Fifth, family-based prevention and control strategies of childhood obesity should focus on more currently identified family-related risk factors of childhood obesity which are not just limited to diet and physical activity. A quantitative analysis on family-based childhood obesity interventions suggested that obesity risk behaviors beyond diet and physical activity inhibit the development and effectiveness of comprehensive, tailored interventions [99]. Some identified risk factor, such as pregnancy complications, pre-pregnancy obesity, gestational weight gain, breastfeeding, eating speed, sleep duration, screen time, ways of raising children, family structure, and parental perception, should be taken into account along with diet and physical activity.

Implication for Family-Based Prevention and Control Strategies of Childhood Obesity

Current cumulative evidence confirms that more attention should be paid to the key roles of mothers in the early growth and development and families in the formation of good behavior habits of their children. Family-related risk factors of obesity, as an integrated framework strongly supported the development of family-based prevention and control strategies of childhood obesity and the implementation of the family-based strategies in practice. The family-based strategies enable provision of flexible and personalized interventions for correcting unhealthy family sharing environment and personal behaviors and lifestyles of the children.

Preschool period is the critical period of energy balance adjustment in human growth and development, and also a key link between infancy and school-age period. From the perspective of life course, more efforts to intervene childhood obesity at younger ages can help to limit more adverse outcomes. Data from literatures suggest that educational interventions toward healthy eating habits and physical activity at school could be a key strategy in the prevention of obesity, because it has been shown that is difficult to treat obesity in adults through changes in the lifestyle rather than during childhood [100-101]. School-based obesity prevention and control strategies have been proved to be effective in reducing the risk of overweight and obesity for school children [102-103]. Schools are an important setting for health promotion for school children, and family environment is an important setting for preschool children. A cluster-randomised controlled trial in China concluded that school- and family-based obesity prevention programme was effective and highly cost effective in reducing BMI z-scores in primary-school children [104]. Developing the family-based strategies is therefore necessary, feasible and operable for preschool children and school children. Integration of clinical and public health systems and integration of family-based and school-based population strategies should be strengthened to more efficiently prevent and control overweight and obesity from infancy through childhood and adolescence.

Successful public health strategies tackling childhood obesity will need to take a holistic approach and target behavior change in multiple aspects of children's lifestyles and their surroundings, including nutritional education, diet, sleep, screen time, parental support and physical activity. Some interventions had the intended effect on the targeted changes in obesity (48%) and obesity-associated behaviors, such as physical activity (73%), diet (87%) and screen time (63%) [105]. To promote the compliance of children, parents and families and the feasibility of practical suggesting intervention measures, differentiating family-based strategies should be developed according to their social, cultural, and environmental characteristics in the countries or regions.

Future suggesting measures for family-based prevention and control strategies of childhood obesity should include but not limited to pregnancy complications, pre-pregnancy obesity, gestational weight gain, caesarean section, breastfeeding, eating speed, sugar-sweetened beverage, fast food, physical activity, sleep duration, screen time, ways of raising children, family structure, and parental perception. Future researches should focus on the development, continuous improvement and implementation effect evaluation of the family-based or school-based strategies.

REFERENCES

[1] Ng M, Fleming T, Robinson M, et al. Global, regional, and national prevalence of overweight and obesity in children and adults during 1980-2013: a systematic analysis for the Global Burden of Disease Study 2013. *Lancet*, 2014, 384: 766-781.

[2] NCD Risk Factor Collaboration (NCD-RisC). Worldwide trends in body-mass index, underweight, overweight, and obesity from 1975 to 2016: a pooled analysis of 2416 population-based measurement studies in 128.9 million children, adolescents, and adults. *Lancet*, 2017, 390: 2627-2642.

[3] Thompson DR, Obarzanek E, Franko DL, et al. Childhood overweight and cardiovascular disease risk factors: the National Heart, Lung, and Blood Institute Growth and Health Study. *J Pediatr*, 2007, 150(1): 18-25.

[4] Kyrgiou M, Kalliala I, Markozannes G, et al. Adiposity and cancer at major anatomical sites: umbrella review of the literature. *BMJ*, 2017, 356: j477.

[5] Office USGA. *Childhood Obesity: Most Experts Identified Physical Activity and the Use of Best Practices as Key to Successful Programs* [Internet]. 2005. https://digital.library.unt.edu/ark:/67531/metadc299223/. [2020-2-14].

[6] Yano Epstein LH, Paluch RA, Roemmich JN, et al. Family-based obesity treatment, then and now: twenty-five years of pediatric obesity treatment. *Health Psychology*, 2007, 26: 381-391.

[7] Yano KB, Ebesutani J, Lu C, et al. Practical Guidelines for Childhood Obesity Interventions. *Handbook of Obesity Intervention for the Lifespan*. Springer New York, 2009.

[8] Wibaek R, Vistisen D, Girma T, et al. Body mass index trajectories in early childhood in relation to cardiometabolic risk profile and body composition at 5 years of age. *Am J Clin Nutr*, 2019, 110:1175-1185.

[9] Gortmaker SL, Swinburn BA, Levy D, et al. Changing the future of obesity: science, policy, and action. *Lancet*, 2011, 378: 838-847.

[10] Reilly JJ, Armstrong J, Dorosty AR, et al. Early life risk factors for obesity in childhood: cohort study. *BMJ*, 2005, 330: 1357.

[11] Cnattingius S, Villamor E, Lagerros YT, et al. High birth weight and obesity--a vicious circle across generations. *Int J Obes* (Lond), 2012, 36):1320-1324.

[12] Rugholm S, Baker JL, Olsen LW, et al. Stability of the association between birth weight and childhood overweight during the development of the obesity epidemic. *Obes Res*, 2005, 13: 2187-2194.

[13] Schellong K, Schulz S, Harder T, et al. Birth weight and long-term overweight risk: systematic review and a meta-analysis including 643,902 persons from 66 studies and 26 countries globally. *PLoS One*, 2012, 7: e47776.

[14] Qiao Y, Ma J, Wang Y, et al. Birth weight and childhood obesity: a 12-country study. *Int J Obes Suppl*, 2015, 5(Suppl 2): S74-79.

[15] Knop MR, Geng TT, Gorny AW, et al. Birth Weight and Risk of Type 2 Diabetes Mellitus, Cardiovascular Disease, and Hypertension in Adults: A Meta-Analysis of 7 646 267 Participants From 135 Studies. *J Am Heart Assoc*, 2018, 7: e008870.

[16] Ye R, Pei L, Ren A, et al. Birth weight, maternal body mass index, and early childhood growth: a prospective birth cohort study in China. *J Epidemiol*, 2010, 20: 421-428.

[17] Mi D, Fang H, Zhao Y, et al. Birth weight and type 2 diabetes: A meta-analysis. *Exp Ther Med*, 2017, 14: 5313-5320.

[18] Zhao H, Song A, Zhang Y, et al. The association between birth weight and the risk of type 2 diabetes mellitus: a systematic review and meta-analysis. *Endocr J*, 2018, 65: 923-933.

[19] Hillier TA, Pedula KL, Vesco KK, et al. Excess gestational weight gain: modifying fetal macrosomia risk associated with maternal glucose. *Obstet Gynecol*, 2008, 112: 1007-1014.

[20] Monasta L, Batty GD, Cattaneo A, et al. Early-life determinants of overweight and obesity: a review of systematic reviews. *Obes Rev*, 2010, 11: 695-708.

[21] Goldstein RF, Abell SK, Ranasinha S, et al. Association of Gestational Weight Gain With Maternal and Infant Outcomes: A Systematic Review and Meta-analysis. *JAMA*, 2017, 317: 2207-2225.

[22] Aune D, Saugstad OD, Henriksen T, et al. Maternal body mass index and the risk of fetal death, stillbirth, and infant death: a systematic review and meta-analysis. *JAMA*, 2014, 311: 1536-1546.

[23] Yu Z, Han S, Zhu J, et al. Pre-pregnancy body mass index in relation to infant birth weight and offspring overweight/obesity: a systematic review and meta-analysis. *PLoS One*, 2013, 8: e61627.

[24] LifeCycle Project-Maternal Obesity and Childhood Outcomes Study Group, Voerman E, Santos S, et al. Association of Gestational Weight Gain With Adverse Maternal and Infant Outcomes. *JAMA*, 2019, 321: 1702-1715.

[25] Patro Golab B, Santos S, Voerman E, et al. Influence of maternal obesity on the association between common pregnancy complications and risk of childhood obesity: an individual participant data meta-analysis. *Lancet Child Adolesc Health*, 2018, 2: 812-821.

[26] Santos S, Voerman E, Amiano P, et al. Impact of maternal body mass index and gestational weight gain on pregnancy complications: an individual participant data meta-analysis of European, North American and Australian cohorts. *BJOG*, 2019, 126: 984-995.

[27] Logan KM, Gale C, Hyde MJ, et al. Diabetes in pregnancy and infant adiposity: systematic review and meta-analysis. *Arch Dis Child Fetal Neonatal Ed*, 2017, 102: F65-F72.

[28] Kawasaki M, Arata N, Miyazaki C, et al. Obesity and abnormal glucose olerance in offspring of diabetic mothers: A systematic review and meta-analysis. *PLoS One*, 2018, 13: e0190676.

[29] Skrypnik D, Bogdański P, Zawiejska A, et al. Role of gestational weight gain, gestational diabetes, breastfeeding, and hypertension in mother-to-child obesity transmission. *Pol Arch Intern Med*, 2019, 129: 267-275.

[30] Zheng JS, Liu H, Ong KK, et al. Maternal Blood Pressure Rise during Pregnancy and Offspring Obesity Risk at 4 to 7 Years Old: The Jiaxing Birth Cohort. *J Clin Endocrinol Metab*, 2017, 102: 4315-4322.

[31] Gu Y, Lu J, Li W, et al. Joint Associations of Maternal Gestational Diabetes and Hypertensive Disorders of Pregnancy with Overweight in Offspring. *Front Endocrinol* (Lausanne), 2019, 10: 645.

[32] Darmasseelane K, Hyde MJ, Santhakumaran S, et al. Mode of delivery and offspring body mass index, overweight and obesity in adult life: a systematic review and meta-analysis. *PLoS One*, 2014, 9: e87896.

[33] Kuhle S, Tong OS, Woolcott CG. Association between caesarean section and childhood obesity: a systematic review and meta-analysis. *Obes Rev*, 2015, 16: 295-303.

[34] Yuan C, Gaskins AJ, Blaine AI, et al. Association between Cesarean Birth and Risk of Obesity in Offspring in Childhood, Adolescence, and Early Adulthood. *JAMA Pediatr*, 2016, 170: e162385.

[35] Rutayisire E, Wu X, Huang K, et al. Cesarean section may increase the risk of both overweight and obesity in preschool children. *BMC Pregnancy Childbirth*, 2016, 16: 338.

[36] Chu S, Zhang Y, Jiang Y, et al. Cesarean section and risks of overweight and obesity in school-aged children: a population-based study. *QJM*, 2018, 111: 859-865.

[37] Bergmann KE, Bergmann RL, Von Kries R, et al. Early determinants of childhood overweight and adiposity in a birth cohort study: role of breast-feeding. *Int J Obes Relat Metab Disord*, 2003, 27: 162-172.

[38] Wang L, Collins C, Ratliff M, et al. Breastfeeding Reduces Childhood Obesity Risks. *Child Obes*, 2017, 13: 197-204.

[39] Lee JW, Lee M, Lee J, et al. The Protective Effect of Exclusive Breastfeeding on Overweight/Obesity in Children with High Birth Weight. *J Korean Med Sci*, 2019, 34: e85.

[40] Owen CG, Martin RM, Whincup PH, et al. Effect of infant feeding on the risk of obesity across the life course: a quantitative review of published evidence. *Pediatrics*, 2005, 115: 1367-1377.

[41] Harder T, Bergmann R, Kallischnigg G, Plagemann A. Duration of breastfeeding and risk of overweight: a meta-analysis. *Am J Epidemiol*, 2005,162: 397-403.

[42] Keino S, Plasqui G, Ettyang G, et al. Determinants of stunting and overweight among young children and adolescents in sub-Saharan Africa. *Food Nutr Bull*, 2014, 35: 167-178.

[43] Liberali R, Kupek E, de Assis MAA. Dietary Patterns and Childhood Obesity Risk: A Systematic Review. *Child Obes*, 2019 Nov 19. [Epub ahead of print].

[44] Shang L, O'Loughlin J, Tremblay A, et al. The association between food patterns and adiposity among Canadian children at risk of overweight. *Appl Physiol Nutr* Metab, 2014, 39: 195-201.

[45] Asghari G, Yuzbashian E, Mirmiran P, et al. Fast Food Intake Increases the Incidence of Metabolic Syndrome in Children and Adolescents: Tehran Lipid and Glucose Study. *PLoS One*, 2015, 10: e0139641.

[46] Taveras EM, Sandora TJ, Shih MC, et al. The association of television and video viewing with fast food intake by preschool-age children. *Obesity* (Silver Spring), 2006, 14: 2034-2041.

[47] Borghese MM, Tremblay MS, Leduc G, et al. Independent and combined associations of total sedentary time and television viewing time with food intake patterns of 9- to 11-year-old Canadian children. *Appl Physiol Nutr Metab*, 2014, 39: 937-943.

[48] Keller A, Bucher Della Torre S. Sugar-Sweetened Beverages and Obesity among Children and Adolescents: A Review of Systematic Literature Reviews. *Child Obes*, 2015, 11: 338-346.

[49] Luger M, Lafontan M, Bes-Rastrollo M, et al. Sugar-Sweetened Beverages and Weight Gain in Children and Adults: A Systematic Review from 2013 to 2015 and a Comparison with Previous Studies. *Obes Facts*, 2017, 10: 674-693.

[50] Gebrie A, Alebel A, Zegeye A, et al. Prevalence and associated factors of overweight/ obesity among children and adolescents in Ethiopia: a systematic review and meta-analysis. *BMC Obes*, 2018, 5: 19.

[51] Frantsve-Hawley J, Bader JD, Welsh JA, et al. A systematic review of the association between consumption of sugar-containing beverages and excess weight gain among children under age 12. *J Public Health Dent*, 2017, 77 Suppl 1: S43-S66.

[52] Zong XN, Li H, Zhang YQ. Family-related risk factors of obesity among preschool children: results from a series of national epidemiological surveys in China. *BMC Public Health*, 2015, 15: 927.

[53] Zeng X, Cai L, Ma J, et al. Eating fast is positively associated with general and abdominal obesity among Chinese children: A national survey. *Sci Rep*, 2018, 8: 14362.

[54] Liu S, Zhang J, Ma J, et al. Synergistic interaction between bedtime and eating speed in predicting overweight and obesity in Chinese preschool-aged children. *Aging* (Albany NY), 2019, 11: 2127-2137.

[55] Ochiai H, Shirasawa T, Ohtsu T, et al. Eating behaviors and overweight among adolescents: a population-based survey in Japan. *J Obes*, 2013, 2013: 717942.

[56] Ohkuma T, Hirakawa Y, Nakamura U, et al. Association between eating rate and obesity: a systematic review and meta-analysis. *Int J Obes* (Lond), 2015, 39: 1589-1596.

[57] World Health Organization. *Information sheet: global recommendations on physical activity for health 5-17 years old* [Internet]. 2011. https://www.who.int/dietphysicalactivity/publications/recommendations5_17years/en/. [2020-2-14].

[58] Te Velde SJ, van Nassau F, Uijtdewilligen L, et al. Energy balance-related behaviours associated with overweight and obesity in preschool children: a systematic review of prospective studies. *Obes Rev*, 2012, 13 Suppl 1: 56-74.

[59] Renninger M, Hansen BH, Steene-Johannessen J, et al. Associations between accelerometry measured physical activity and sedentary time and the metabolic syndrome: A meta-analysis of more than 6000 children and adolescents. *Pediatr Obes*, 2020, 15: e12578.

[60] Wang Y, Wu Y, Wilson RF, et al. *Childhood Obesity Prevention Programs: Comparative Effectiveness Review and Meta-Analysis* [Internet]. 2013. https://www.ncbi.nlm.nih.gov/pubmed/23865092. [2020-2-14].

[61] Carson V, Hunter S, Kuzik N, et al. Systematic review of sedentary behaviour and health indicators in school-aged children and youth: an update. *Appl Physiol Nutr Metab*, 2016, 41(6 Suppl 3):S240-265.

[62] Fang K, Mu M, Liu K, et al. Screen time and childhood overweight/obesity: A systematic review and meta-analysis. *Child Care Health Dev*, 2019, 45: 744-753.

[63] Xu H, Wen LM, Rissel C. Associations of parental influences with physical activity and screen time among young children: a systematic review. *J Obes*, 2015, 2015: 546925.

[64] Wu L, Sun S, He Y, et al. The effect of interventions targeting screen time reduction: A systematic review and meta-analysis. *Medicine* (Baltimore), 2016, 95: e4029.

[65] *American Academy of Pediatrics Announces New Recommendations for Children's Media Use* [Internet]. [2016]. https://www.aap.org/en-us/about-the-aap/aap-press-room/pages/american-academy-of-pediatrics-announces-new-recommendations-for-childrens-media-use.aspx. [2020-2-14].

[66] Miller MA, Kruisbrink M, Wallace J, et al. Sleep duration and incidence of obesity in infants, children, and adolescents: a systematic review and meta-analysis of prospective studies. *Sleep*, 2018, 41(4).

[67] Felső R, Lohner S, Hollódy K, et al. Relationship between sleep duration and childhood obesity: Systematic review including the potential underlying mechanisms. *Nutr Metab Cardiovasc Dis*, 2017, 27: 751-761.

[68] Hale L, Guan S. Screen time and sleep among school-aged children and adolescents: a systematic literature review. *Sleep Med Rev*, 2015, 21:50-58.

[69] Paruthi S, Brooks LJ, D'Ambrosio C, et al. Recommended Amount of Sleep for Pediatric Populations: A Consensus Statement of the American Academy of Sleep Medicine. *J Clin Sleep Med*, 2016, 12: 785-786.

[70] Fesinmeyer MD, North KE, Ritchie MD, et al. Genetic risk factors for BMI and obesity in an ethnically diverse population: Results from the population architecture using genomics and epidemiology (PAGE) study. *Obesity*, 2013, 21: 835-846.

[71] Turcot V, Lu Y, Highland HM, et al. Protein-altering variants associated with body mass index implicate pathways that control energy intake and expenditure in obesity. *Nat Genet*, 2018, 50: 26-41.

[72] Tyrrell J, Richmond RC, Palmer TM, et al. Genetic Evidence for Causal Relationships Between Maternal Obesity-Related Traits and Birth Weight. *JAMA*, 2016, 315: 1129-1140.

[73] Wang Y, Min J, Khuri J, et al. A Systematic Examination of the Association between Parental and Child Obesity across Countries. *Adv Nutr*, 2017, 8: 436-448.

[74] Han TS, Hart CL, Haig C, et al. Contributions of maternal and paternal adiposity and smoking to adult offspring adiposity and cardiovascular risk: the Midspan Family Study. *BMJ Open*, 2015, 5: e007682.

[75] Mistry SK, Puthussery S. Risk factors of overweight and obesity in childhood and adolescence in South Asian countries: a systematic review of the evidence. *Public Health*, 2015, 129: 200-209.

[76] Dinsa GD, Goryakin Y, Fumagalli E, et al. Obesity and socioeconomic status in developing countries: a systematic review. *Obes Rev*, 2012, 13: 1067-1079.

[77] Jin Y, Jones-Smith JC. Associations between family income and children's physical fitness and obesity in California, 2010-2012. *Prev Chronic Dis*, 2015, 12: E17.

[78] Chung A, Backholer K, Wong E, et al. Trends in child and adolescent obesity prevalence in economically advanced countries according to socioeconomic position: a systematic review. *Obes Rev*, 2016, 17: 276-295.

[79] Wang Y, Lim H. The global childhood obesity epidemic and the association between socio-economic status and childhood obesity. *Int Rev Psychiatry*, 2012, 24: 176-188.

[80] Duriancik DM1, Goff CR. Children of single-parent households are at a higher risk of obesity: A systematic review. *J Child Health Care*, 2019, 23: 358-369.

[81] Hohwü L, Zhu JL, Graversen L, et al. Prenatal parental separation and body weight, including development of overweight and obesity later in childhood. *PLoS One*, 2015, 10: e0119138.

[82] Belcher BR, Maher JP, Lopez NV, et al. Dual versus Single Parental Households and Differences in Maternal Mental Health and Child's Overweight/Obesity. *Matern Child Health J*, 2019, 23: 547-556.

[83] He Q, Li X, Wang R. Childhood obesity in China: Does grandparents' coresidence matter? *Econ Hum Biol*, 2018, 29: 56-63.

[84] Ikeda N, Fuse K, Nishi N. Changes in the effects of living with no siblings or living with grandparents on overweight and obesity in children: Results from a national cohort study in Japan. *PLoS One*, 2017, 12: e0175726.

[85] Bramsved R, Regber S, Novak D, et al. Parental education and family income affect birthweight, early longitudinal growth and body mass index development differently. *Acta Paediatr*, 2018, 107: 1946-1952.

[86] Ruiz M, Goldblatt P, Morrison J, et al. Impact of Low Maternal Education on Early Childhood Overweight and Obesity in Europe. *Paediatr Perinat Epidemiol*, 2016, 30: 274-284.

[87] Ahrens W, Pigeot I, Pohlabeln H, et al. Prevalence of overweight and obesity in European children below the age of 10. *Int J Obes* (Lond), 2014, 38 Suppl 2: S99-107.

[88] Massion S, Wickham S, Pearce A, et al. Exploring the impact of early life factors on inequalities in risk of overweight in UK children: findings from the UK Millennium Cohort Study. *Arch Dis Child*, 2016, 101:724-730.

[89] Carrillo-Larco RM, Bernabe-Ortiz A, Miranda JJ, et al. Children's weight changes according to maternal perception of the child's weight and health: A prospective cohort of Peruvian children. *PLoS One*, 2017, 12: e0175685.

[90] Chaparro MP, Langellier BA, Kim LP, et al. Predictors of accurate maternal perception of their preschool child's weight status among Hispanic WIC participants. *Obesity* (Silver Spring), 2011, 19: 2026-2030.

[91] Watson JL. Food as a lens: the past, present and future of family life in China. In Jing J, editor. *Feeding China's little emperors: food, children and social change*. Stanford, CA: Stanford University Press, 2000.

[92] Archer E. The childhood obesity epidemic as a result of nongenetic evolution: the maternal resources hypothesis. *Mayo Clin Proc*, 2015, 90: 77-92.

[93] Richardson SS, Daniels CR, Gillman MW, et al. Society: Don't blame the mothers. *Nature*, 2014, 512: 131-132.

[94] Xi B, Mi J, Duan J, et al. Familial clustering of obesity and the role of lifestyle factors among children in Beijing. *Chin J Prev Med*, 2009, 43: 122-127.

[95] Capital Institute of Pediatrics; Coordinating Study Group of Nine Cities on the Physical Growth and Development of Children. A national epidemiological survey on obesity of children under seven years of age in nine cities of China in 2016. *Zhonghua Er Ke Za Zhi*, 2018, 56: 745-752.

[96] Hebestreit A, Intemann T, Siani A, et al. Dietary Patterns of European Children and Their Parents in Association with Family Food Environment: Results from the I.Family Study. *Nutrients*, 2017, 9. pii: E126.

[97] Chai LK, Collins C, May C, et al. Effectiveness of family-based weight management interventions for children with overweight and obesity: an umbrella review. *JBI Database System Rev Implement Rep*, 2019, 17: 1341-1427.

[98] Alulis S, Grabowski D. Theoretical frameworks informing family-based child and adolescent obesity interventions: A qualitative meta-synthesis. *Obes Res Clin Pract*, 2017, 11: 627-639.

[99] Ash T, Agaronov A, Young T, et al. Family-based childhood obesity prevention interventions: a systematic review and quantitative content analysis. *Int J Behav Nutr Phys Act*, 2017, 14: 113.

[100] Verrotti A, Penta L, Zenzeri L, et al. Childhood obesity: prevention and strategies of intervention. A systematic review of school-based interventions in primary schools. *J Endocrinol Invest*, 2014, 37: 1155-1164.

[101] Dudley DA, Cotton WG, Peralta LR. Teaching approaches and strategies that promote healthy eating in primary school children: a systematic review and meta-analysis. *Int J Behav Nutr Phys Act*, 2015, 12: 28.

[102] Dobbins M, Husson H, DeCorby K, LaRocca RL: School-based physical activity programs for promoting physical activity and fitness in children and adolescents aged 6 to 18. *Cochrane Database Syst Rev* 2013, 2: CD007651.

[103] Katz DL, O'Connell M, Njike VY, Yeh MC, Nawaz H: Strategies for the prevention and control of obesity in the school setting: systematic review and meta-analysis. *Int J Obes* (Lond), 2008, 32: 1780-1789.

[104] Li B, Pallan M, Liu WJ, et al. The CHIRPY DRAGON intervention in preventing obesity in Chinese primary-school--aged children: A cluster-randomised controlled trial. *PLoS Med*, 2019, 16: e1002971.

[105] Sisson SB, Krampe M, Anundson K, et al. Obesity prevention and obesogenic behavior interventions in child care: A systematic review. *Prev Med*, 2016, 87: 57-69.

In: Childhood Obesity
Editor: Roya Kelishadi

ISBN: 978-1-53618-158-6
© 2020 Nova Science Publishers, Inc.

Chapter 6

Simple Interactive Tools Supporting the Diagnosis of Obesity, Hypertension and Low Physical Fitness in Children and Adolescents

***Tadeusz Nawarycz*[1], *Krzysztof Pytel*[2] and *Lidia Ostrowska-Nawarycz*[1]**

[1]Department of Biophysics, Chair of Experimental and Clinical Physiology, Medical University of Lodz, Poland

[2]Faculty of Physics and Applied Informatics, University of Lodz, Poland

Abstract

Introduction: Obesity, elevated blood pressure and low physical activity among children and adolescents are well-documented risk factors for CVD and the development of vascular disease in adulthood. In addition, their early identification is complex, and often results in misdiagnosis. However, modern Internet technologies are promising.

Aim: The study presents the concept of a multi-criterial online calculator supporting the interpretation and classification of (i) general and central obesity, (ii) blood pressure (BP) measurements and (iii) physical fitness (PF) in pediatric subjects.

Project elements: The calculator consists of three similar blocks:

- A block for the interpretation and classification of anthropometric measurements, such as height and body mass, BMI, WC and AC (arm circuit). It allows independent classification of BMI and WC according to both national (PL) and international (IOTF, INT) criteria.

– A block for the interpretation and classification of BP measurements. BP measurements can be interpreted according to national (PL), European (2016-ESH), American (2017-AAP) and International (2017-INT) criteria.
– A block for the interpretation and classification of PF measurements based on: (i) national references (according to EUROFIT-PL battery tests) and (ii) the international Alpha-fit test.

Each block contains a detailed description of the methodology of performing individual measurements, as well as a simple interpretation/graphical classification of the results using the traffic light principle.

Summary: The developed calculator has several advantages: (i) it is a friendly solution supporting the identification of children/adolescents with both general obesity and AO, as well as with elevated BP; (ii) it contains a wide range of local and international criteria for BMI and WC as well as BP and PF measurements, (iii) it interprets the obtained data according to recommended original normative tables.

Keywords: obesity, children and adolescents, blood pressure, physical fitness, interactive tools

INTRODUCTION

Cardiovascular diseases (CVD) are the leading cause of morbidity and mortality in many countries of the world and their development started already in the early periods of ontogenesis [1, 2]. Despite the identification of many new biomarkers of atherosclerosis in recent years, great importance is also attributed to traditional, modifiable risk factors, which are dominated by: obesity, hypertension (HT) and low physical fitness (PF) [3-5]. Many recently developed new guidelines, both country- and international- specific, related to obesity, hypertension and low PF in children and adolescents, can improve the effectiveness of early CVD prevention [6-9]. Correct early identification and monitoring of these classic risk factors in children and adolescents have become a major public health challenge in many countries around the world in recent decades.

Overweight and obesity in adults and children are a global public health problem [10]. The prevalence of obesity in children and adolescents varies considerably worldwide, likely reflecting socio-economic, ethnic and lifestyle differences [11].

Although body mass index (BMI) is commonly used to evaluate weight status and obesity, other indices such as abdominal obesity (AO) may better predict risk of chronic diseases [12]. Compared with BMI as a measure of general fatness, AO is more strongly correlated to an increased risk of cardiometabolic complications, insulin resistance and metabolic syndrome [13, 14]. Both, in clinical practice and epidemiological studies, anthropometric measures such as waist circumference (WC) and waist-to-height ratio (WHtR) are actually the two most frequently used measures of AO in pediatric populations [15, 16]. National/local WC and BMI reference curves have been developed in Poland and in many other counties [17-22]. In international, comparative epidemiological studies of both overweight and general obesity, the use of BMI distributions developed by IOTF is most often recommended [23].

In the case of AO, recently developed international WC standard for children and adolescents aged 6-18 years with normal weight (data from eight countries in different world regions) deserves attention [24].

In Poland, as in many other European countries, the prevalence of overall and central obesity is increasing, both in rural and urban areas. Over the last 20-30 years, 3-fold increase in the number of children with abnormal body weight and elevated blood pressure is estimated. Depending on the studied region of Poland, obesity (BMI > 95th centile) is diagnosed in 3.5-5% of children and adolescents, but it is mainly simple obesity caused by excessive calorie supply in relation to the body's energy expenditure [25].

Elevated blood pressure (BP) in early childhood, together with frequently coexisting excessive body weight, are considered the main factors initiating the development of atherosclerosis and increased risk of target organ damage [26, 27]. Furthermore, elevated BP in childhood tracks into adulthood, which increases long-term risk of subclinical atherosclerosis and premature death at adulthood [28].

The evaluation of arterial BP in children and adolescents constitutes an important element not only of the pediatric examination of sick children, but also of preventive medical tests. Elevated BP in children and adolescents is usually defined based on the distribution of BP in the reference population. In general, it is considered that children and adolescents have elevated BP if their BP values are in the upper range of the distribution (eg, hypertension if BP is >95th percentile) [26, 29]. However, hypertension screening is generally performed less regularly in clinical practice, and hypertension is frequently underdiagnosed in children whose BP is measured.

In 2004, the Fourth Report (IVR) of the US National High Blood Pressure Education Program Working Group on High Blood Pressure in Children and Adolescents recommended that pediatric hypertension be defined as systolic/diastolic BP (SBP/DBP) above the 95th percentile by sex, age, and height measured on 3 different occasions [29]. Country - specific BP reference curves have been developed in many counties around the world [30-32] as well as in Poland [27, 33]. Particularly noteworthy are the recent recommendations developed by experts of the European Society of Hypertension (2016-ESH) [34], the recommendations of the American Pediatric Association (2017-AAP) [35] as well as globally harmonized international BP references for children and adolescents (2017-INT) by using 7 nationally representative data sets [36]. The worldwide trends in the prevalence of pediatric elevated BP in the past decades, though varied due to geografic location, age range and methodology, demonstrate a steady ongoing rise [37]. In Poland the prevalence of HT has doubled over the past decade. The overall prevalence of HT for systolic and/or diastolic BP combined was about 4% in 2000 and 8,9% in 2010 [26, 27, 37].

Physical fitness (PF) is nowadays considered as a powerful marker of health and quality of life in childhood [38]. PF is determined both genetically and environmentally with the key role of the individual level of physical activity (PA). PA is a key factor in the harmonious motor development of a child and obtaining an adequate level of PF.

The protective effect of intentional PA on CVD risk factors has been reported in people of all ages [39, 40]. Low PA of children and adolescents in many countries assumes alarming proportions. In Poland for instance, only about 10-24% of children meet the recommended level of daily physical activity i.e., minimum 60 min of moderate-to-vigorous PA (MVPA) daily.

In the recently promoted concept of Health-Related Fitness (H-RF), the results of individual fitness tests should primarily support changes in health-related behavior patterns, create a healthy lifestyle and not solely concentrate on their numerical figures. The physiological and medical components of H-RF and the system energy efficiency are both of great importance. In practice, the H-RF components are evaluated using various tests which sometimes hinder comparative analysis [41]. Currently, there are more fifteen PF batteries for assessing children and adolescents based on the concept of H-RF worldwide.

The percentile values of PF for Polish school age children and youths (7-19 y), according to EUROFIT test battery, the International Physical Fitness Test (IPFT) and Cooper Test of PF, were developed in 2015 at the University of Physical Education in Warsaw [42]. Recently, PF norms (Alpha - Fit) have also been developed for European children and adolescents aged 5-18 [43].

It should be emphasized that early diagnosis of both obesity and elevated BP and PF in developmental age is complex. Recommended by leading scientific societies, country- or international- specific, normative systems in the form of extended reference tables or centile charts are in practice cumbersome and time-consuming. Interactive medical calculators, which are becoming increasingly popular, can be helpful in solving these problems.

New Information and Communication Technologies (ICTs) and Internet – based tools are an inseparable element of modern medicine. Dynamically developing e-Health and m-Health sectors as well as many other newer technology solutions (e.g., Wearable Technology, Internet of Things: IoT, Videogames for health: G4H, Intelligent Technologies, smartwatches and many others) have a great potential for effective prophylaxis of many Non-Communicable Diseases (NCDs), including the prevention of obesity complications [44].

Different types of calculators (interactive tools), intended for both medical personnel and patients, are an integral part of many portals and websites of leading societies and scientific organizations or medical universities.

Examples of such modern tool solutions are:

- IDEFICS MetS Score Tool: for supporting the pediatricians in the assessment of Methabolic Syndrom in children aged 3-11. The calculator determines the percentile/z-score position of the examined child and enables graphic presentation of the following: Height, BMI, WC, glucose, insulin, HOMA, TG, HDL-C and SBP/DBP according to gender and age [45].
- Ped(z) Pediatric calculator: contains a wide range of interactive tools that may be useful in daily work of a German pediatrician implemented for both PC and App [46].
- MedCalc: a website containing a large number of the latest clinical calculators, including pediatric ones (among others, BP calculator according to 2017-AAP) [47]

Pediatric calculators for children and adolescents are most often a component of larger web tools designed to diagnose the MetS which, unfortunately, do not include the PA or PF assessment.

The paper presents the concept of a pediatric interactive calculator supporting independent identification and monitoring of children with: (i) obesity, including abdominal obesity (AO), (ii) hypertension and (iii) reduced PF. The main purpose of the developed calculator is to support school medical staff (school nurses, physical education teachers, health educators, instructors).

The Concept of a Web-Based Calculator - Project Elements

During designing the calculator, the following assumptions were made:

- it should have a universal structure and low hardware requirements as well as allow easy upgrades,
- it should be based on the latest reference systems of the analyzed parameters, both country- and international- specific,
- it should have a uniform form of interpretation of measurement results and a simple and friendly user interface,
- it should contain easily accessible methodological information on the procedures for individual tests.

The presented calculator solution is another modification of our earlier studies intended mainly for medical school staff (school nurses) and physical education teachers [48]

The block diagram of the calculator and the screenshot of the main window are shown in Figure 1 and Figure 2 respectively.

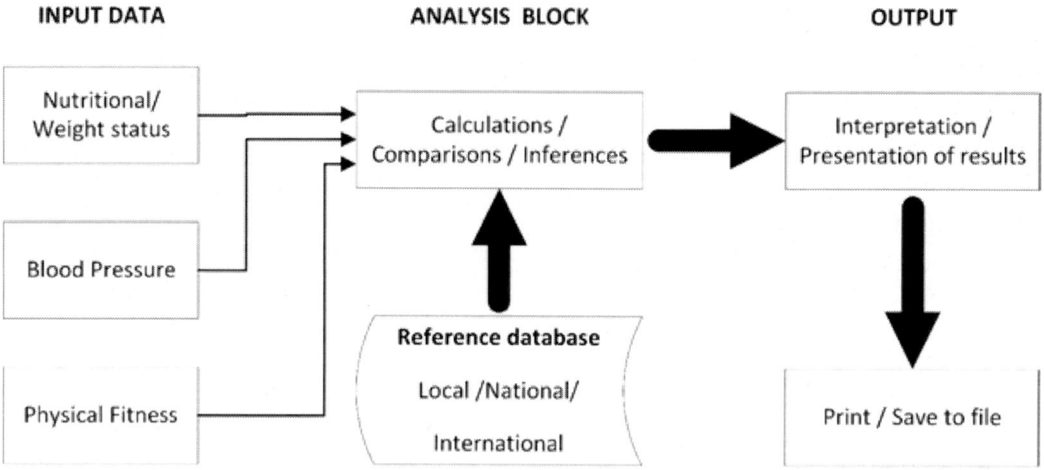

Figure 1. The concept of internet- based calculator supporting diagnosis of obesity, elevated blood pressure and low physical fitness in pediatric subjects.

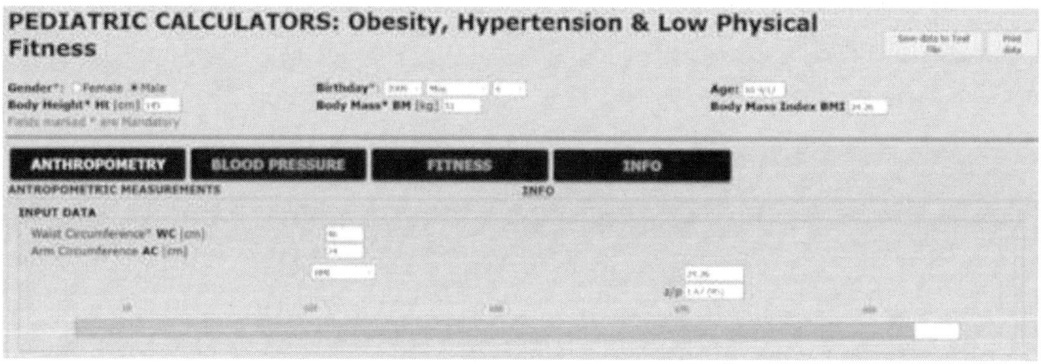

Figure 2. The main window of the developed calculator.

The main window allows to enter the basic input data of the examined child (gender, date of birth, Ht-height, BM-weight, WC-waist circumference and AC-arm circumference, as well as allows you to select sections of the analyzed parameters (buttons: Anthropometry, Blood Pressure and Fitness). In addition, in the main window, you can quickly assess the child's basic development parameters (percentile / z-score of: Ht, BM, WC, BMI) according to current national guidelines.

For all three sections (Anthropometry, Blood Pressure and Fitness), a uniform form of interpretation of the results was adopted in the form of a reference table fragment appropriate for the examined child. The "traffic light" model was used to indicate the level of disturbance of a given parameter. This approach was adopted due to the universal access to reference systems of the analyzed features in a tabular form.

In the current version of the calculator, the "Anthropometry" section enables independent classification of BMI and WC according to both national (PL [18]) and international (IOTF [23], INT [24]) protocols.

Section "Blood Pressure", in turn, allows the analysis of SBP and DBP of the examinated child, according to national (PL [27]), European (2016-ESH [34]), American (2017-AAP) [30] and International (2017-INT [36]) criteria.

The current version of the "Fitness" section allows the assessment of a child's PF according to national reference systems (EUROFIT-PL battery test [42] as well as based on the Alpha-Fit test recently developed for European children [43]. Each block contains a detailed description of the methodology of performing individual measurements, as well as a simple interpretation/graphical classification of results using the traffic light principle.

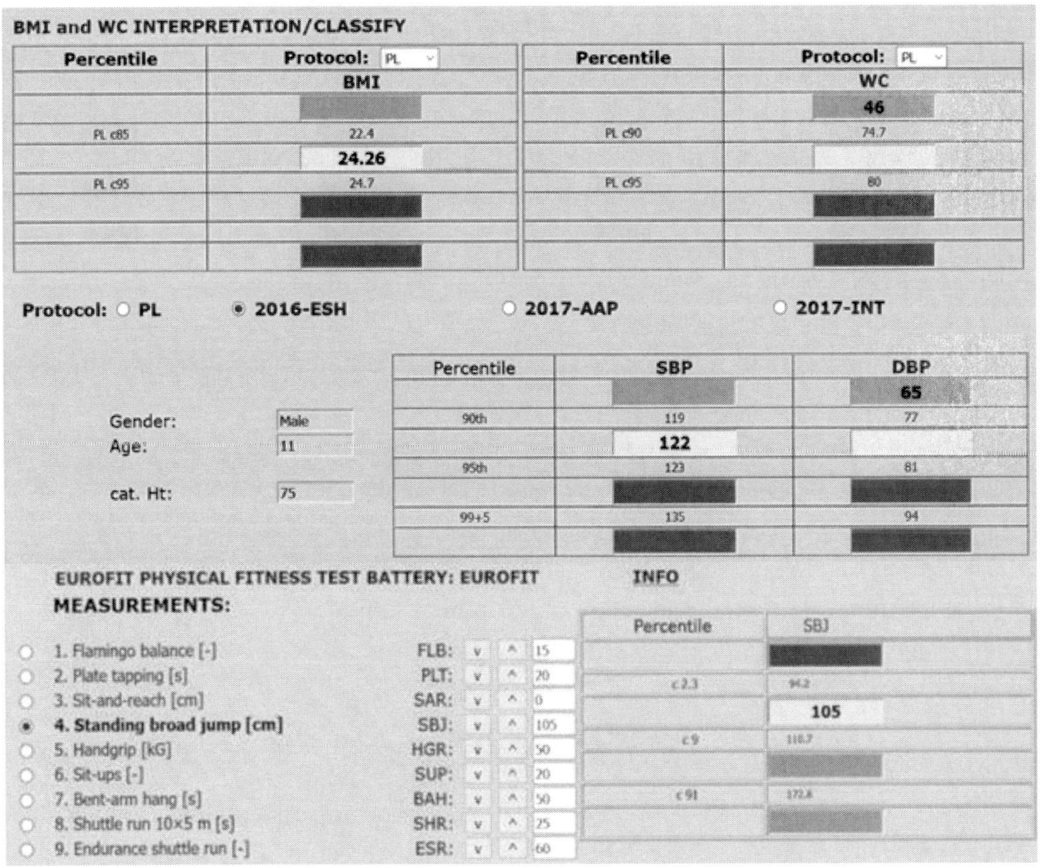

Figure 3. An example assessment of the nutritional status, blood pressure, and physical fitness for an 11 year old boy; A/ BMI and WC assessment using the protocol developed for Polish children (PL), B/ SBP and DBP according to the protocol ESH-2016, C/ Standing broad jump (SBJ) according to EUROFIT battery tests.

Figure 3 presents examples of interpretation of BMI, WC, BP and PF measurement results using a developed calculator.

SUMARY AND PERSPECTIVES

The rapid progress of civilization, including the development of new technologies, has contributed to the change in the lifestyle of modern societies, especially regarding the level of daily physical activity and diet. Technological processes and tools are being developed and implemented more and more often (mainly mhealth Apps) to consolidate correct healthy lifestyle patterns. A report published in 2015 by the IMS Institute for Healthcare Informatics shows that the largest percentage of applications relates to fitness is - 36%, followed by lifestyle and stress reduction - 17%, and nutrition and diet - 12% [49].

Many papers also point to the huge potential of various modern technologies in the prevention of CVD by monitoring and controlling traditional risk factors, which include obesity and improper diet, smoking, hypertension, and low PA. Proper assessment of CVD risk factors in developmental age is an important aspect of early prophylaxis of cardio-metabolic complications in adults.

It seems that the calculator presented in the paper meets all the assumptions presented at the beginning. The most important adventages of the interactive tool presented are the following:

- A simple form of identification of children and adolescents with obesity, hypertension or reduced PF
- Great flexibility in selection of an optimal diagnostic protocol that best suits the purpose of the study.
- Easy upgrades which can be easily extended to a registered version that will allow the history of measurements to be saved in a database.

The current version of the calculator has an experimental character and we treat it as a "voice in the discussion" on the selection of an optimal solution.

REFERENCES

[1] WHO. *Global Health Observatory (GHO): NCD mortality and morbidity*. Available at: www.who.int/gho/ncd/mortality_morbidity/en. Accessed 16 Sept 2014.

[2] Berenson GS, Srinivasan SR, Bao W, Newman 3rd WP, Tracy RE, Wattigney WA. Association between multiple cardiovascular risk factors and atherosclerosis in children and young adults. The Bogalusa heart study. *N. Engl. J. Med.* 1998;338 (23):1650–6.

[3] McGill Jr HC, McMahan CA, Gidding SS. Preventing heart disease in the 21st century: implications of the pathobiological determinants of atherosclerosis in youth (PDAY) study. *Circulation.* 2008;117(9):1216–27.

[4] Chen X, Wang Y. Tracking of blood pressure from childhood to adulthood: a systematic review and meta-regression analysis. *Circulation.* 2008;117(25):3171–80.

[5] Telama R, Yang X, Viikari J, Välimäki I, Wanne O, Raitakari O. Physical activity from childhood to adulthood: a 21-year tracking study. *Am. J. Prev. Med.* 2005; 28(3):267–73.

[6] Freedman DS, Mei Z, Srinivasan SR, Berenson GS, Dietz WH. Cardiovascular risk factors and excess adiposity among overweight children and adolescents: the Bogalusa heart study. *J. Pediatr.* 2007;150(1):12–7. e2.

[7] National Heart, Lung, and Blood Institute (NHLBI). *Integrated guidelines for cardiovascular health and risk reduction in children and adolescents.* 2012.

[8] Falkner B. Monitoring and management of hypertension with obesity in adolescents. *Integr. Blood Press Control.* 2017 Nov 20;10:33-39.

[9] Lobstein T, Baur LA. Policies to prevent childhood obesity in the European Union, *European Journal of Public Health*, Vol. 15, No. 6f, 576–579.

[10] Worldwide trends in body-mass index, underweight, overweight, and obesity from 1975 to 2016: a pooled analysis of 2416 population-based measurement studies in 128·9 million children, adolescents, and adults. *WHO raport.*

[11] Moreno LA, Pigeot I, Ahrens W. *Epidemiology of Obesity in Children and Adolescents Prevalence and Etiology.* Springer-Verlag New York, 2011.

[12] Mahadevan S, Ali I. Is body mass index a good indicator of obesity? *Int. J. Diabetes Dev. Countries.* 2016;36:140–142.

[13] Kelishadi R, Mirmoghtadaee P, Najafi H, et al. Systematic review on the association of abdominal obesity in children and adolescents with cardio-metabolic risk factors. *J. Res. Med. Sci.* 2015;20:294–307.

[14] Marcovecchio ML, Mohn A, Chiarelli F. Obesity and insulin resistance in children. *J. Pediatr. Gastroenterol. Nutr.* 2010;51:S149–S150.

[15] Ochoa SC, Ochoa-Brezmes J. Waist-to-height ratio as a risk marker for metabolic syndrome in childhood. *A metaanalysis. Pediatr. Obes.* 2018.

[16] Ashwell M, Hsieh SD. Six reasons why the waist-to-height ratio is a rapid and effective global indicator for health risks of obesity and how its use could simplify the international public health message on obesity. *Int. J. Food Sci. Nutr.* 2005; 56:303-7.

[17] Ostrowska-Nawarycz L et.al: Percentile distributions of waist circumference for 7–19-year-old Polish children and adolescents. *Obesity Reviews* (2010) 11, 281–288.

[18] Kułaga Z, Litwin M, Tkaczyk M, et al. Polish 2010 growth references for school-aged children and adolescents. *Eur J Pediatr.* 2011; 170:599-609.

[19] Hatipoglu N, Ozturk A, Mazicioglu MM, Kurtoglu S, Seyhan S, Lokoglu F. Waist circumference percentiles for 7- to 17-year-old Turkish children and adolescents. *Eur. J. Pediatr.* 2008; 167: 383– 389.

[20] Schwandt P, Kelishadi R, Haas G-M. First reference curves of waist circumference for German children in comparison to international values: the PEP Family Heart Study. *World J. Pediatr.* 2008; 4: 259–266.

[21] Fredriks AM, van Buuren S, Fekkes M, Verloove-Vanhorick SP, Wit JM. Are age references for waist circumference, hip circumference and waist-hip ratio in Dutch children useful in clinical practice? *Eur. J. Pediatr.* 2005; 164: 216–222.

[22] Inokuchi M, Matsuo N, Anzo M, Takayama JI, Hasegawa T. Age-dependent percentile for waist circumference for Japanese children based on the 1992–1994 cross-sectional national survey data. *Eur. J. Pediatr.* 2007; 166: 655–661.

[23] Cole TJ, Lobstein T. Extended international (IOTF) body mass index cut-offs for thinness, overweight and obesity. *Pediatr. Obes.* 2012; 7: 284 - 94. https://dx.doi.org/10.1111/ijpo.12285.

[24] Xi B, Zong X, Kelishadi R, Litwin M, et al. International Waist Circumference Percentile Cutoffs for Central Obesity in Children and Adolescents Aged 6 to 18 Years. *J. Clin. Endocrinol. & Metab.* 2020; 105: e1569–e1583.

[25] Małecka-Tendera E, Klimek K, Matusik P, Olszanecka-Glinianowicz M, Lehingue Y. Obesity prevalence in Polish 7- to 9-year old children. *Obes Res* 2005; 13: 964–968.

[26] Litwin M, Niemirska A, Śladowska-Kozlowska J, et al. Regression of target organ damage in children and adolescents with primary hypertension. *Pediatr Nephrol.* 2010; 25(12): 2489–2499.

[27] Krzyzaniak A, Krzywińska-Wiewiorowska M, Stawińska-Witoszyńska B, et. al. 2009: Blood pressure references for Polish children and adolescents. *Eur. J. Pediatr.* 168:1335–1342.

[28] Litwin M, Niemirska A. Intima-media thickness measurements in children with cardiovascular risk factors. *Pediatr. Nephrol.* 2009; 24(4): 707–719.

[29] National High Blood Pressure Education Program Working Group of High Blood Pressure in Children Adolescents. 2004. The fourth report on the diagnosis, evaluation and treatment of high blood pressure in children and adolescents. *Pediatrics* 114(2 Suppl 4th Report): 555–576.

[30] Rosner B, Cook N, Portman R et. al. Determination of Blood Pressure Percentiles in Normal-Weight Children: Some Methodological Issues, *American Journal of Epidemiology*. 2008; 167(6): 653–666.

[31] Schwandt P, Scholze JE, Bertsch T. et al. Blood Pressure Percentiles in 22,051 German Children and Adolescents: The PEP Family Heart Study, *American Journal of Hypertension*. 2015; 28(5): 672–679.

[32] Neuhauser, HK Thamm M, Ellert U. et al. Blood Pressure Percentiles by Age and Height From Nonoverweight Children and Adolescents in Germany, *Pediatrics*. 2011; 127(4): e978-e988.

[33] Litwin M, Niemirska A, Łukasz Obrycki Ł. Et al. Guidelines of the Pediatric Section of the Polish Society of Hypertension on diagnosis and treatment of arterial hypertension in children and adolescents. *Arterial Hypertension.* 2018; 22(2):45-73.

[34] Lurbe E, Agabiti-Rosei E, Cruickshank JK, Dominiczak A. et al. 2016 European Society of Hypertension guidelines for the management of high blood pressure in children and adolescents. *J. Hypertens*. 2016; 34(10):1887-920.

[35] Flynn JT, Kaelber DC, Baker-Smith CM. et al. Clinical Practice Guideline for Screening and Management of High Blood Pressure in Children and Adolescents, *Pediatrics*. 2017; 140 (3): e20171904.

[36] Xi B, Zong X, Kelishadi R. et al.Establishing International Blood Pressure References Among Nonoverweight Children and Adolescents Aged 6 to 17 Years. *Circulation.* 2016;133:398-408.

[37] Krzyzaniak A, Krzywińska-Wiewiorowska M, Stawińska-Witoszyńska B, et. al. Percentile distribution of blood pressure readings in relation to body mass index: a populationbased cross-sectional study ADOPOLNOR. *Anthropol. Review.* 2015; 78(1): 91–106.

[38] Ortega FB, Ruiz JR, Castillo MJ, Sjöström M. Physical fitness in childhood and adolescence: a powerful marker of health. Int J Obes (Lond). 2008 Jan;32(1):1-11. Pedersen and Saltin 2006, WHO. *Global recommendations on Physical Activity for Health- 5-17 years old.* Geneva: WHO; 2011.

[39] Strong WB, Malina RM, Blimkie CJ, Daniels SR. et all. Evidence based physical activity for school-age youth. *J. Pediatr.* 2005;146(6):732-7.

[40] Skinner, J.S., Oja, P.: Laboratory and field tests for assessing health- related fitness. In: Bouchard, C., Shephard, R.J., Stephens, T. (eds.) *Physical activity, fitness and health.* Human Kinetics Publishers (1994).

[41] Joschtel, B., Gomersall, S.R., Tweedy, S. et al. Objectively measured physical activity and sedentary behaviour in children with bronchiectasis: a cross-sectional study. *BMC Pulm Med.* 2019; 19: 7. https://doi.org/10.1186/s12890-018-0772-8

[42] Dobosz J. Mayorga-VegaD, Jesús Viciana J. Percentile values of physical fitness levels among Polish children aged 7 to 19 years – a population -based study. *Cent. Eur. J. Public Health* 2015; 23 (4): 340–351.

[43] Kolimechkov S, Petrov L, Albena A. *Alpha-fit test battery norms for children and adolescents from 5 to 18 years of age obtained by a linear interpolation of existing European physical fitness references.* 2019; Eur. J. Physic. Edu. Sport Scie. 5: 1-14.

[44] Baranowski T, Blumberg F, BudayR et al. Games for Health for Children—Current Status and Needed Research, *GAMES FOR HEALTH JOURNAL*: Research, Development, and Clinical Applications Volume 5, Number 1, 2016.

[45] *IDEFICS Metabolic Syndrome Score Tool*: https://mets-score.bips.eu/.

[46] Grafe D. *Ped(z) - Pediaatric Calculator*. https://www.pedz.de/en .

[47] *MedCalc*: https://www.mdcalc.com/ .

[48] Nawarycz T, Pytel K, Ostrowska-Nawarycz L. The concept of a web-based calculator for supporting waist circumference interpretation among pediatric subjects. In: Watson RR (Ed), *Nutrition in the prevention and treatment of abdominal obesity*. 2019; chapter 9: 95-105.

[49] Top mHealth Apps with the Highest Number of Downloads (Android only) Patient Adoption of mHealth. *Report by the IMS Institute for Healthcare Informatics*, 2015.

In: Childhood Obesity
Editor: Roya Kelishadi
ISBN: 978-1-53618-158-6
© 2020 Nova Science Publishers, Inc.

Chapter 7

Sleep Patterns and Sedentary Behaviors: Is the Association with Obesity Already Evident in Childhood?

Cézane Priscila Reuter[1,*], PhD, Silvia Isabel Rech Franke[1], PhD, Aline Rosso Lehnhard[2], Ana Paula Sehn[2], João Francisco de Castro Silveira[2], Jane Dagmar Pollo Renner[3], PhD and Roya Kelishadi[4], MD

[1]Department of Health Sciences and Graduate Program in Health Promotion, University of Santa Cruz do Sul, Santa Cruz do Sul, Rio Grande do Sul, Brazil
[2]Graduate Program in Health Promotion, University of Santa Cruz do Sul, Santa Cruz do Sul, Rio Grande do Sul, Brazil
[3]Department of Life Sciences and Graduate Program in Health Promotion, University of Santa Cruz do Sul, Santa Cruz do Sul, Rio Grande do Sul, Brazil
[4]Child Growth and Development Research Center, Research Institute for Primordial Prevention of Non-Communicable Disease, Isfahan University of Medical Sciences, Isfahan, Iran

Abstract

There is an escalating trend of weight excess amongst children and adolescents in the last decades. It has become a common public health problem worldwide once the increasing rates of obesity are higher in the pediatric age group than in the adulthood.

* Corresponding Author's Email: cezanereuter@unisc.br.

Evidence shows that less time spent in unhealthy habits during childhood is a strongly associated factor with an overweight or obesity condition development, which in turn would affect general health. Childhood obesity is associated with markers of worse cardiovascular and metabolic outcomes, which augments long-term morbidity and mortality later in life. Sleep patterns and sedentary behaviors are important factors to be highlighted because it is documented that they are associated with excess body weight. However, still the association between sleep duration and weight excess is not well established; it may be affected by other habits, which consequently increase weight. Furthermore, current evidence shows that the causal relationship between sedentary behavior and childhood obesity are also unclear. However, the detrimental effect of sedentary behaviors on cardiometabolic and obesity-related outcomes is independent of physical activity levels. Thus, daily life habits in childhood and youth are as important as periods of regular health-related physical activity. Therefore, a better understanding of the impact caused by sleep duration and sedentary habits in the pediatric age group could help to prioritize intervention targets to prevent, manage, and treat obesity. This chapter aims to discuss whether various aspects of the association of sleep patterns and sedentary behavior with obesity is already evident in children and adolescents or not. In general, this chapter indicates that such an evidence is still scarce in the pediatric age group, but life-course interventions for healthy lifestyle should be underscored at individual and public health levels.

Keywords: sleep, sedentary behavior, obesity, prevention, control, children

INTRODUCTION

The prevalence of weight excess has increased worldwide in the last decades, affecting not only the adult population (Abarca-Gómez et al. 2017; Kelishadi et al. 2015). The evidence shows that the rates of obesity increasing in childhood are higher than the adult ones. Also, the current weight excess rates estimate a total of 107.7 million obese children (Afshin et al. 2017). Despite this estimation, evidence shows that more children and adolescents are underweight than obese. However, if the current trends of weight excess growth continue, there will be more obese children and adolescents than underweight by 2022 (Abarca-Gómez et al. 2017). Therefore, the alarming weight excess growth has become a common problem amongst children and adolescents, and a major public health problem worldwide which affects social and health care systems (Faienza et al. 2016; McCrindle 2015).

The consequences of pediatric weight excess development have many adverse health effects and it also affects markers of worse cardiovascular and metabolic outcomes, including hypertension, metabolic syndrome, and type 2 diabetes, which amplifies long-term morbidity and mortality implications in adulthood (Chung, Onuzuruike, and Magge 2018; Faienza et al. 2016; Güngör 2014; Khan et al. 2018), once pediatric weight excess has a moderate chance to track into adulthood (Singh et al. 2008). Therefore, there is a need to start efforts on preventing overweight and obesity as early as possible (Ortega, Lavie, and Blair 2016), because most children and adolescents do not have cardiovascular diseases but are already in the initial stages of metabolic risk factors development (Andersen et al. 2015).

An identification of evolving behavioral risk factors from early childhood is needed to foment changes in these habits that may avoid the development of premature obesity. Sleep patterns and sedentary behaviors are important factors to be highlighted because the literature demonstrates their association with high levels of body weight. Therefore, a better understanding of the impact caused by sleep duration and sedentary habits on childhood and youth health could help prioritize intervention targets to prevent, manage, and treat obesity.

Sleep Patterns and Sedentary Behaviors in Childhood

Children and adolescents should meet the recommendations of sleep duration for their physical and psychological development. However, the childhood and youth population is already presenting changes in their sleep pattern, and this may be related to higher exposure to sedentary behaviors, interpersonal and social relationships (Ciampo 2012), and food consumption (Hoefelmann et al. 2014). Therefore, it is important to highlight that both insufficient or prolonged hours of sleep are harmful to health (Krittanawong et al. 2019; Liu et al. 2017).

Regarding sedentary behavior, first, it is necessary to understand that sedentary behavior and physical inactivity are different constructs, although both are harmful to health. Physical inactivity is a behavioral risk related to performing insufficient amounts of moderate-to-vigorous daily, while sedentary behavior is any waking behavior characterized by low energy expenditure (Tremblay 2012) and movement lack during an ordinary day (Cristi-Montero et al. 2015). The evidence shows that highly sedentary (more than 9.5 hours per day) subjects present higher values of Body Mass Index (BMI), percentage of body fat, and waist circumference, besides lower cardiorespiratory fitness and higher levels of physical inactivity (Leiva et al. 2017).

Sleep Patterns

The prevalence of individuals sleeping less than recommended and presenting changes in their sleep habits has generally increased. Also, the amount of sleep, especially insufficient sleep, seems to be affecting children's and adolescents' overall health (Ogilvie and Patel 2017). Evidence indicates that insufficient sleep may be associated with childhood obesity development (Gong et al. 2018; 2019; Li et al. 2017; Miller et al. 2018; Sluggett, Wagner, and Harris 2019; Sun et al. 2018) and body weight increase throughout time (Anton-Paduraru, Teslariu, and Mocanu 2016; Fatima, Doi, and Mamun 2015). However, there is evidence indicating that prolonged hours of sleep seem to associate with overweight/obesity as well. Therefore, only the ideal amount of sleep would be beneficial to prevent obesity development (Wang et al. 2016; Wu et al. 2015).

The inadequate quality and amount of sleep makes the subject eat more often, especially unhealthy foods, which facilitates the weight body gain (Atar, Pirgon, and Buyukgebiz 2019; Kracht et al. 2019). Furthermore, it is possible to verify that the more problems related to sleep patterns the individual has, the higher the chances of developing obesity. Parallel factors may also influence the relationship between sleep and obesity, such as sedentary behavior itself and the consumption of sugary drinks (Morrissey, Allender, and Strugnell 2019; Sluggett, Wagner, and Harris 2019) and high-calorie foods (Tambalis et al. 2018). Also, the effects of insufficient sleep on obesity may present different responses for sex (Cao et al. 2015; Jiang et al. 2015) and years of age (Cao et al. 2015; Sun et al. 2018).

The human body is adapted to perform tasks that require more movement during the day and calmer and peaceful activities at night while sleeping. The circadian rhythm systems improved to adapt to daily changes of movement. These rhythms are timed according to the light-dark cycle, which considers the 24 hours of the day. The intrinsic oscillatory system is responsible for the organism's synchronization to the physiological and behavioral rhythms every 24 hours (Maury 2019). However, the constant lighting of the environment is compromising this synchronization because it omits light and dark changes. These modifications alter the body's functioning and result in metabolic disorders like obesity. Therefore, the body activities need to meet the circadian rhythm system to reduce negative health consequences (Covassin, Singh, and Somers 2016; Maury 2019).

The role of sleep patterns on obesity development is still not clear (Felső et al. 2017). Further longitudinal and intervention studies are essential to verify a cause and effect relationship between sleep patterns and obesity (Kim et al. 2019). There researches should aim at sleep patterns to reverse and reduce cases of obesity (Ogilvie and Patel 2017; Rosi et al. 2017). Furthermore, children should be encouraged to meet sleep duration recommendations to prevent harmful effects on health. Lastly, parents should know the importance of adequate sleep duration (Kim et al. 2019; Li et al. 2017; Miller et al. 2018).

Sedentary Behaviors

The literature shows that both physical inactivity and sedentary behaviors amongst children and adolescents are harmful to overall health and obesity development (Ferrari et al. 2019; Werneck et al. 2019; Santos et al. 2019; Keane et al. 2017; Leiva et al. 2017; Mann et al. 2017; Norman et al. 2017).

A study with Brazilian adolescents verified that shorter sedentary bouts (less than 4 minutes) were associated with less adiposity. The authors suggested a higher number of breaks on the daily sedentary behaviors to prevent obesity (Werneck et al. 2019). A similar research with Portuguese children verified an inverse association between shorter sedentary bouts and adiposity, while more than five minutes were positively associated with adiposity, regardless of the time spent in moderate-to-vigorous activities (Santos et al. 2019). Additionally, a study examining Irish children showed that only 10.8% of waking time was spent with moderate-to-vigorous activities, while 61.3% on sedentary behaviors. The time of moderate-to-vigorous activities was inversely associated to overweight/obesity development, regardless of total sedentary bouts. Also, screen time was associated with higher risk of overweight/obesity, regardless of physical activity (Keane et al. 2017).

The screen time is one of the most investigated sedentary behaviors (Ferrari et al. 2019) and has been inversely associated with several metabolic indicators (Keane et al. 2017). A study examining the relationship between sedentary time and metabolic health amongst obese American children and adolescents demonstrated an association of higher screen time and obesity, blood pressure and lipid indicators, regardless of time spent on moderate-to-vigorous activities (Norman et al. 2017). Besides, an 8-year longitudinal research verified that the more the time spent in front of screen, the higher the levels of adiposity. The authors also suggested that intervention programs would be more effective if they consider the age-group, in which there is an increase in screen time (Mann et al. 2017). The main focus of interventions could be to limit or replace the amount higher of 3 hours in front of screens for physically active tasks to prevent childhood obesity and comorbidities (Norman et al. 2017).

The alarming reality concerning the metabolic health of children and adolescents is possible to change once both physical inactivity and sedentary behaviors are modifiable factors, especially at this stage of life. Intervention strategies are extremely relevant, urgent, and achievable as 20 minutes per day spent with moderate-to-vigorous activities could impact behavior patterns and anthropometry levels of overweight and obese children (Keane et al. 2017). Additionally, these intervention programs aiming to improve moderate-to-vigorous activities should be a priority once they also improve the cardiorespiratory fitness of children and adolescents (Santos et al. 2019).

In Brazil, a systematic review verified a lack of evidence concerning sedentary behaviors amongst children and adolescents. There is also a need for more longitudinal studies plus standardized and validated measurement instruments and cut off points to identify those at risk (Guerra, Farias Júnior, and Florindo 2016). The authors still found associations between higher sedentary behaviors and higher levels of body composition and lower levels of physical activity.

The associations of causality and effect between sedentary behavior and obesity are still weak and low, mostly because of the different methods in different researches (Biddle, García Bengoechea, and Wiesner 2017). Therefore, further studies to provide a better understanding of the impact caused by sedentary behaviors on children's and adolescents' metabolic health are essential to identify targets of intervention (Norman et al. 2017).

COMBINED EFFECT OF SLEEP DISORDERS AND SEDENTARY BEHAVIORS ON OBESITY RISK: ARE THERE EVIDENCES IN CHILDHOOD?

Few studies have evaluated the combined effect of sleep patterns and sedentary behaviors with the risk of developing obesity, especially in children (Laurson et al. 2014). In adolescents, a study conducted with 9866 adolescents aged 11-17 years evaluated the integrated role of multiple healthy weight behaviors, including MVPA, screen time, sleep, and fruit and vegetable consumption. The results showed that 2% and 33% of adolescents met all and none recommendations, respectively. However, only MVPA demonstrated association with obesity after adjustments for age, sex, social status, parental education, and ethnicity (odds ratio: 1.29; confidence interval: 1.03 to 1.62). Also, in the model with the four behaviors, there was no significant association of any variable with obesity. These results suggest that not complying with the recommendations of physical activity seems to be the main factor associated with the risk of obesity in adolescents (Menon et al. 2019).

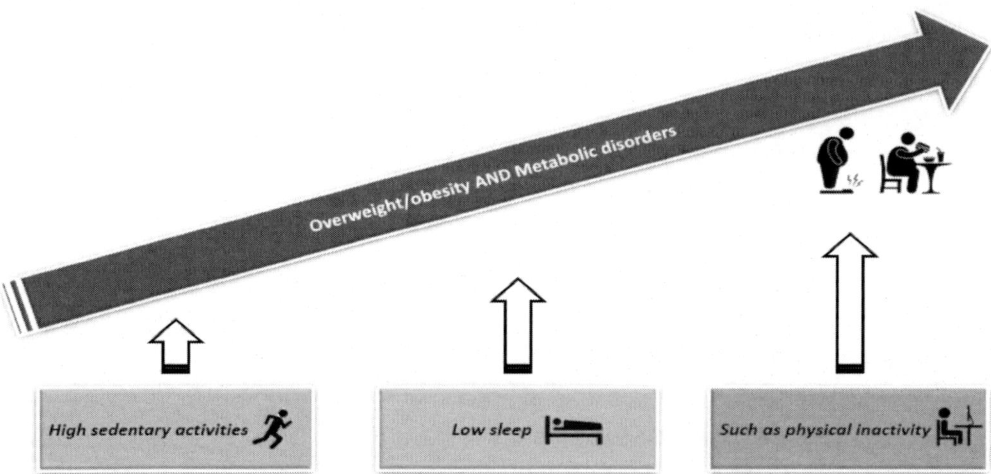

Figure 1. Modifiable behaviors associated with metabolic disorders.

In children from the United States, the concurrent associations between physical activity, screen time, and sleep duration with childhood obesity were tested. The results showed that children who complied with the recommendations of the three behaviors (9.2%) were less likely to be obese. For comparison, 11.3% of boys and girls achieving all recommendations were overweight or obese; among children who did not comply with any recommendation, the value was approximately 50.0%. When analyzing the interaction between behavioral variables with BMI percentile, any significant predictors were found. However, when physical activity, screen time, and sleep patterns were included in the regression model, both physical activity and sleep patterns were the strongest predictors associated with BMI, while screen time was not associated (Laurson et al. 2014).

In a systematic review with 13 cross-sectional studies and a single prospective cohort study, children and youth with a combination of healthy behaviors (high physical activity, high sleep, and low sedentary behavior) showed a more desirable metabolic profile compared to those with all behaviors considered unhealthy (low physical activity, low sleep, and high sedentary behavior) (Saunders et al. 2016).

Although still little explored together in the child population, the behavioral variables are dependent on each other and cannot be explained alone. Thus, current approaches, like compositional data analysis (Chastin et al. 2015), demonstrate that messages that physical activity can offset the adverse effects of other inappropriate behaviors, such as poor eating habits or sleep deprivation, for example, are not the best strategies. All behaviors are important to maintaining and promote metabolic and overall health (Chaput and Dutil 2016), as shown in Figure 1.

CONCLUSION

The association of inappropriate behaviors, including time in front of screens, physical inactivity, and reduced sleep time, in isolation, are already well documented in the literature, including in childhood. However, we must consider that these factors alone are not part of real life. Individuals have a set of behaviors that must be considered. Thus, the combination of inappropriate behaviors, such as physical inactivity, low sleep, and high sedentary activities would increase the risk of developing excess weight and related metabolic disorders. Evidence is still scarce in the pediatric age group, but it already demonstrates the importance of intervention programs from an early age, with a focus on life-course reduction of inappropriate lifestyle behaviors.

REFERENCES

Abarca-Gómez, L., Abdeen, Z. A., Hamid, Z. A., Abu-Rmeileh, N. M., Acosta-Cazares, B., Acuin, C., Adams, R. J. et al. (2017). Worldwide Trends in Body-Mass Index, Underweight, Overweight, and Obesity from 1975 to 2016: A Pooled Analysis of 2416 Population-Based Measurement Studies in 128·9 Million Children, Adolescents, and Adults. *The Lancet* 390 (10113): 2627–42.

Afshin, A., Forouzanfar, M. H., Reitsma, M. H., Sur, P., Estep, K., Lee, A., Marczak, L. et al. (2017). Health Effects of Overweight and Obesity in 195 Countries over 25 Years. *New England Journal of Medicine* 377 (1): 13–27.

Andersen, L. B., Lauersen, J. B., Brønd, J. C., Anderssen, S. A., Sardinha, L. B., Steene-Johannessen, J., McMurray, R. G. et al. (2015). A New Approach to Define and Diagnose Cardiometabolic Disorder in Children. *Journal of Diabetes Research*, 1–10.

Anton-Paduraru, D. T., Teslariu, O., and Mocanu, V. (2016). Influence of Sleep on Obesity in Children. *Revista Medico-Chirurgicala a Societatii de Medici Si Naturalisti Din Iasi* 120 (2): 239–43.

Atar, M., Pirgon, Ö., and Buyukgebiz, A. (2019). Sleep Disorders and Obesity in Childhood: A New Component in Solving Obesity. *Pediatric Endocrinology Reviews* 16 (4): 441–51.

Biddle, S. J. H., Bengoechea, E. G., and Wiesner, G. (2017). Sedentary Behaviour and Adiposity in Youth: A Systematic Review of Reviews and Analysis of Causality. *International Journal of Behavioral Nutrition and Physical Activity* 14 (1).

Cao, M., Zhu, Y., He, B., Yang, W., Chen, Y., Ma, J., and Jing, J. (2015). Association between Sleep Duration and Obesity Is Age-and Gender-Dependent in Chinese Urban Children Aged 6-18 Years: A Cross-Sectional Study. *BMC Public Health* 15 (1).

Chaput, J. P., and Dutil, C. (2016). "Lack of Sleep as a Contributor to Obesity in Adolescents: Impacts on Eating and Activity Behaviors." *International Journal of Behavioral Nutrition and Physical Activity* 13 (1).

Chastin, S. F. M., Palarea-Albaladejo, J., Dontje, M. L., and Skelton, D. A. (2015). Combined Effects of Time Spent in Physical Activity, Sedentary Behaviors and Sleep on Obesity and Cardio-Metabolic Health Markers: A Novel Compositional Data Analysis Approach. *PLOS ONE* 10 (10).

Chung, S. T., Onuzuruike, A. U., and Magge, S. N. (2018). Cardiometabolic Risk in Obese Children. *Annals of the New York Academy of Sciences* 1411 (1): 166–83.

Ciampo, L. A. D. (2012). O Sono Na Adolescência. *Adolescência & Saúde* 9 (2): 60–6. [Sleep in adolescence. *Adolescence & Health* 9 (2): 60–6].

Covassin, N., Singh, P., and Somers, V. K. (2016). Keeping up with the Clock: Circadian Disruption and Obesity Risk. *Hypertension* 68 (5): 1081–90.

Cristi-Montero, C., Celis-Morales, C., Ramírez-Campillo, R., Aguilar-Farías, N., Álvarez, C., and Rodríguez-Rodríguez, F. (2015). ¡Sedentarismo e Inactividad Física No Son Lo Mismo!: Una Actualización de Conceptos Orientada a La Prescripción Del Ejercicio Físico Para La Salud. *Revista Medica de Chile* 143 (8): 1089–90. [Sedentary behaviour and physical inactivity is not the same!: An update of concepts oriented towards the prescription of physical exercise for health. *Journal of Chile Medicine* 143 (8): 1089–90].

Faienza, M. F., Wang, D. Q. H., Frühbeck, G., Garruti, G., and Portincasa, P. (2016). The Dangerous Link between Childhood and Adulthood Predictors of Obesity and Metabolic Syndrome. *Internal and Emergency Medicine* 11 (2): 175–82.

Fatima, Y., Doi, S. A. R., and Mamun, A. A. (2015). Longitudinal Impact of Sleep on Overweight and Obesity in Children and Adolescents: A Systematic Review and Bias-Adjusted Meta-Analysis. *Obesity Reviews* 16 (2): 137–49.

Felső, R., Lohner, S., Hollódy, K., Erhardt, É., and Molnár, D. (2017). Relationship between Sleep Duration and Childhood Obesity: Systematic Review Including the Potential Underlying Mechanisms. *Nutrition, Metabolism and Cardiovascular Diseases* 27 (9): 751–61.

Ferrari, G. L. M., Pires, C., Solé, D., Matsudo, V., Katzmarzyk, P. T., and Fisberg, M. (2019). Factors Associated with Objectively Measured Total Sedentary Time and Screen Time in Children Aged 9–11 Years. *Jornal de Pediatria* 95 (1): 94–105.

Gong, Q. H., Li, S. X., Li, H., Cui, J., and Xu, G. Z. (2018). Insufficient Sleep Duration and Overweight/Obesity among Adolescents in a Chinese Population. *International Journal of Environmental Research and Public Health* 15 (5).

Gong, Q. H., Li, S. X., Wang, S. J., Wu, Y. H., Han, L. Y., and Li, H. (2019). Sleep Duration and Overweight in Chinese Adolescents: A Prospective Longitudinal Study with 2-Year Follow-Up. *Sleep and Breathing*.

Guerra, P. H., Farias Júnior, J. C., and Florindo, A. A. (2016). Comportamento Sedentário Em Crianças e Adolescentes Brasileiros: Revisão Sistemática. *Revista de Saúde Pública* 50 (9): 1–15. [Sedentary Behavior in Brazilian children and adolescents: systematic review. *Journal of Public Health* 50 (9): 1–15].

Güngör, N. K. (2014). Overweight and Obesity in Children and Adolescents. *Journal of Clinical Research in Pediatric Endocrinology* 6 (3): 129–43.

Hoefelmann, L. P., Silva, K. S., Barbosa Filho, V. C., Silva, J. A., and Nahas, M. V. (2014). Behaviors Associated to Sleep among High School Students: Cross-Sectional and Prospective Analysis. *Revista Brasileira de Cineantropometria e Desempenho Humano* 16: 68–78.

Jiang, Y. R., Spruyt, K., Chen, W. J., Mei, H., Sun, W. Q., Wang, Y., Li, S. H., et al. (2015). Associations between Parent-Reported Sleep Duration and Adiposity in Chinese Early Adolescents. *Journal of Public Health (United Kingdom)* 37 (2): 277–85.

Keane, E., Li, X., Harrington, J. M., Fitzgerald, A. P., Perry, I. J., and Kearney, P. M. (2017). Physical Activity, Sedentary Behavior and the Risk of Overweight and Obesity in School-Aged Children. *Pediatric Exercise Science* 29 (3): 408–18.

Kelishadi, R., Mirmoghtadaee, P., Najafi, H., and Keikha, M. (2015). Systematic Review on the Association of Abdominal Obesity in Children and Adolescents with Cardio-Metabolic Risk Factors. *Journal of Research in Medical Sciences* 20 (3): 294–307.

Khan, S. S., Ning, H., Wilkins, J. T., Allen, N., Carnethon, M., Berry, J. D., Sweis, R. N., et al. (2018). Association of Body Mass Index with Lifetime Risk of Cardiovascular Disease and Compression of Morbidity. *JAMA Cardiology* 3 (4): 280–87.

Kim, J., Noh, J. W., Kim, A., and Kwon, Y. D. (2019). Relationships between Sleep Patterns, Health Risk Behaviors, and Health Outcomes among School-Based Population of Adolescents: A Panel Analysis of the Korean Children and Youth Panel Survey. *International Journal of Environmental Research and Public Health* 16 (13).

Kracht, C. L., Chaput, J. P., Martin, C. K., Champagne, C. M., Katzmarzyk, P. T., and Staiano, A. E. (2019). Associations of Sleep with Food Cravings, Diet, and Obesity in Adolescence. *Nutrients* 11 (12).

Krittanawong, C., Tunhasiriwet, A., Wang, Z., Zhang, H., Farrell, A. M., Chirapongsathorn, S., Sun, T., et al. (2019). Association between Short and Long Sleep Durations and Cardiovascular Outcomes: A Systematic Review and Meta-Analysis. *European Heart Journal: Acute Cardiovascular Care* 8 (8): 762–70.

Laurson, K. R., Lee, J. A., Gentile, D. A., Walsh, D. A., and Eisenmann, J. C. (2014). Concurrent Associations between Physical Activity, Screen Time, and Sleep Duration with Childhood Obesity. *ISRN Obesity* 2014: 1–6.

Leiva, A. M., Martínez, M. A., Cristi-Montero, C., Salas, C., Ramírez-Campillo, R., Martínez, X. D., Aguilar-Farías, N., et al. (2017). El Sedentarismo Se Asocia a Un Incremento de Factores de Riesgo Cardiovascular y Metabólicos Independiente de Los Niveles de Actividad Física. *Revista Medica de Chile* 145 (4): 458–67. [Sedentary lifestyle is associated with metabolic and cardiovascular risk factors independent of physical activity. *Journal of Chile Medicine* 145 (4): 458–67].

Li, L., Zhang, S., Huang, Y., and Chen, K. (2017). Sleep Duration and Obesity in Children: A Systematic Review and Meta-Analysis of Prospective Cohort Studies. *Journal of Paediatrics and Child Health* 53 (4): 378–85.

Liu, T. Z., Xu, C., Rota, M., Cai, H., Zhang, C., Shi, M. J., Yuan, R. X. et al. (2017). Sleep Duration and Risk of All-Cause Mortality: A Flexible, Non-Linear, Meta-Regression of 40 Prospective Cohort Studies. *Sleep Medicine Reviews* 32: 28–36.

Mann, K. D., Howe, L. D., Basterfield, L., Parkinson, K. N., Pearce, M. S., Reilly, J. K., Adamson, A. J., et al. (2017). Longitudinal Study of the Associations between Change in Sedentary Behavior and Change in Adiposity during Childhood and Adolescence: Gateshead Millennium Study. *International Journal of Obesity* 41 (7): 1042–47.

Maury, E. (2019). Off the Clock: From Circadian Disruption to Metabolic Disease. *International Journal of Molecular Sciences* 20 (7).

McCrindle, B. W. (2015). Cardiovascular Consequences of Childhood Obesity. *Canadian Journal of Cardiology* 31 (2): 124–30.

Menon, S., Philipneri, A., Ratnasingham, S., and Manson, H. (2019). The Integrated Role of Multiple Healthy Weight Behaviours on Overweight and Obesity among Adolescents: A Cross-Sectional Study. *BMC Public Health* 19 (1).

Miller, M. A., Kruisbrink, M., Wallace, J., Ji, C., and Cappuccio, F. P. (2018). Sleep Duration and Incidence of Obesity in Infants, Children, and Adolescents: A Systematic Review and Meta-Analysis of Prospective Studies. *Sleep* 41 (4).

Morrissey, B., Allender, S., and Strugnell, C. (2019). Dietary and Activity Factors Influence Poor Sleep and the Sleep-Obesity Nexus among Children. *International Journal of Environmental Research and Public Health* 16 (10).

Norman, G. J., Carlson, J. A., Patrick, K., Kolodziejczyk, J. K., Godino, J. G., Huang, J., and Thyfault, J. (2017). Sedentary Behavior and Cardiometabolic Health Associations in Obese 11-13-Year Olds. *Childhood Obesity* 13 (5): 425–32.

Ogilvie, R. P., and Patel, S. R. (2017). The Epidemiology of Sleep and Obesity. *Sleep Health* 3 (5): 383–88.

Ortega, F. B., Lavie, C. J., and Blair, S. N. (2016). Obesity and Cardiovascular Disease. *Circulation Research* 118 (11): 1752–70.

Rosi, A., Calestani, M. V., Parrino, L., Milioli, G., Palla, L., Volta, E., Brighenti, F., et al. (2017). Weight Status Is Related with Gender and Sleep Duration but Not with Dietary Habits and Physical Activity in Primary School Italian Children. *Nutrients* 9 (6): 1–10.

Santos, D. A., Magalhães, J. P., Júdice, P. B., Correia, I. R., Minderico, C. S., Ekelund, U., and Sardinha, L. B. (2019). Fitness Mediates Activity and Sedentary Patterns Associations with Adiposity in Youth. *Medicine and Science in Sports and Exercise* 51 (2): 323–29.

Saunders, T. J., Gray, C. E., Poitras, V. J., Chaput, J. P., Janssen, I., Katzmarzyk, P. T., Olds, T., et al. (2016). Combinations of Physical Activity, Sedentary Behaviour and Sleep: Relationships with Health Indicators in School-Aged Children and Youth. *Applied Physiology, Nutrition and Metabolism* 41 (6): 283–93.

Singh, A. S., Mulder, C., Twisk, J. W. R., Van Mechelen, W., and Chinapaw, M. J. M. (2008). Tracking of Childhood Overweight into Adulthood: A Systematic Review of the Literature. *Obesity Reviews* 9 (5): 474–88.

Sluggett, L., Wagner, S. L., and Harris, R. L. (2019). Sleep Duration and Obesity in Children and Adolescents. *Canadian Journal of Diabetes* 43 (2): 146–52.

Sun, Q., Ba, Y., Zhai, L., Wei, W. and Jia, L. (2018). Association between Sleep Duration and Overweight/Obesity at Age 7-18 in Shenyang, China in 2010 and 2014. *International Journal of Environmental Research and Public Health* 15 (5).

Tambalis, K. D., Panagiotakos, D. B., Psarra, G., and Sidossis, L. S. (2018). Insufficient Sleep Duration Is Associated with Dietary Habits, Screen Time, and Obesity in Children. *Journal of Clinical Sleep Medicine* 14 (10): 1689–96.

Tremblay, M. (2012). Letter to the Editor: Standardized Use of the Terms 'Sedentary' and 'Sedentary Behaviours.' *Applied Physiology, Nutrition and Metabolism* 37 (3): 540–2.

Wang, F., Liu, H., Wan, Y., Li, J., Chen, Y., Zheng, J., Huang, T., et al. (2016). Sleep Duration and Overweight/Obesity in Preschool-Aged Children: A Prospective Study of up to 48,922 Children of the Jiaxing Birth Cohort. *Sleep* 39 (11): 2013–19.

Werneck, A. O., Silva, E. C. A., Bueno, M. R. O., Vignadelli, L. Z., Oyeyemi, A. L., Romanzini, C. L. P., Ronque, E. R. V., et al. (2019). Association(s) between Objectively Measured Sedentary Behavior Patterns and Obesity among Brazilian Adolescents. *Pediatric Exercise Science* 31 (1): 37–41.

Wu, J., Wu, H., Wang, J., Guo, L., Deng, X., and Lu, C. (2015). Associations between Sleep Duration and Overweight/Obesity: Results from 66,817 Chinese Adolescents. *Scientific Reports* 5.

In: Childhood Obesity
Editor: Roya Kelishadi

ISBN: 978-1-53618-158-6
© 2020 Nova Science Publishers, Inc.

Chapter 8

PARENTAL FACTORS ASSOCIATED WITH CHILDHOOD OBESITY

Sara Jalali-Farahani, PhD, Hasti Masihay-Akbar, MD and Parisa Amiri, PhD*

Research Center for Social Determinants of Health,
Research Institute for Endocrine Sciences,
Shahid Beheshti University of Medical Sciences, Tehran, Iran

ABSTRACT

Childhood obesity is a complex and multifactorial health problem with an alarming and rising trend in recent years. Obesity related behaviors including dietary intakes, eating habits, sedentary and physical activity patterns are mainly developed during childhood. Several parental factors including parental age, working status, education, weight status, feeding practice and lifestyle found to be associated with shaping obesity related behaviors and consequently childhood overweight and obesity. Additionally, parental perception regarding their offspring's weight status found to be another factor that can contribute to development of childhood obesity. Considering the important role of parents in shaping their offspring's lifestyle and consequently their future weight, it is important to identify and consider parental correlates of childhood obesity in childhood obesity prevention and treatment programs. Therefore, this chapter aims to introduce and describe what is known regarding the main parental correlates of childhood obesity which will be reviewed in four main sections including 1) parental socio-demographic characteristics, 2) parental weight status, 3) parental perception of child's weight status, and 4) parenting styles and feeding practices.

* Corresponding Author's Email: amiri@endocrine.ac.ir.

1. Parental Socio-Demographic Characteristics

Previous studies have shown different socio-demographic factors including parental age, marital status, education and maternal employment have been associated with childhood obesity (Keane et al. 2012, Valerio et al. 2006, Jalali-Farahani, Amiri, et al. 2017). Regarding parental age, findings of a systematic reviews found no association between maternal age at birth and childhood overweight (Weng et al. 2012); however, findings of a study conducted in Iran to investigate the effects of different risk clusters on the incidence of overweight in children through more than a decade follow-up, indicated that mean maternal and paternal age were significantly higher in high-risk cluster compared to medium and low-risk clusters (Jalali-Farahani, Amiri, et al. 2017). Besides, another evidence from Sweden indicating that those children who were born from older mothers were more likely to be overweight or obese; moreover, they were less likely to exercise which can result in excessive weight gain in the long term (Barclay and Myrskylä 2016). Existing findings limit the possibility of making a definitive conclusion and suggest more investigation on this topic in future studies.

Regarding marital status, several studies investigated the role of family structure in offspring's overweight and obesity (Biehl et al. 2014, Chaparro et al. 2017, Yannakoulia et al. 2008). In this regard, in a cross-sectional study conducted in Greece, parent's divorce was significantly associated with higher BMI and overweight in 9-11 year old children; however, such difference in mean BMI was not significant in unmarried or widowed parents compared to married ones (Yannakoulia et al. 2008). Other cross-sectional findings from Norway indicated prevalence of overweight and abdominal obesity were more in offspring from divorced compared to married parents (Biehl et al. 2014). Furthermore, a longitudinal research conducted in Sweden to investigate the association between maternal history of marital status and risk of overweight and obesity in women's adulthood. The findings revealed that compared to those women whose mothers belonged to stable marriage category, women whose mothers belonged to the stable cohabitation, the cohabiting then separating, married then divorcing, the not with father, and varied transitions categories were at higher risk of overweight and obesity in adulthood (Chaparro et al. 2017). Findings of UK Millennium Cohort which aimed to indicate the association between divorce and children's BMI and risk of overweight/obesity demonstrated no association between parental separation and increases in children's BMI and their risk of overweight/obesity pre-separation and short-term after separation; however, this association was significant in long-term and specifically in children under 6 years (Goisis, Özcan, and Van Kerm 2019). Findings of another longitudinal study entitled as Fragile Families and Child Wellbeing Study revealed a higher risk of becoming overweight/obese in children who belonged to families in which mothers dissolved a union recently and had been living without a partner for at least 2 years compared to those belonged to married families. Furthermore, better BMI trajectories were reported for the offspring of those single mothers who entered a new union compared to those single mothers who remained single or recently became single. These findings emphasized the importance of stable family structure (Schmeer 2012). In conclusion, results from the above-mentioned studies implying higher risk for overweight and obesity in offspring from unstable families.

Considering parental education, in Tehran Lipid and Glucose Study (TLGS), considering importance level of factors in the classification of parental risk clusters, maternal education found to be the most influential factor among studied socio-demographic factors (Jalali-Farahani, Amiri, et al. 2017). Findings of a study using data from 12 countries (Kenya, South Africa, Brazil, Colombia, Canada, USA, Finland, Portugal, United Kingdom (UK), China, Australia and India) indicated positive association between maternal education and childhood overweight in Colombia and Kenya as well as paternal education and childhood overweight in Kenya and a negative association between paternal education and overweight in Brazil and USA (Muthuri et al. 2016). Results of a longitudinal study conducted in European region including 11countries (Italy, Spain, Portugal, UK, Sweden, France, Netherlands, Czech Republic, Ukraine, Greece and Finland) on 45413 children aged 4-7 years indicated higher risk of overweight and obesity in early childhood among children born to mothers with low education (Ruiz et al. 2016). Another data from Millennium Cohort Study in UK indicated higher risk for overweight and abdominal obesity in offspring of mothers with the lowest level of education (Noonan and Fairclough 2018). Besides, findings of a longitudinal study conducted in Australia demonstrated that higher maternal education was found to be associated with lower risk of becoming overweight/obese (Kerr et al. 2017). However, findings of the China Health Nutrition Survey (CHNS) demonstrated that a negative association between maternal education and overweight in school-aged children and children with higher maternal education levels were more likely to be overweight/obese (Feng et al. 2019). Similarly, findings of a cohort study including 672 mother-baby pairs conducted in Brazil indicated that lower maternal education had a protective role (Portela et al. 2015). Considering above-mentioned findings, it seems that the association between parental education and childhood overweight-obesity differs in various countries, and potentially it may associate with their developmental stage.

A substantial body of evidence documented association between maternal employment and childhood obesity. In this regard, using cross-sectional nationally representative data from 38 low- and middle-income countries, it is found that the risk of childhood overweight was higher in offspring of formally employed mothers compared to non-employed ones and magnitude of this association in 14 countries depend on maternal level of education (Oddo et al. 2017). From the longitudinal perspective, findings of a longitudinal study conducted in the UK revealed maternal employment significantly associated with higher children's BMI during childhood specifically in the offspring of single mothers (Fitzsimons and Pongiglione 2019). This results were in agreement with findings of another study conducted in UK, in which three main mechanisms including mean number of daily meals, reading/talking/listening to music, and watching TV were suggested for the observed association between maternal employment and childhood BMI (Fertig, Glomm, and Tchernis 2009). However, using data of the China Health and Nutrition Survey (CHNS), no association was found between maternal employment and childhood obesity (Nie and Sousa-Poza 2014). Similarly, findings of another study conducted in eight European countries provide little evidence for association of maternal employment and childhood obesity. As the findings indicated this association was only significant in Italy and Cyprus. In terms of part-time employment, no significant association was observed between part-time maternal employment and any measure of fatness in children (Gwozdz et al. 2013). Considering findings of abovementioned studies, we cannot come to a consensus conclusion regarding association between maternal employment and childhood obesity.

2. Parental Weight Status

Parental weight is one of the main predictors of obesity in children and adolescents that is likely due to a combination of genetic predisposition and environmental factors (da Costa Ribeiro, Taddei, and Colugnatti 2003). Familial aggregation of obesity seen in different studies is due to interactions between mentioned factors (Lobsetin, Baur, and Uauy 2004, Xi et al. 2009). Family environment moderates expression of obesity genes. In other words, genes define the tendency to develop overweight, and behaviors (e. g. diet and physical activity) determine to what extent the obesity-related phenotype and genotype match (Silventoinen et al. 2016).

There is a correlation between parental and their offspring weight status from the intrauterine period onwards. From the limited number of studies that have analyzed this correlation in early years of life, most yielded inconsistent results (Stunkard et al. 2004, Zalbahar et al. 2016), some reported a positive association between maternal BMI and their offspring's weight at birth (Knight et al. 2007, Regnault et al. 2010), and only one reported paternal BMI as an influencing factor on child's birth weight (Xue et al. 2008). Mei et al. (Mei et al. 2018) found maternal weight effective on child's growth from the intrauterine stage up to two years of age, while paternal weight status was only slightly effective on child's growth after birth. However, studies focusing on children aged 2-18 years, including cohort studies (Andriani, Liao, and Kuo 2015, Jaaskelainen et al. 2011, Naess et al. 2018, Whitaker et al. 2010), have more consistent results across different countries, whether in preschoolers (Andriani, Liao, and Kuo 2015, Bingham et al. 2013, Dev et al. 2013, Jaaskelainen et al. 2011, Manios et al. 2010, Menezes et al. 2011, Ntenda, Mhone, and Nkoka 2019, Warkentin et al. 2018, Whitaker et al. 2010, Zhang et al. 2014) or school-age children (Andegiorgish et al. 2012, Bahreynian et al. 2017, Bingham et al. 2013, Bjelland et al. 2010, Bushnik, Garriguet, and Colley 2017, Drenowatz et al. 2014, Ejtahed et al. 2018, Fasting et al. 2011, Greene-Cramer et al. 2018, Jaaskelainen et al. 2011, Jiang et al. 2013, Lazzeri et al. 2011, Liu et al. 2013, Maddah and Nikooyeh 2010, Martinovic et al. 2015, McCarthy et al. 2015, Naess et al. 2018, Shafaghi et al. 2014, Warkentin et al. 2018, Whitaker et al. 2010, Zhang et al. 2014). Warkentin et al. found that higher maternal BMI predicts greater body weight in both preschool and school-aged children (Bammann et al. 2017, Dev et al. 2013, Jiang et al. 2013, Lazzeri et al. 2011, Stettler et al. 2000, Zong, Li, and Zhang 2015) and this association becomes even stronger as child ages (Warkentin et al. 2018). There are two hypothesis suggested to explain this age differences. First, an overweight mother further exposes her child with an obesogenic environment which have a greater cumulative effect on child's weight over time. Second, the influence of genetic factors on child's weight increases throughout childhood (Haworth et al. 2008). Researchers have mostly focused on the mother-child weight relationship; however, Warkentin et al. (Warkentin et al. 2018) also observed an influence of father weight, but just among school-aged children. They suggested that as opposed to earlier stages of childhood when mothers are most influential on their children, the whole family becomes important as child ages (Warkentin et al. 2018). In conclusion, parental weight is amongst factors associated with childhood obesity specifically maternal weight, but the strength of the relationship differs with child's age.

3. Parental Perception of Child's Weight Status

Parents play a key role in prevention and treatment of childhood obesity through supporting and modeling of a healthy lifestyle and setting rules for obesity-related behaviors (Bauer et al. 2011, Ostbye et al. 2013) and parental involvement was among the features of effective lifestyle modification interventions (Golley et al. 2011). Parental low levels of concern and misperception regarding children's weight status can influence prevention of childhood obesity in different ways. Based on existing evidence, expressing concern by parents regarding child's weight was associated with more engaging in regulatory strategies such as restrictive and monitoring feeding practices to decrease daily energy intake (Seburg et al. 2014). In another study, maternal concerns about children's excessive weight also found to influence their feeding practice and more concerns regarding child's weight status is associated with a higher chance of food restriction by mothers (Crouch, O'dea, and Battisti 2007). Based on the findings of study by Moore et al. in the United States, parental concern regarding child's weight was significantly related to limiting screen time viewing, increasing physical activity and taking measures to improve family's diet (Moore, Harris, and Bradlyn 2012). Parental concern is closely tied to their perception of their offspring's weight status (Mulder et al. 2009, Moore, Harris, and Bradlyn 2012). For example, Mulder et al. indicated that mothers of overweight boys and girls were more concerned regarding their children's weight compared to mothers of normal-weight children. In this regard, their findings demonstrated, perceived child's weight and concern for child's weight by parents were significant determinants of BMI z score at age 12. (Mulder et al. 2009). In another study, parental perception of overweight/obesity and children's obesity were factors that influenced parental concern regarding their offspring's weight (Moore, Harris, and Bradlyn 2012).

A body of evidence indicates that a considerable number of parents cannot correctly and accurately determine their offspring's weight status (Crouch, O'dea, and Battisti 2007, Jalali-Farahani, Chin, et al. 2017, Regber et al. 2013, McDonald et al. 2016, Vallejo, Cortes-Rodríguez, and Colin-Ramirez 2015, Lydecker and Grilo 2016, Min et al. 2017, Ashraf, Shamsi, and Ashraf 2017, Cheng et al. 2016, Robinson and Sutin 2016, Al-Mohaimeed 2016, Zhang et al. 2018, Nemecek et al. 2017, AlRodhan et al. 2019, Christofaro et al. 2016, Hong et al. 2017, Ling and Stommel 2019, Caraza et al. 2016, Manios et al. 2015, Leppers et al. 2017, Gregori et al. 2018, Berggren et al. 2018). This misperception of children's weight status by parents has been reported in both pre-school (Crouch, O'dea, and Battisti 2007, Regber et al. 2013, Vallejo, Cortes-Rodríguez, and Colin-Ramirez 2015, Cheng et al. 2016, Robinson and Sutin 2016, Caraza et al. 2016, Berggren et al. 2018) and school children (Jalali-Farahani, Chin, et al. 2017, Regber et al. 2013, McDonald et al. 2016, Min et al. 2017, Al-Mohaimeed 2016, Zhang et al. 2018, AlRodhan et al. 2019, Christofaro et al. 2016, Manios et al. 2015, Leppers et al. 2017). Misclassifying children's weight status is common across various cultures and different groups of children's body weight status. The findings of some of the most recent studies from different countries are summarized in Table 1.

Table 1. Rates of misclassification of children's weight status by parents

Country, Year of publication, Number of participants (n)	Children's age (year)	Children's weight status	Misclassification rates
Region of the Americas			
Mexico, 2015, n=140 (Vallejo, Cortes-Rodríguez, and Colin-Ramirez 2015)	Age range: 2-6	Normal weight: 46.4% Overweight: 53.6%	49.2 and 61.3% of parents of normal weight and overweight children
Canada, 2016, n=450 (McDonald et al. 2016)	Age range: 6-8 Mean age: 7.4±0.6	Thin: 9.7% Normal weight: 74.1% Overweight: 9.0% Obese: 7.2%	27.2% of all parents (82.1, 8.1, 91.7 and 69% of parents of underweight, normal weight, overweight and obese children)
USA, 2016, n=1007 (Lydecker and Grilo 2016)	Age range: 5-15 Mean age: 10.2±3.0	Not reported	51.0% of all parents (47.7, 24.3, 73.1 and 89.8% of parents of underweight, normal weight, overweight and obese children)
Mexico, 2016, n= 605 (Caraza et al. 2016)	Age range: 2-6 Mean age: 4.2±1.2	Underweight or Normal weight: 73.5% Overweight: 12.2% Obese: 14.3%	98.8% of parents of overweight and obese children

Country, Year of publication, Number of participants (n) | Children's age (year) | Children's weight status | Misclassification rates

Brazil, 2016, n=1231 (Christofaro et al. 2016)	Age range: 14-17 Mean age: 15.6 ±1.1	Underweight: 1.5% Normal weight: 79.1% Overweight: 14.1% Obese: 5.3%	12.3 and 12.2% of all mothers and fathers respectively
USA, 2017, n= 1571 (Hong et al. 2017)	Age range: 3-15 Mean age: 8.9±3.7	Healthy weight: 63.7% Overweight: 36.3%	0.8 and 61.3% of parents of healthy weight and overweight children
USA, 2019, n=16869 (Ling and Stommel 2019)	Age range: 2-17	Underweight: 3.3% Healthy weight: 64.8% Overweight: 15.1% Obese: 16.9%	28% of all parents (61.2% of parents of overweight children)
European Region			
8 European countries (Belgium, Greece, Hungary, Netherlands, Norway, Slovenia, Spain and Switzerland), 2015, n=6113 (Manios et al. 2015)	Age range: 10-12	-	14.2 and 27.6%* of parents of normal weight and overweight or obese children *(Underestimation rates)
Ireland, 2016, n=8568 (Shiely et al. 2017)	Age range: 9 years	Not reported	59.4, 13.7 and 52.7% of parents of underweight, normal weight and overweight children
Germany, 2017, n=3408 (Leppers et al. 2017)	Age range: 8-12 Mean age: 9.7±0.3	Underweight: 7.1% Normal weight: 78.2% Overweight: 12.3% Obese: 2.3%	22.6, 20.7, 48.6 and 79.7% of parents of underweight, normal weight, overweight and obese children
Austria, 2017, n= 600 (Nemecek et al. 2017)	Age range: 0-14 Mean age: 4.7±2.9	Underweight: 10.2% Normal weight: 76.0% Overweight: 10.7% Obese: 3.2%	24.3% of all parents (68.9, 7.5, 90.6 and 63.2% parents of underweight, normal weight, overweight and obese children)
Sweden, 2018, At age 2: (n=2133) & At age 5: (n=1862) (Berggren et al. 2018)	Age range: 2-5	At age 2: Underweight: 7.4% Normal weight: 77.8% Overweight: 12.7% Obese: 2.2% At age 5: Underweight: 9.4% Normal weight: 78.8% Overweight: 9.5% Obese: 2.3%	At age 2: 0.1 and 96.4% of parents of normal weight and overweight children At age 5: 0.4 and 87.1% of parents of normal weight and overweight children
Western Pacific Region			
Australia, 2016, n=3557 (Robinson and Sutin 2016)	Age range: 4-5	Underweight: 4.8% Normal weight: 75.4% Overweight/obese: 19.7%	55.2, 14.6 and 81.4% of parents of underweight, normal weight and overweight/obese children
Singapore, 2016, n=821 (Cheng et al. 2016)	Age range: 3 years	Underweight: 19.6% Normal weight: 72.0% Overweight: 5.5% Obese: 2.9%	16.8, 75.6 and 95.9% of parents of normal weight, overweight and obese children
New Zealand, 2016, n=1093(Meredith-Jones, Williams, and Taylor 2016)	Age range: 4-8 Mean age: 6.5±1.4	Underweight: 1.0% Normal weight: 74.0% Overweight: 15.0% Obese: 10.0%	15% of all parents

Table 1. (Continued)

Country, Year of publication, Number of participants (n)	Children's age (year)	Children's weight status	Misclassification rates
China, 2017, n=816 (Min et al. 2017)	Age range: 6-18 Mean age: 10.5±2.7	Underweight: 20.0% Normal weight: 66.4% Overweight: 13.6%	36.2% of parents (55.2%, 25.6% and 59.5% parents of underweight, normal weight and overweight children)
China, 2017, n=47417 (Zhang et al. 2018)	Age range: 6-17 Mean age: ±	Underweight: 6.6% Normal weight: 68.7% Overweight/obese: 24.7%	39.2% of all parents
Eastern Mediterranean Region			
Saudi Arabia, 2016, n=601 (Al-Mohaimeed 2016)	Age range: 6-10 Mean age: 8.4±1.3	Normal weight: 78.0% Overweight: 12.7% Obese: 9.3%	90.0 and 64.3% of parents of overweight and obese children
Pakistan, 2017, n=305 (Ashraf, Shamsi, and Ashraf 2017)	Age range: 5-14 Mean age: 8.4 ± 2.7	Normal weight: 83.9% Overweight: 7.5% Obese: 8.5%	58.7% of all parents (54.0%, 78.0% and 81.0% of parents of normal weight, overweight and obese children)
Iran, 2017, n=465 (Jalali-Farahani, Chin, et al. 2017)	Mean age: 15.6 ± 0.9	Thin: 2.8% Normal weight: 58.7% Overweight/obese: 38.5%	43.5% of parents
Kuwait, 2019, n= 1002 (AlRodhan et al. 2019)	Age range: 6-8	Underweight: 4.3% Normal weight: 54.8% Overweight: 13.5% Obese: 27.4%	92.2% of parents of overweight children
Multi regions			
10 countries (Chile, Mexico, Argentina, Brazil, Germany, Italy, France, United Kingdom, Georgia and India), 2018, n= 2714 (Gregori et al. 2018)	Age range: 3-11	Underweight: 12.6% Normal weight: 58.9% Overweight: 15.9% Obese: 12.6%	73.0, 15.0, 92.0 and 54.0% of parents of underweight, normal weight, overweight and obese children

Based on existing evidence, underestimation of children's body weight status by parents is more common compared to overestimation (Jalali-Farahani, Chin, et al. 2017, Regber et al. 2013, Vallejo, Cortes-Rodríguez, and Colin-Ramirez 2015, Lydecker and Grilo 2016, Min et al. 2017, Cheng et al. 2016, Robinson and Sutin 2016, Zhang et al. 2018, AlRodhan et al. 2019, Christofaro et al. 2016, Hong et al. 2017, Ling and Stommel 2019, Caraza et al. 2016, Leppers et al. 2017). Considering children's actual weight, parental misclassification rates were more common in parents of overweight and obese children compared to underweight and normal-weight ones (Regber et al. 2013, Lydecker and Grilo 2016, Jalali-Farahani, Chin, et al. 2017, Vallejo, Cortes-Rodríguez, and Colin-Ramirez 2015, Ashraf, Shamsi, and Ashraf 2017, Robinson and Sutin 2016, Al-Mohaimeed 2016, AlRodhan et al. 2019, Hong et al. 2017, Ling and Stommel 2019,

Manios et al. 2015, Leppers et al. 2017, Berggren et al. 2018). In some studies, by increasing children's weight, the rates of parental misperception regarding their children's weight status worsened (Jalali-Farahani, Chin, et al. 2017, Regber et al. 2013, Ashraf, Shamsi, and Ashraf 2017, Hong et al. 2017, Manios et al. 2015, Berggren et al. 2018). Findings of study conducted by Regber et al. in eight European countries demonstrated that 19.1%, 66.3% and 88.2% of parents of normal weight, overweight and obese children misclassified their children's weight status respectively (Regber et al. 2013). In agreement with this finding, another report from eight European countries indicated higher underestimation rates in by parents of overweight/obese children compared to parents of normal weight ones (14.2%) (Manios et al. 2015). In another study from Iran, Jalali-Farahani et al. reported the percentages of parental incorrect perception of adolescents' body weight status in severely thin, thin, normal weight, overweight and obese adolescents were 0.0%, 18.2%, 30.9%, 53.8% and 86.0% respectively (Jalali-Farahani, Chin, et al. 2017). In Pakistan, Ashraf et al. reported 54.0, 78.0 and 81.0% of misclassification rates by parents in normal weight, overweight and obese children (Ashraf, Shamsi, and Ashraf 2017). In the USA, substantial difference was observed in misclassification rates reported by parents of healthy weight (0.8%) and overweight children (61.3%) (Hong et al. 2017). Two studies applied two methods of verbal description and schematic body images to assess parental perception regarding offspring's weight status (Cheng et al. 2016, Vallejo, Cortes-Rodríguez, and Colin-Ramirez 2015). In one study conducted by Vallejo et al. in Mexico, using verbal description same pattern was observed; while when schematic body images method was used, parental misperception rates in overweight children (57.3%) was less than normal-weight children (72.3%) (Vallejo, Cortes-Rodríguez, and Colin-Ramirez 2015). In the other study conducted by Cheng et al. in Singapore, using verbal method, misclassification rates were more in overweight and obese children compared to underweight ones, while using visual method, misclassification rates were more in underweight group compared to overweight/obese group (Cheng et al. 2016). However, in some studies, parental misperception rates were fairly equal in both underweight and overweight children. For instance, McDonald et al. reported 82.1%, 91.7% and 69% of parents of underweight, overweight and obese children tended to misperceive their offspring's weight status (McDonald et al. 2016). In China, 55.2 and 59.5% of parents of underweight and overweight children, misclassified their children's weight status (Min et al. 2017). Similarly, in Ireland, Shiely et al. reported relatively equal misperception rates in underweight (59.4%) and overweight children (52.7%) by parents (Shiely et al. 2017). Considering children's overweight and obesity status, findings of number of studies implying better ability of parents in detection of obesity compared to overweight (Crouch, O'dea, and Battisti 2007, McDonald et al. 2016, Al-Mohaimeed 2016). In this regard, based on results of study by Crouch et al., mother's ability to correctly detect children's obesity was better than overweight (Crouch, O'dea, and Battisti 2007). Similarly, based on McDonald et al. report, more parents of obese children (31.0%) believed that their child should weigh less compared to overweight ones (8.3%) (McDonald et al. 2016). Al-Mohaimeed reported more misclassification rates in overweight children (90.0%) compared to obese ones (64.3%) in Saudi Arabia (Al-Mohaimeed 2016).

Existing evidence indicates that correct detection of excessive weight in children may influence lifestyle modification and consequently weight management in children. In this regard, findings of study by Park et al. indicated that parental recognition of overweight in their offspring was associated with intention to change behavior and providing feedback regarding children's overweight status was related to positive change in health-related behaviors in more than half of the parents (Park et al. 2014). In addition, the detection of overweight status in children found to be associated with encouraging children for improvement of their lifestyle by parents; however, this inspiration did not associated with child's BMI (Min et al. 2017). In conclusion, in prevention and treatments of childhood obesity, parental concern and early identification of overweight and obesity in children is required to motivate and incline parents for facilitating and supporting lifestyle modification in their overweight/obese offspring. Weight screening in school setting by trained school staff can help parents to correctly recognize overweight and obesity in their offspring.

4. Parenting Styles and Feeding Practices

Parenting style as a function of the parents' attitudes, beliefs, and behaviors is a general behavioral construct that sets the emotional context for parent-child interaction (Darling and Steinberg 1993). Parenting style has been conceptualized by Baumrind (Baumrind 1966, Baumrind 1967) based on two important elements of parenting: *(1) parental demandingness* (the rules which parents set to control their children's behavior, parental demands and expectations of their children regarding those rules, and the consequences of breaking those rules); and *(2) parental responsiveness* (the degree to which parents respond to their children's needs in a warm, supportive and accepting manner to foster individuality, self-regulation, and self-assertion). Based on the aforementioned domains, three initial parenting styles could be identified:

1) *Authoritative parenting*, associated with being both demanding and responsive. Authoritative parents place limits but not as strict as authoritarian parents, they explain different situations in a warm and nurturing way and encourage their children to decide and act independently. In case of any misbehavior, authoritative parents try to discuss, allowing the child to explain him/herself and learn why his/her behavior was inappropriate. If the child is to be punished, the punishment would be appropriate to his/her shortcoming. Authoritative parents place limits, encourage independence and demand maturity but they are forgiving as well.

2) *Authoritarian parenting,* characterized by high demandingness but low responsiveness. Authoritarian parents set strict rules in the family environment which is not open to children's feelings and opinions. Verbal and non-verbal punishments are commonly used in this parenting style, believing to prepare the child for a future hard life in society, even without any learning feedback from the child.
3) *Indulgent or permissive parenting*, linked with high responsiveness and low demandingness. This parenting style is referred to as child-centered parenting in which parents respond to all their children's needs without any expectations or controlling rules. Permissive parents allow their children to make their own decisions but do not provide enough information and therefore do not expect their child to behave properly and with discipline. Children of permissive parents learn to live independently but not in a mature way.

   Maccoby and Martin (McCoby 1983) expanded upon Baumrind's typology by providing a two-dimensional framework for parenting style and suggested a fourth style of parenting:
4) *Neglectful or uninvolved parenting,* associated with not being demanding nor responsive. They neither place any rules to control their children' behavior, nor make any demands of them. They are ignorant of their children's needs and feeling and do not offer any behavioral guidance and support. Characteristics of four main categories of parenting style based on two dimensions of demandingness and responsiveness are illustrated in Figure 1.

The feeding style is considered as a sub-category of parenting style which is specific to food-related situations. It was derived (differentiated) from general parenting style by Hughes et al. (Hughes et al. 2005), thus the same dimensions as of parenting style (demandingness and responsiveness) applies to feeding style, but in the feeding context (Blissett 2011, Hughes et al. 2005, Ventura and Birch 2008). In feeding styles, demandingness refers to the extent parents place demands on their children to control their eating (Hughes et al. 2005). Responsiveness refers to the ways of carrying out eating-related demands. In the responsive style, the parent knows the child's needs and feeling towards eating and respond to them in a supportive way (Hughes et al. 2005). Based on these two dimensions, authoritative, authoritarian, indulgent, and uninvolved feeding styles were identified. For example, in the feeding context, in an authoritative style, rules are placed and fully explained by parents in a supportive way to change children's eating behaviors.

<table>
<tr><td></td><td colspan="3">Responsiveness
The degree to which:
-Parents respond to the children's needs in a supportive manner
-Parents foster individuality and self-regulation in the children</td></tr>
<tr><td rowspan="3">Demandingness
The extent to which:
-Parents set rules to control the children's behaviors
-Parents expect the children to follow the rules
-Parents punish the children when breaking the rules</td><td></td><td>High</td><td>Low</td></tr>
<tr><td>High</td><td>Authoritative parents
-Place limits and rules
-Explain those rules in a nurturing way
-Encourage independent decision-making
-Either forgive child's shortcomings or punish him/her appropriately</td><td>Authoritarian parents
-Set strict rules in the family environment
-Punish the children when breaking those rules
-Ignorant children's feelings and needs
- Suppress independence in children</td></tr>
<tr><td>Low</td><td>Permissive parents
-Respond to children's needs and feelings
-Have low or zero expectations from the children
-Permit children to decide independently but without proper guidance</td><td>Neglectful parents
-Place no rules and regulations for the children
-Have no expectations of the children to behave properly
-Ignore children's feelings and needs
-Do not offer behavioral guidance</td></tr>
</table>

Figure 1. Parenting styles based on levels of demandingness and responsiveness.

4.1. Parenting/Feeding Styles in Relation to Children Weight Status

Researchers have mostly investigated children's behaviors and body weight through feeding practices and only a small proportion of literature has focused on the influence of parenting and feeding style on children's body weight (Shloim et al. 2015). Parenting styles, feeding styles, and feeding practices exert their effect on children's weight status both directly and indirectly through modifying childhood obesogenic behaviors such as dietary intakes, physical activity, and sedentary behaviors (Faith et al. 2012). Previous studies support the fact that the authoritative parenting style is related to more desirable behaviors in children, including more healthy food consumption and physical activity and less unhealthy eating habits (Lohaus, Vierhaus, and Ball 2009). Regarding diet, children of authoritative parents show a higher capacity for regulating their eating behaviors while in an authoritarian parenting style, children's developmental abilities are ignored so they exercise less self-control overeating (Sokol, Qin, and Poti 2017). Regarding physical activity patterns, compared to children living with highly demanding parents, children of parents with high levels of responsiveness are naturally more interested in physical activity, for they are not under strict rules (Rhee et al. 2006).

The direct relationship between parenting style and weight status has been reviewed in both cross-sectional (Sleddens et al. 2011, Vollmer and Mobley 2013) and longitudinal studies (Berge et al. 2010, Olvera and Power 2010, Rhee et al. 2006). It is suggested that children raised in authoritative homes have lower body mass index (BMI) compared to children raised with other styles (Sleddens et al. 2011, Vollmer and Mobley 2013). Neglectful and indulgent parenting styles more predicted high BMI in children compared to authoritative and authoritarian ones (Olvera and Power 2010, Rodenburg et al. 2012). Findings of a recent review of longitudinal studies (Sokol, Qin, and Poti 2017) also suggested that authoritative parenting is associated with a lower likelihood of overweight/obesity, but with a high level of heterogeneity. This suggests that obesity and weight gain are dynamic, and the relationship between parenting style experienced in childhood and later weight status may change over time. Hancock et al. (Hancock, Lawrence, and Zubrick 2014), have also demonstrated that high maternal protectiveness is also associated with overweight or obesity in 10-11 years compared to 4-5 years, showing that negative or positive effects of some parenting styles may emerge or vanish as a child grows up.

A more consistent relationship between feeding style and risk of obesity is revealed by cross-sectional studies, compared to general parenting style (Shloim et al. 2015). It seems that children of parents with indulgent and permissive feeding style have higher BMI and are more at risk of developing overweight or obesity and there is gender and ethnic differences evident in this relationship (Hughes et al. 2011).

As parenting styles and feeding styles do not always agree in one family, they could have different influences on child dietary intake, activity behaviors and weight status (Hennessy et al. 2010). Overall, due to differences in conceptualization and measurement, results for feeding styles are much more consistent than for parenting style. Weak evidence in the literature to describe the interactions between parenting and feeding styles and child obesity risk could be one reason. Another reason for these heterogeneous findings may be due to the age-differences in different studies. While the studies on parenting style focus mostly on adolescence and school-age children, preschool children make up the majority of target population in feeding style literature. Obesity and weight gain are dynamic phenomena whose relationship with parenting and feeding styles may change over time. Negative or positive effects of some parenting styles may emerge or vanish as child grows up. As an example, authoritarian feeding style which might be beneficial for preschool children loses its effects as child grows older. It is explained that preschool children respond to demands placed to eat healthy food and restrict unhealthy food even without thorough explanations, while as the child ages, without warm and reasonable explanation, he/she may not be able to gauge hunger or fullness and grows preference for the foods that were previously restricted (Fuemmeler et al. 2012, Vollmer and Baietto 2017).

4.2. Parenting and Feeding Practices

Parenting practices are general behaviors or actions performed by parents to influence their children's attitudes, behaviors, or beliefs. As opposed to styles, practices are defined by and changed in different contexts (Darling and Steinberg 1993). Feeding practices are parental behaviors in food-related situations that control what, how much, or when their children eat (Hughes et al. 2013). This might include attempts to increase or decrease intake of certain foods. Common feeding practices include: restrictive guidance, active guidance, modeling, control of availability, pressure to eat, food as reward for positive behavior, rewarding food consumption and verbal praise (Gevers et al. 2014).

Feeding and other context-specific parenting practices happen in a broader and more complex environment, namely parenting styles which moderates the effectiveness of those specific practices (Tschann et al. 2015). Therefore examining feeding practices is only reasonable when these other factors are taken into account (Darling and Steinberg 1993). Specific feeding practices used in different family contexts and parenting styles, can affect children's eating behaviors in different ways (Koerner and Fitzpatrick 2006). As an example, this mediator effect of the parenting style is noted when restrictive guidance helps less permissive parents lower unhealthy food intake in their children (Hennessy et al. 2012). De Bourdeaudhuij et al. also shows that vegetable intake in children of authoritative families is increased more than authoritarian families when using restrictive guidance (De Bourdeaudhuij et al. 2009).

4.3. Types of Feeding Practices in Relation to Children Weight Status

4.3.1. Restrictive Guidance

Restrictive guidance is defined as the limits, rules, or restrictions set by parents regarding food consumption in children. A recent review conducted by Yee et al. (Yee, Lwin, and Ho 2017) revealed a large amount of heterogeneity in the relationship between restrictive guidance and both healthy and unhealthy food consumption behaviors in children. However, in their review restricting behaviors showed a small negative correlation with unhealthy food consumption which was stronger among older children (Yee, Lwin, and Ho 2017); suggesting that although restrictive guidance might be ineffective in promoting desirable food choices among older children, its negative effects in unhealthy food consumption become even more pronounced, as child grows. Regarding child weight status, restricting intake is associated with higher BMI in preschoolers, meaning that parents use restrictions when they perceive their child is fat (Dev et al. 2013); while helpful in short-term, it may have opposite effects which are even larger on BMI as child grows up (Vollmer and Baietto 2017, Warkentin et al. 2018).

4.3.2. Active Guidance

Active guidance or education is defined as active and verbal discussions and interactions between parents and children to guide their child regarding food. Few researches that have focused on this area of feeding practices are mostly inconclusive. In a recent meta-analysis (Yee, Lwin, and Ho 2017), utilizing active guidance by parents could increase healthy eating in their children but had no significant effect on unhealthy eating behaviors.

4.3.3. Modeling

Based on social cognitive theory, children adapt and change their beliefs and behaviors through observing behaviors of significant others including parents, the process which is commonly referred to as modeling (Bandura 1998, 2001). Modeling is measured in two ways across the literature. The first way is based on parental intake of a specific food; in this way of measurement, whenever a positive relationship between parent and child is seen in terms of what they eat, a significant modeling effect exists. In the second way, modeling is measured as the frequency in which parents eat healthily and demonstrate the benefits and pleasure of healthy eating in front of children. In both cases, modeling is consistently found to be associated with child-eating. Yee et al. in their review found a homogenous and significant effect for modeling on children's eating behaviors. It suggests that children eat what they see their parents are eating whether healthy or unhealthy (Yee, Lwin, and Ho 2017).

It is mostly hypothesized that modeling can be used more easily and effectively in older children. Warkentin et al. (Warkentin et al. 2018) showed that, contrary to this common perception which makes parents less likely to use modeling methods on preschoolers, these practices have shown stronger effects on child weight in this age. It can be explained by the fact that as children get older, gradually, the direct impact of parents over their child's food intake gives place to the becoming influence of teachers, peers, and media (de Lauzon-Guillain et al. 2009).

4.3.4. Parental Control of Availability

Parental control of availability simply refers to whether a particular food is available at home. Researchers suggest that control of food availability can be a consistent predictor of child food consumption, meaning that healthy or unhealthy foods that are accessible to the child are more frequently consumed. Availability also has a stronger association with healthy food consumption among older children (Yee, Lwin, and Ho 2017).

4.3.5. Pressure to Eat

This practice refers to when parents verbally communicate or physically struggle with their children to consume more food. In this feeding practice, children are asked to empty their plate even if they are not hungry (Birch et al. 2001). Contrary to the intentions of parents who want to increase their child's consumption of healthy food, this method has shown opposite effects and lowered fruits and vegetables intake (Fisher et al. 2002, Galloway et al. 2005). Parents who use pressure to peruse healthy eating in their children get negative results and their pressure pushes their children more toward unhealthy food, than healthy ones. Comparing modeling to pressure, it seems that "do as I do" approach has been proven to be more successful in changing children's dietary habits than "do as I say," especially in fruit and vegetable intakes, trying unfamiliar or disliked foods (Duncker 1938, Harper and Sanders 1975, Birch 1980). Regarding weight status, pressure to eat is mostly related to lower BMI in children (Afonso et al. 2016, Galloway et al. 2006, Wardle and Carnell 2007), not that this practice is effective against weight gain, but that parents of thinner children pressure them to eat more (Vaughn et al. 2016). The undesirable effects of parental pressure on healthy food consumption are greater among younger children (Warkentin et al. 2018), whose eating habits are just beginning to develop and are more peaky and neophobic regarding their food (Galloway et al. 2006).

4.3.6. Food as a Reward

Parents might utilize food as a reward when children behave as desired. Using healthy food as a reward shows no significant effect on encouraging children to eat more healthy food. On the contrary, rewarding children with snacks further leads kids to unhealthy food (Yee, Lwin, and Ho 2017). As parents usually use unhealthy food and snacks as a reward, this practice shown to increase the use of unhealthy food in children (Birch and Fisher 1998, Savage, Fisher, and Birch 2007).

4.3.7. Rewarding Food Consumption Materially and Verbally

Parents sometimes use rewards either materially such as playtime or toys, or verbally to modify their child's eating behavior. Verbal praise demonstrates promising effects in increasing healthy food intake as well as decreasing unhealthy ones. whereas material rewards have no significant effects on eating behaviors, whether healthy or unhealthy (Yee, Lwin, and Ho 2017). It might be explained by the fact that eating certain food loses its value through time as the child is offered a reward every time (Birch, Marlin, and Rotter 1984). Age-based examinations showed positive associations between verbal praise and healthy food consumption only among younger children, and not older children (Yee, Lwin, and Ho 2017).

References

Afonso, Lisa, Carla Lopes, Milton Severo, Susana Santos, Helena Real, Catarina Durao, Pedro Moreira, and Andreia Oliveira. 2016. "Bidirectional association between parental child-feeding practices and body mass index at 4 and 7 y of age." *The American journal of clinical nutrition* no. 103 (3):861-867.

Al-Mohaimeed, Abdulrahman A. 2016. "Parents' perception of children's obesity, in Al-Qassim, Saudi Arabia." *Journal of family & community medicine* no. 23 (3):179.

AlRodhan, Yousif, Yousef AlAbdeen, Eisa Saleh, Naser AlFodari, Hamad AlSaqer, Farah Alhumoud, and Lukman Thalib. 2019. "Obesity and maternal perception: a cross-sectional study of children aged 6 to 8 years in Kuwait." *Eastern Mediterranean Health Journal* no. 25 (7).

Andegiorgish, A. K., J. Wang, X. Zhang, X. Liu, and H. Zhu. 2012. "Prevalence of overweight, obesity, and associated risk factors among school children and adolescents in Tianjin, China." *Eur J Pediatr* no. 171 (4):697-703. doi: 10.1007/s00431-011-1636-x.

Andriani, H., C. Y. Liao, and H. W. Kuo. 2015. "Parental weight changes as key predictors of child weight changes." *BMC Public Health* no. 15:645. doi: 10.1186/s12889-015-2005-x.

Ashraf, Hiba, Nida Ilyas Shamsi, and Ruhma Ashraf. 2017. "Parental perception and childhood obesity: Contributors to incorrect perception." *Journal of the Pakistan Medical Association* no. 67 (2):214.

Bahreynian, M., M. Qorbani, B. M. Khaniabadi, M. E. Motlagh, O. Safari, H. Asayesh, and R. Kelishadi. 2017. "Association between Obesity and Parental Weight Status in Children and Adolescents." *J Clin Res Pediatr Endocrinol* no. 9 (2):111-117. doi: 10. 4274/jcrpe.3790.

Bammann, Karin, Wencke Gwozdz, Claudia Pischke, Gabriele Eiben, Juan M. Fernandez-Alvira, Stefaan De Henauw, Lauren Lissner, Luis A. Moreno, Yannis Pitsiladis, and L. Reisch. 2017. "The impact of familial, behavioural and psychosocial factors on the SES gradient for childhood overweight in Europe. A longitudinal study." *International Journal of Obesity* no. 41 (1):54-60.

Bandura, Albert. 1998. "Health promotion from the perspective of social cognitive theory." *Psychology and health* no. 13 (4):623-649.

Bandura, Albert. 2001. "Social cognitive theory: An agentic perspective." *Annual review of psychology* no. 52 (1):1-26.

Barclay, Kieron, and Mikko Myrskylä. 2016. "Maternal age and offspring health and health behaviours in late adolescence in Sweden." *SSM-population health* no. 2:68-76.

Bauer, K. W., D. Neumark-Sztainer, J. A. Fulkerson, P. J. Hannan, and M. Story. 2011. "Familial correlates of adolescent girls' physical activity, television use, dietary intake, weight, and body composition." *Int J Behav Nutr Phys Act* no. 8:25. doi: 10.1186/1479-5868-8-25.

Baumrind, D. 1967. "Child care practices anteceding three patterns of preschool behavior." *Genet Psychol Monogr* no. 75 (1):43-88.

Baumrind, Diana. 1966. "Effects of authoritative parental control on child behavior." *Child development*:887-907.

Berge, Jerica M, Melanie Wall, Katie Loth, and Dianne Neumark-Sztainer. 2010. "Parenting style as a predictor of adolescent weight and weight-related behaviors." *Journal of Adolescent Health* no. 46 (4):331-338.

Berggren, S., J. Roswall, B. Alm, S. Bergman, J. Dahlgren, and G. Almquist-Tangen. 2018. "Parents with overweight children two and five years of age did not perceive them as weighing too much." *Acta Paediatr* no. 107 (6):1060-1064. doi: 10.1111/apa.14174.

Biehl, Anna, Ragnhild Hovengen, Else-Karin Grøholt, Jøran Hjelmesæth, Bjørn Heine Strand, and Haakon E. Meyer. 2014. "Parental marital status and childhood overweight and obesity in Norway: a nationally representative cross-sectional study." *BMJ open* no. 4 (6):e004502.

Bingham, D. D., M. I. Varela-Silva, M. M. Ferrao, G. Augusta, M. I. Mourao, H. Nogueira, V. R. Marques, and C. Padez. 2013. "Socio-demographic and behavioral risk factors associated with the high prevalence of overweight and obesity in Portuguese children." *Am J Hum Biol* no. 25 (6):733-42. doi: 10.1002/ajhb.22440.

Birch, Leann L., and Jennifer O. Fisher. 1998. "Development of eating behaviors among children and adolescents." *Pediatrics* no. 101 (Supplement 2):539-549.

Birch, Leann L., Jennifer O. Fisher, Karen Grimm-Thomas, Charlotte N. Markey, Richard Sawyer, and Susan L. Johnson. 2001. "Confirmatory factor analysis of the Child Feeding Questionnaire: a measure of parental attitudes, beliefs and practices about child feeding and obesity proneness." *Appetite* no. 36 (3):201-210.

Birch, Leann Lipps. 1980. "Effects of peer models' food choices and eating behaviors on preschoolers' food preferences." *Child development*: 489-496.

Birch, Leann Lipps, Diane Wolfe Marlin, and Julie Rotter. 1984. "Eating as the" means" activity in a contingency: Effects on young children's food preference." *Child development*: 431-439.

Bjelland, M., N. Lien, I. H. Bergh, M. Grydeland, S. A. Anderssen, K. I. Klepp, Y. Ommundsen, and L. F. Andersen. 2010. "Overweight and waist circumference among Norwegian 11-year-olds and associations with reported parental overweight and waist circumference: The HEIA study." *Scand J Public Health* no. 38 (5 Suppl):19-27. doi: 10.1177/1403494810385036.

Blissett, Jackie. 2011. "Relationships between parenting style, feeding style and feeding practices and fruit and vegetable consumption in early childhood." *Appetite* no. 57 (3):826-831.

Bushnik, T., D. Garriguet, and R. Colley. 2017. "Parent-Child association in body weight status." *Health Rep* no. 28 (6):12-19.

Caraza, Karla L. Chávez, Julieta Rodríguez de Ita, Jesús Santos Guzmán, J. G. Segovia Aguirre, D. C. Altamirano Montealvo, and V. M. Matías Barrios. 2016. "Altered perception of the nutritional status of preschoolers by their parents: A risk factor for overweight and obesity." *Arch Argent Pediatr* no. 114 (3):237-242.

Chaparro, M. Pia, Xavier De Luna, Jenny Häggström, Anneli Ivarsson, Urban Lindgren, Karina Nilsson, and Ilona Koupil. 2017. "Childhood family structure and women's adult overweight risk: A longitudinal study." *Scandinavian journal of public health* no. 45 (5):511-519.

Cheng, Tuck Seng, See Ling Loy, Yin Bun Cheung, Jerry Kok Yen Chan, Mya Thway Tint, Keith M. Godfrey, Peter D. Gluckman, Kenneth Kwek, Seang Mei Saw, and Yap-Seng Chong. 2016. "Singaporean mothers' perception of their three-year-old child's weight status: a cross-sectional study." *PLoS One* no. 11 (1):e0147563.

Christofaro, D. G. D., S. M. Andrade, R. A. Fernandes, M. A. S. Cabrera, F. Rodríguez-Artalejo, and A. E. Mesas. 2016. "Overweight parents are twice as likely to underestimate the weight of their teenage children, regardless of their sociodemographic characteristics." *Acta Paediatrica* no. 105 (10):e474-e479.

Crouch, Patrick, Jennifer A. O'dea, and Robert Battisti. 2007. "Child feeding practices and perceptions of childhood overweight and childhood obesity risk among mothers of preschool children." *Nutrition & Dietetics* no. 64 (3):151-158.

da Costa Ribeiro, Isabela, José Augusto A. C. Taddei, and Fernando Colugnatti. 2003. "Obesity among children attending elementary public schools in Sao Paulo, Brazil: a case–control study." *Public Health Nutrition* no. 6 (7):659-663.

Darling, Nancy, and Laurence Steinberg. 1993. "Parenting Style as Context: An Integrative Model." *Psychological Bulletin* no. 113:487-496. doi: 10.1037/0033-2909.113.3.487.

De Bourdeaudhuij, Ilse, Saskia J. Te Velde, Lea Maes, Carmen Pérez-Rodrigo, Maria D. V. de Almeida, and Johannes Brug. 2009. "General parenting styles are not strongly associated with fruit and vegetable intake and social–environmental correlates among 11-year-old children in four countries in Europe." *Public health nutrition* no. 12 (2):259-266.

de Lauzon-Guillain, Blandine, Dara Musher-Eizenman, Emeline Leporc, Shayla Holub, and Marie Aline Charles. 2009. "Parental feeding practices in the United States and in France: relationships with child's characteristics and parent's eating behavior." *Journal of the American Dietetic Association* no. 109 (6):1064-1069.

Dev, Dipti A., Brent A. McBride, Barbara H. Fiese, Blake L. Jones, and on behalf of the STRONG Kids Research Team Cho, Hyunkeun. 2013. "Risk factors for overweight/obesity in preschool children: an ecological approach." *Childhood obesity* no. 9 (5):399-408.

Drenowatz, C., N. Erkelenz, O. Wartha, S. Brandstetter, and J. M. Steinacker. 2014. "Parental characteristics have a larger effect on children's health behaviour than their body weight." *Obes Facts* no. 7 (6):388-98. doi: 10.1159/000369984.

Duncker, Karl. 1938. "Experimental modification of children's food preferences through social suggestion." *The Journal of Abnormal and Social Psychology* no. 33 (4):489.

Ejtahed, H. S., R. Heshmat, M. E. Motlagh, S. Hasani-Ranjbar, H. Ziaodini, M. Taheri, Z. Ahadi, T. Aminaee, G. Shafiee, A. Goodarzi, M. Qorbani, and R. Kelishadi. 2018. "Association of parental obesity with cardiometabolic risk factors in their children: The CASPIAN-V study." *PLoS One* no. 13 (4):e0193978. doi: 10.1371/journal.pone. 0193978.

Faith, Myles S., Linda Van Horn, Lawrence J. Appel, Lora E. Burke, Jo Ann S. Carson, Harold A. Franch, John M. Jakicic, Tanja V. E. Kral, Angela Odoms-Young, and Brian Wansink. 2012. "Evaluating parents and adult caregivers as "agents of change" for treating obese children: evidence for parent behavior change strategies and research gaps: a scientific statement from the American Heart Association." *Circulation* no. 125 (9):1186-1207.

Fasting, M. H., T. I. Nilsen, T. L. Holmen, and T. Vik. 2011. "Changes in parental weight and smoking habits and offspring adiposity: data from the HUNT-study." *Int J Pediatr Obes* no. 6 (2-2):e399-407. doi: 10.3109/17477166.2010.518238.

Feng, Yuejing, Lulu Ding, Xue Tang, Yi Wang, and Chengchao Zhou. 2019. "Association between Maternal Education and School-Age Children Weight Status: A Study from the China Health Nutrition Survey, 2011." *International journal of environmental research and public health* no. 16 (14):2543.

Fertig, Angela, Gerhard Glomm, and Rusty Tchernis. 2009. "The connection between maternal employment and childhood obesity: Inspecting the mechanisms." *Review of Economics of the Household* no. 7 (3):227.

Fisher, Jennifer Orlet, Diane C Mitchell, Helen Smiciklas-Wright, and Leann Lipps Birch. 2002. "Parental influences on young girls' fruit and vegetable, micronutrient, and fat intakes." *Journal of the American dietetic association* no. 102 (1):58-64.

Fitzsimons, Emla, and Benedetta Pongiglione. 2019. "The impact of maternal employment on children's weight: Evidence from the UK." *SSM-population health* no. 7:100333.

Fuemmeler, Bernard F., Chongming Yang, Phil Costanzo, Rick H. Hoyle, Ilene C. Siegler, Redford B. Williams, and Truls Østbye. 2012. "Parenting styles and body mass index trajectories from adolescence to adulthood." *Health Psychology* no. 31 (4):441.

Galloway, Amy T., Laura Fiorito, Yoonna Lee, and Leann L. Birch. 2005. "Parental pressure, dietary patterns, and weight status among girls who are "picky eaters." *Journal of the American Dietetic Association* no. 105 (4):541-548.

Galloway, Amy T., Laura M. Fiorito, Lori A. Francis, and Leann L. Birch. 2006. "'Finish your soup': counterproductive effects of pressuring children to eat on intake and affect." *Appetite* no. 46 (3):318-323.

Gevers, D. W. M., S. P. J. Kremers, N. K. De Vries, and P. Van Assema. 2014. "Clarifying concepts of food parenting practices. A Delphi study with an application to snacking behavior." *Appetite* no. 79:51-57.

Goisis, Alice, Berkay Özcan, and Philippe Van Kerm. 2019. "Do children carry the weight of divorce?" *Demography* no. 56 (3):785-811.

Golley, Rebecca K., G. A. Hendrie, Amy Slater, and N. Corsini. 2011. "Interventions that involve parents to improve children's weight-related nutrition intake and activity patterns–what nutrition and activity targets and behaviour change techniques are associated with intervention effectiveness?" *Obesity reviews* no. 12 (2):114-130.

Greene-Cramer, B., M. B. Harrell, D. M. Hoelscher, S. Sharma, N. Ranjit, V. Gupta, G. Nazar, and M. Arora. 2018. "Association between parent and child weight status among private school children in Delhi, India." *Glob Health Promot* no. 25 (2):67-74. doi: 10.1177/1757975916658002.

Gregori, Dario, Alexander Hochdorn, Danila Azzolina, Paola Berchialla, Giulia Lorenzoni, and OBEY-AD Study Consortium. 2018. "Does love really make mothers blind? A large transcontinental study on mothers' awareness about their children's weight." *Obesity* no. 26 (7):1211-1224.

Gwozdz, Wencke, Alfonso Sousa-Poza, Lucia A. Reisch, Wolfgang Ahrens, Gabriele Eiben, Juan M. Fernandéz-Alvira, Charalampos Hadjigeorgiou, Stefaan De Henauw, Eva Kovács, and Fabio Lauria. 2013. "Maternal employment and childhood obesity–A European perspective." *Journal of Health Economics* no. 32 (4):728-742.

Hancock, Kirsten J., David Lawrence, and Stephen R. Zubrick. 2014. "Higher maternal protectiveness is associated with higher odds of child overweight and obesity: a longitudinal Australian study." *PLoS One* no. 9 (6).

Harper, Lawrence V., and Karen M. Sanders. 1975. "The effect of adults' eating on young children's acceptance of unfamiliar foods." *Journal of experimental child psychology* no. 20 (2):206-214.

Haworth, Claire M. A., Susan Carnell, Emma L. Meaburn, Oliver S. P. Davis, Robert Plomin, and Jane Wardle. 2008. "Increasing heritability of BMI and stronger associations with the FTO gene over childhood." *Obesity* no. 16 (12):2663-2668.

Hennessy, Erin, Sheryl O. Hughes, Jeanne P. Goldberg, Raymond R. Hyatt, and Christina D. Economos. 2010. "Parent behavior and child weight status among a diverse group of underserved rural families." *Appetite* no. 54 (2):369-377.

Hennessy, Erin, Sheryl O. Hughes, Jeanne P. Goldberg, Raymond R. Hyatt, and Christina D. Economos. 2012. "Permissive parental feeding behavior is associated with an increase in intake of low-nutrient-dense foods among American children living in rural communities." *Journal of the Academy of Nutrition and Dietetics* no. 112 (1):142-148.

Hong, Ickpyo, Cynthia Brown Dodds, Patty Coker-Bolt, Annie N. Simpson, and Craig A. Velozo. 2017. "How Accurately Do Both Parents and Health Professionals Assess Overweight in Children?" *Pediatric Physical Therapy* no. 29 (3):283-285.

Hughes, Sheryl O., Leslie A. Frankel, Alicia Beltran, Eric Hodges, Sharon Hoerr, Julie Lumeng, Alison Tovar, and Stef Kremers. 2013. "Food parenting measurement issues: Working group consensus report." *Childhood obesity* no. 9 (s1):S-95-S-102.

Hughes, Sheryl O., Thomas G. Power, Jennifer Orlet Fisher, Stephen Mueller, and Theresa A. Nicklas. 2005. "Revisiting a neglected construct: parenting styles in a child-feeding context." *Appetite* no. 44 (1):83-92.

Hughes, Sheryl O., Thomas G. Power, Maria A. Papaioannou, Matthew B. Cross, Theresa A. Nicklas, Sharon K. Hall, and Richard M. Shewchuk. 2011. "Emotional climate, feeding practices, and feeding styles: an observational analysis of the dinner meal in Head Start families." *International Journal of Behavioral Nutrition and Physical Activity* no. 8 (1):60.

Jaaskelainen, A., J. Pussinen, O. Nuutinen, U. Schwab, J. Pirkola, M. Kolehmainen, M. R. Jarvelin, and J. Laitinen. 2011. "Intergenerational transmission of overweight among Finnish adolescents and their parents: a 16-year follow-up study." *Int J Obes (Lond)* no. 35 (10):1289-94. doi: 10.1038/ijo.2011.150.

Jalali-Farahani, Sara, Parisa Amiri, Behnood Abbasi, Mehrdad Karimi, Leila Cheraghi, Maryam Sadat Daneshpour, and Fereidoun Azizi. 2017. "Maternal characteristics and incidence of overweight/obesity in children: a 13-year follow-up study in an Eastern Mediterranean population." *Maternal and child health journal* no. 21 (5):1211-1220.

Jalali-Farahani, Sara, Yit Siew Chin, Mohd Nasir Mohd Taib, and Parisa Amiri. 2017. "Parental Correlates of Body Weight Status Among High School Students in Tehran." *International journal of endocrinology and metabolism* no. 15 (2).

Jiang, Mo-han, Yang Yang, Xiao-fan Guo, and Ying-xian Sun. 2013. "Association between child and adolescent obesity and parental weight status: a cross-sectional study from rural North China." *Journal of international medical research* no. 41 (4):1326-1332.

Keane, Eimear, Richard Layte, Janas Harrington, Patricia M. Kearney, and Ivan J. Perry. 2012. "Measured parental weight status and familial socio-economic status correlates with childhood overweight and obesity at age 9." *PloS one* no. 7 (8).

Kerr, Jessica A., Catherine Long, Susan A. Clifford, Joshua Muller, Alanna N. Gillespie, Susan Donath, and Melissa Wake. 2017. "Early-life exposures predicting onset and resolution of childhood overweight or obesity." *Archives of Disease in Childhood* no. 102 (10):915-922.

Knight, Bridget, Beverley M. Shields, Anita Hill, Roy J. Powell, David Wright, and Andrew T. Hattersley. 2007. "The impact of maternal glycemia and obesity on early postnatal growth in a nondiabetic Caucasian population." *Diabetes Care* no. 30 (4):777-783.

Koerner, Ascan F., and Mary Anne Fitzpatrick. 2006. "Family communication patterns theory: A social cognitive approach." *Engaging theories in family communication: Multiple perspectives*:50-65.

Lazzeri, Giacomo, Andrea Pammolli, Valentina Pilato, and Mariano V. Giacchi. 2011. "Relationship between 8/9-yr-old school children BMI, parents' BMI and educational level: a cross sectional survey." *Nutrition journal* no. 10 (1):76.

Leppers, Iris, Henning Tiemeier, Sonja A. Swanson, Frank C. Verhulst, Vincent W. V. Jaddoe, Oscar H. Franco, and Pauline W. Jansen. 2017. "Agreement between weight status and perceived body size and the association with body size satisfaction in children." *Obesity* no. 25 (11):1956-1964.

Ling, Jiying, and Manfred Stommel. 2019. "Parental and Self-Weight Perceptions in US Children and Adolescents, NHANES 2005-2014." *Western journal of nursing research* no. 41 (1):42-57.

Liu, Y., H. J. Chen, L. Liang, and Y. Wang. 2013. "Parent-child resemblance in weight status and its correlates in the United States." *PLoS One* no. 8 (6):e65361. doi: 10. 1371/journal.pone.0065361.

Lobsetin, T., L. Baur, and R. Uauy. 2004. "IASO International Obesity Task Force. Obesity in children and young people: a crisis in public health." *Obesity Reviews* no. 5 (4,104).

Lohaus, Arnold, Marc Vierhaus, and Juliane Ball. 2009. "Parenting styles and health-related behavior in childhood and early adolescence: Results of a longitudinal study." *The Journal of Early Adolescence* no. 29 (4):449-475.

Lydecker, Janet A., and Carlos M. Grilo. 2016. "The apple of their eye: Attitudinal and behavioral correlates of parents' perceptions of child obesity." *Obesity* no. 24 (5):1124-1131.

Maddah, M., and B. Nikooyeh. 2010. "Factors associated with overweight in children in Rasht, Iran: gender, maternal education, skipping breakfast and parental obesity." *Public Health Nutr* no. 13 (2):196-200. doi: 10.1017/s1368980009990589.

Manios, Y., G. Moschonis, E. Grammatikaki, A. Anastasiadou, and T. Liarigkovinos. 2010. "Determinants of childhood obesity and association with maternal perceptions of their children's weight status: the "GENESIS" study." *J Am Diet Assoc* no. 110 (10):1527-31. doi: 10.1016/j.jada.2010.07.004.

Manios, Yannis, George Moschonis, Kalliopi Karatzi, Odysseas Androutsos, Mai Chinapaw, Luis A Moreno, Elling Bere, Denes Molnar, Natasha Jan, and Alain Dössegger. 2015. "Large proportions of overweight and obese children, as well as their parents, underestimate children's weight status across Europe. The ENERGY (EuropeaN Energy balance Research to prevent excessive weight Gain among Youth) project." *Public health nutrition* no. 18 (12):2183-2190.

Martinovic, M., G. Belojevic, G. W. Evans, D. Lausevic, B. Asanin, M. Samardzic, N. Terzic, S. Pantovic, M. Jaksic, and J. Boljevic. 2015. "Prevalence of and contributing factors for overweight and obesity among Montenegrin schoolchildren." *Eur J Public Health* no. 25 (5):833-9. doi: 10.1093/eurpub/ckv071.

McCarthy, K., Y. L. Ye, S. Yuan, and Q. Q. He. 2015. "Parental weight status and offspring cardiovascular disease risks: a cross-sectional study of Chinese children." *Prev Chronic Dis* no. 12:E01. doi: 10.5888/pcd12.140384.

McCoby, E. E. 1983. "Socialization in the context of the family: Parent-child interaction." *Handbook of child psychology* no. 4:1-101.

McDonald, Sheila W., Heather K. Ginez, Angela E. Vinturache, and Suzanne C. Tough. 2016. "Maternal perceptions of underweight and overweight for 6–8 years olds from a Canadian cohort: reporting weights, concerns and conversations with healthcare providers." *BMJ open* no. 6 (10):e012094.

Mei, Hong, Siyu Guo, Hongyan Lu, Yunhong Pan, Wenhua Mei, Bin Zhang, and Jianduan Zhang. 2018. "Impact of parental weight status on children's body mass index in early life: evidence from a Chinese cohort." *BMJ open* no. 8 (6):e018755.

Menezes, R. C., P. I. Lira, J. S. Oliveira, V. S. Leal, S. C. Santana, S. L. Andrade, and M. Batista Filho. 2011. "Prevalence and determinants of overweight in preschool children." *J Pediatr (Rio J)* no. 87 (3):231-7. doi: 10.2223/jped.2092.

Meredith-Jones, Kim, Sheila Williams, and Rachael Taylor. 2016. "Agreement between parental perception of child weight status and actual weight status is similar across different ethnic groups in New Zealand." *Journal of primary health care* no. 8 (4):316-324.

Min, Jungwon, Vivian H. C. Wang, Hong Xue, Jie Mi, and Youfa Wang. 2017. "Maternal perception of child overweight status and its association with weight-related parenting practices, their children's health behaviours and weight change in China." *Public health nutrition* no. 20 (12):2096-2103.

Moore, L. C., C. V. Harris, and A. S. Bradlyn. 2012. "Exploring the relationship between parental concern and the management of childhood obesity." *Matern Child Health J* no. 16 (4):902-8. doi: 10.1007/s10995-011-0813-x.

Mulder, Christiaan, Juliana Kain, Ricardo Uauy, and Jaap C. Seidell. 2009. "Maternal attitudes and child-feeding practices: relationship with the BMI of Chilean children." *Nutrition journal* no. 8 (1):37.

Muthuri, Stella K., Vincent O. Onywera, Mark S. Tremblay, Stephanie T. Broyles, Jean-Philippe Chaput, Mikael Fogelholm, Gang Hu, Rebecca Kuriyan, Anura Kurpad, and Estelle V. Lambert. 2016. "Relationships between parental education and overweight with childhood overweight and physical activity in 9–11 year old children: Results from a 12-country study." *PloS one* no. 11 (8).

Naess, M., E. R. Sund, T. L. Holmen, and K. Kvaloy. 2018. "Implications of parental lifestyle changes and education level on adolescent offspring weight: a population based cohort study - The HUNT Study, Norway." *BMJ Open* no. 8 (8):e023406. doi: 10.1136/bmjopen-2018-023406.

Nemecek, Daniela, Christian Sebelefsky, Astrid Woditschka, and Peter Voitl. 2017. "Overweight in children and its perception by parents: cross-sectional observation in a general pediatric outpatient clinic." *BMC pediatrics* no. 17 (1):212.

Nie, Peng, and Alfonso Sousa-Poza. 2014. "Maternal employment and childhood obesity in China: evidence from the China Health and Nutrition Survey." *Applied Economics* no. 46 (20):2418-2428.

Noonan, R. J., and S. J. Fairclough. 2018. "Is there a deprivation and maternal education gradient to child obesity and moderate-to-vigorous physical activity? Findings from the Millennium Cohort Study." *Pediatric obesity* no. 13 (7):458-464.

Ntenda, P. A. M., T. G. Mhone, and O. Nkoka. 2019. "High Maternal Body Mass Index Is Associated with an Early-Onset of Overweight/Obesity in Pre-School-Aged Children in Malawi. A Multilevel Analysis of the 2015-16 Malawi Demographic and Health Survey." *J Trop Pediatr* no. 65 (2):147-159. doi: 10.1093/tropej/fmy028.

Oddo, Vanessa M., Sara N. Bleich, Keshia M. Pollack, Pamela J. Surkan, Noel T. Mueller, and Jessica C. Jones-Smith. 2017. "The weight of work: the association between maternal employment and overweight in low-and middle-income countries." *International Journal of Behavioral Nutrition and Physical Activity* no. 14 (1):66.

Olvera, Norma, and Thomas G. Power. 2010. "Brief report: parenting styles and obesity in Mexican American children: a longitudinal study." *Journal of pediatric psychology* no. 35 (3):243-249.

Ostbye, T., R. Malhotra, M. Stroo, C. Lovelady, R. Brouwer, N. Zucker, and B. Fuemmeler. 2013. "The effect of the home environment on physical activity and dietary intake in preschool children." *Int J Obes (Lond)* no. 37 (10):1314-21. doi: 10. 1038/ijo.2013.76.

Park, Min Hae, Catherine L. Falconer, Helen Croker, Sonia Saxena, Anthony S. Kessel, Russell M. Viner, and Sanjay Kinra. 2014. "Predictors of health-related behaviour change in parents of overweight children in England." *Preventive medicine* no. 62:20-24.

Portela, Daniel S., Tatiana O. Vieira, Sheila M. A. Matos, Nelson F. de Oliveira, and Graciete O. Vieira. 2015. "Maternal obesity, environmental factors, cesarean delivery and breastfeeding as determinants of overweight and obesity in children: results from a cohort." *BMC pregnancy and childbirth* no. 15 (1):94.

Regber, Susann, Masuma Novak, Gabriele Eiben, Karin Bammann, Stefaan De Henauw, Juan M. Fernández-Alvira, Wencke Gwozdz, Yiannis Kourides, Luis Alberto Moreno, and Dénes Molnar. 2013. "Parental perceptions of and concerns about child's body weight in eight E uropean countries–the IDEFICS study." *Pediatric obesity* no. 8 (2):118-129.

Regnault, Nolwenn, Jérémie Botton, Anne Forhan, Régis Hankard, Olivier Thiebaugeorges, Teresa A. Hillier, Monique Kaminski, Barbara Heude, and Marie-Aline Charles. 2010. "Determinants of early ponderal and statural growth in full-term infants in the EDEN mother-child cohort study." *The American journal of clinical nutrition* no. 92 (3):594-602.

Rhee, Kyung E., Julie C. Lumeng, Danielle P. Appugliese, Niko Kaciroti, and Robert H. Bradley. 2006. "Parenting styles and overweight status in first grade." *Pediatrics* no. 117 (6):2047-2054.

Robinson, Eric, and Angelina R. Sutin. 2016. "Parental perception of weight status and weight gain across childhood." *Pediatrics* no. 137 (5):e20153957.

Rodenburg, Gerda, Stef P. J. Kremers, Anke Oenema, and Dike van de Mheen. 2012. "Associations of children's appetitive traits with weight and dietary behaviours in the context of general parenting." *PloS one* no. 7 (12).

Ruiz, Milagros, Peter Goldblatt, Joana Morrison, Daniela Porta, Francesco Forastiere, Daniel Hryhorczuk, Youriy Antipkin, Marie-Josèphe Saurel-Cubizolles, Sandrine Lioret, and Martine Vrijheid. 2016. "Impact of low maternal education on early childhood overweight and obesity in Europe." *Paediatric and perinatal epidemiology* no. 30 (3):274-284.

Savage, Jennifer S., Jennifer Orlet Fisher, and Leann L. Birch. 2007. "Parental influence on eating behavior: conception to adolescence." *The Journal of law, medicine & ethics* no. 35 (1):22-34.

Schmeer, Kammi K. 2012. "Family structure and obesity in early childhood." *Social Science Research* no. 41 (4):820-832.

Seburg, Elisabeth M., Alicia Kunin-Batson, Meghan M. Senso, A. Lauren Crain, Shelby L. Langer, and Nancy E. Sherwood. 2014. "Concern about child weight among parents of children at-risk for obesity." *Health behavior and policy review* no. 1 (3):197-208.

Shafaghi, K., Z. M. Shariff, M. N. Taib, H. A. Rahman, M. G. Mobarhan, and H. Jabbari. 2014. "Parental body mass index is associated with adolescent overweight and obesity in Mashhad, Iran." *Asia Pac J Clin Nutr* no. 23 (2):225-31. doi: 10.6133/apjcn. 2014.23.2.11.

Shiely, F., H. Y. Ng, E. M. Berkery, C. Murrin, C. Kelleher, and K. Hayes. 2017. "The association between weight perception and BMI: report and measurement data from the growing up in Ireland cohort study of 9-year olds." *International Journal of Obesity* no. 41 (1):46-53.

Shloim, Netalie, Lisa R Edelson, Nathalie Martin, and Marion M Hetherington. 2015. "Parenting styles, feeding styles, feeding practices, and weight status in 4–12 year-old children: A systematic review of the literature." *Frontiers in psychology* no. 6:1849.

Silventoinen, Karri, Charlotte Huppertz, Catharina E. M. van Beijsterveldt, Meike Bartels, Gonneke Willemsen, and Dorret I. Boomsma. 2016. "The genetic architecture of body mass index from infancy to adulthood modified by parental education." *Obesity* no. 24 (9):2004-2011.

Sleddens, Ster F. C., Sanne M. P. L. Gerards, Carel Thijs, Nanne K. De Vries, and Stef P. J. Kremers. 2011. "General parenting, childhood overweight and obesity-inducing behaviors: a review." *International journal of pediatric obesity* no. 6 (sup3):e12-27.

Sokol, Rebeccah L., Bo Qin, and Jennifer M. Poti. 2017. "Parenting styles and body mass index: a systematic review of prospective studies among children." *Obesity Reviews* no. 18 (3):281-292.

Stettler, Nicolas, Andrew M. Tershakovec, Babette S. Zemel, Mary B. Leonard, Raymond C. Boston, Solomon H. Katz, and Virginia A. Stallings. 2000. "Early risk factors for increased adiposity: a cohort study of African American subjects followed from birth to young adulthood." *The American journal of clinical nutrition* no. 72 (2):378-383.

Stunkard, A. J., R. I. Berkowitz, D. Schoeller, G. Maislin, and V. A. Stallings. 2004. "Predictors of body size in the first 2 y of life: a high-risk study of human obesity." *International journal of obesity* no. 28 (4):503-513.

Tschann, Jeanne M., Suzanna M. Martinez, Carlos Penilla, Steven E. Gregorich, Lauri A. Pasch, Cynthia L. De Groat, Elena Flores, Julianna Deardorff, Louise C. Greenspan, and Nancy F. Butte. 2015. "Parental feeding practices and child weight status in Mexican American families: a longitudinal analysis." *International Journal of Behavioral Nutrition and Physical Activity* no. 12 (1):66.

Valerio, Giuliana, Osvaldo D'Amico, Michele Adinolfi, Anna Munciguerra, Rosa D'Amico, and Adriana Franzese. 2006. "Determinants of weight gain in children from 7 to 10 years." *Nutrition, metabolism and cardiovascular diseases* no. 16 (4):272-278.

Vallejo, Maite, Beatriz A. Cortes-Rodríguez, and Eloisa Colin-Ramirez. 2015. "Maternal underestimation of child's weight status and health behaviors as risk factors for overweight in children." *Journal of pediatric nursing* no. 30 (6):e29-e33.

Vaughn, Amber E., Dianne S. Ward, Jennifer O. Fisher, Myles S. Faith, Sheryl O. Hughes, Stef P. J. Kremers, Dara R. Musher-Eizenman, Teresia M. O'Connor, Heather Patrick, and Thomas G. Power. 2016. "Fundamental constructs in food parenting practices: a content map to guide future research." *Nutrition reviews* no. 74 (2):98-117.

Ventura, Alison K., and Leann L. Birch. 2008. "Does parenting affect children's eating and weight status?" *International Journal of Behavioral Nutrition and Physical Activity* no. 5 (1):15.

Vollmer, Rachel L., and Jamey Baietto. 2017. "Practices and preferences: Exploring the relationships between food-related parenting practices and child food preferences for high fat and/or sugar foods, fruits, and vegetables." *Appetite* no. 113:134-140.

Vollmer, Rachel L., and Amy R. Mobley. 2013. "Parenting styles, feeding styles, and their influence on child obesogenic behaviors and body weight. A review." *Appetite* no. 71:232-241.

Wardle, Jane, and Susan Carnell. 2007. "Parental feeding practices and children's weight." *Acta Paediatrica* no. 96:5-11.

Warkentin, Sarah, Laís A. Mais, Maria do Rosário Dias de Latorre, Susan Carnell, and José Augusto de Aguiar Carrazedo Taddei. 2018. "Parents matter: associations of parental BMI and feeding behaviors with child BMI in Brazilian preschool and school-aged children." *Frontiers in nutrition* no. 5:69.

Weng, Stephen Franklin, Sarah A. Redsell, Judy A. Swift, Min Yang, and Cristine P. Glazebrook. 2012. "Systematic review and meta-analyses of risk factors for childhood overweight identifiable during infancy." *Archives of disease in childhood* no. 97 (12): 1019-1026.

Whitaker, K. L., M. J. Jarvis, R. J. Beeken, D. Boniface, and J. Wardle. 2010. "Comparing maternal and paternal intergenerational transmission of obesity risk in a large population-based sample." *Am J Clin Nutr* no. 91 (6):1560-7. doi: 10.3945/ajcn. 2009.28838.

Xi, B, J Mi, JL Duan, SJ Yan, Hong Cheng, DQ Hou, and XY Zhao. 2009. "Familial clustering of obesity and the role of lifestyle factors among children in Beijing." *Zhonghua yu fang yi xue za zhi [Chinese journal of preventive medicine]* no. 43 (2):122-127.

Xue, Fei, Walter C. Willett, Bernard A. Rosner, Michele R. Forman, and Karin B. Michels. 2008. "Parental characteristics as predictors of birthweight." *Human reproduction* no. 23 (1):168-177.

Yannakoulia, Mary, Katerina Papanikolaou, Ioanna Hatzopoulou, Eleftheria Efstathiou, Constantina Papoutsakis, and George V. Dedoussis. 2008. "Association between family divorce and children's BMI and meal patterns: the GENDAI Study." *Obesity* no. 16 (6):1382-1387.

Yee, Andrew Z. H., May O. Lwin, and Shirley S. Ho. 2017. "The influence of parental practices on child promotive and preventive food consumption behaviors: a systematic review and meta-analysis." *International Journal of Behavioral Nutrition and Physical Activity* no. 14 (1):47.

Zalbahar, Nurzalinda, Hamid Jan B. Jan Mohamed, See Ling Loy, Jake Najman, Harold David McIntyre, and Abdullah Mamun. 2016. "Association of parental body mass index before pregnancy on infant growth and body composition: evidence from a pregnancy cohort study in Malaysia." *Obesity Research & Clinical Practice* no. 10:S35-S47.

Zhang, Q., R. Lamichhane, H. J. Chen, H. Xue, and Y. Wang. 2014. "Does child-parent resemblance in body weight status vary by sociodemographic factors in the USA?" *J Epidemiol Community Health* no. 68 (11):1034-42. doi: 10.1136/jech-2013-203476.

Zhang, Ting, Li Cai, Jin Jing, Lu Ma, Jun Ma, and Yajun Chen. 2018. "Parental perception of child weight and its association with weight-related parenting behaviours and child behaviours: a Chinese national study." *Public health nutrition* no. 21 (9):1671-1680.

Zong, Xin-Nan, Hui Li, and Ya-Qin Zhang. 2015. "Family-related risk factors of obesity among preschool children: results from a series of national epidemiological surveys in China." *BMC Public Health* no. 15 (1):927.

In: Childhood Obesity
Editor: Roya Kelishadi
ISBN: 978-1-53618-158-6
© 2020 Nova Science Publishers, Inc.

Chapter 9

CARDIOVASCULAR SYSTEM IN CHILDHOOD OBESITY

Bahar Dehghan**, MD

Pediatric Cardiology Research Center, Cardiovascular Research Institute,
Isfahan University of Medical Sciences, Isfahan, Iran

ABSTRACT

Childhood obesity is well-known to be associated with established risk factors for cardiovascular diseases including hypertension, atherosclerosis, and cardiac structural and functional changes, especially in the left ventricle. Because of these serious consequences, it is very important for health professionals to find children at risk and provide proper help as needed. Most studies have confirmed that childhood and adulthood obesity, as risk factors of cardiovascular diseases, origin from fetal life. Some environmental stimuli or insults during critical periods in early life might affect later health.

By 2020, the prevalence of heart disease and die of heart disease will rise in young adults, if nothing would be done. Several investigators have demonstrated that certain pharmacologic and/or non-pharmacologic treatments may have an influence on some of these risk factors. Thus, appropriate interventions from early life may reduce these risks.

Several investigators have evaluated the effects of obesity on vascular and myocardial performance all around the world; echocardiography is a non-invasive tool to measure cardiac function and dimensions. Some of these changes are reversible with weight reduction.

In this chapter we will review this correlation between obesity indices and cardiac and vascular measures in different ages from childhood to adolescence and the effect of weight loss on these parameters.

Keywords: childhood obesity, coronary artery disease, atherosclerosis, prevention

---

* Corresponding Author's Email: dr.bahardehghan@gmail.com.

INTRODUCTION

Childhood obesity is already a global epidemic. No age group is safe from this danger; it has been estimated that 1 in 10 children *under the age of 5* are obese in US [1]. By 2030, cardiovascular diseases are expected to account for more than 30% of deaths worldwide [2]. While the mortality rate in high-income countries has declined in recent years, it remains about 50% in low- and middle-income countries mostly in the Eastern Mediterranean Region [3]. Therefore, planning for prevention and control of cardiovascular disease and its risk factors, such as obesity, are the most important measures.

Childhood obesity is well-known to be associated with established risk factors for cardiovascular diseases, including hypertension, atherosclerosis, and cardiac structural and functional changes principally of the left ventricle. Because of these serious consequences, it is very important for health professionals to find children at risk and provide proper help as needed. The American Heart Association (AHA) and the American Academy of Pediatrics (AAP) have put emphasis on the primordial and primary prevention to reduce coronary vascular disease (CVD) risks from an early age [4, 5]. According to the recent AHA scientific statement 2019, there are multiple CVD risk factors which present in childhood (for example: familial hypercholesterolemia, hypertension, severe obesity, diabetes mellitus, chronic renal failure, childhood tumor managements, and chronic inflammatory diseases such as juvenile inflammatory arthritis, systemic lupus erythematous). In addition, children and adolescents with underlying heart disease, whether structural (Coarctation of aorta, Tetralogy of Fallot) or after certain surgeries (arterial switch for Transposition of great arteries, Ross procedure for Bicuspid aortic valve, Fontan), are also prone to future CVD [6]. Those with underlying coronary artery abnormalities, either congenital (anomalous origin of left coronary artery from pulmonary artery) or acquired (Kawasaki disease, sickle cell disease), should be considered as high-risk conditions that promote atherosclerosis as well [7].

Several studies have confirmed that child and adulthood obesity as risk factors for cardiovascular diseases, origin from fetal life. Maternal diet during pregnancy is an important factor that affects the programming of the fetus genes. In the status of maternal malnutrition, changes in production of fetal and placental hormones adjust metabolism, distribution of blood flow to the fetus and body growth [8, 9]. In this chapter we review this correlation between obesity and cardiovascular measures in different periods of life and the effect of weight loss on these parameters.

CHILDHOOD OBESITY AND CARDIOVASCULAR EFFECTS

Hypertension

Research from different countries have revealed that the prevalence of increased blood pressure in (non-selected) pediatric population aged 3–18 years with normal weight is 3–5%, in overweight 4–14%, and in obese 11–33% [10]. It is quite well known that body weight and blood pressure are closely correlated and long-term high blood pressure will increase the risk of end-organ damage. That is why prevention of obesity is so strongly emphasized. Current guidelines endorse regular screening of high blood pressure in all children from 3 years old and at least once a year [4, 5]. In at risk individuals ambulatory monitoring is more preferred because it can better detect changes in blood pressure throughout the day [11].

Elevated childhood arterial blood pressure predicts worse carotid artery intima-media thickness and coronary artery calcification, which are specific markers of arterial insults and coronary atherosclerosis in middle age as well [12-14]. In a study, Magnussen et al., [15] showed that in young patients who could lessen their high blood pressures, carotid intima media thickness also returned to measures similar to adults with normal blood pressure. As a result, treatment should begin as soon as the diagnosis is made. Literatures show changes in lifestyle for blood pressure and weight control may have not been successful in children in the long run [16]. Accordingly antihypertensive treatment is recommended for children who have persistent hypertension despite nonpharmacologic treatments [17]. Current research suggests that adiposity and blood pressure have a greater effect on left ventricular geometry when present together than each alone. Normalization of left ventricular mass in obese hypertensive individuals is achieved when both the person's blood pressure normalizes and their weight decreases [18].

In this regard, treatment of hypertension in pediatric population should include modification of lifestyle and pharmacotherapy to decrease both short and long term complications. According to the Dietary Approaches to Stop Hypertension (DASH) recommendations, for therapeutic lifestyle, patients need to have a diet rich in fruit and vegetables, whole grains and lean proteins combining to low or no fat dairy. Diet low in sodium (< 2300 mg/d) is recommended as well. Moderate to vigorous physical activity (≥ 5 hour/week) is advised. Pharmacotherapy choices should be personalized to each individual. The aim is reduction of blood pressure to below 90% of the age-sex-height–referenced norm or < 130/80 mm Hg, whichever is less [6, 19].

Cardiac Structural and Functional Changes

Obesity in childhood and adolescent periods has robust impacts on structure and function of the heart, especially the left ventricle (LV) which can be proved by echocardiography and cardiac magnetic resonance [20].

Several studies confirmed that increased body mass index (BMI) and adiposity cause left ventricular hypertrophy and dilation (Figure 1) which will increase cardiac work [21]. This may lead to increased LV mass, lower ejection fraction (EF), decreased myocardial contractility, and inability of the left atrium (LA) to fill the left ventricle completely [22]. Taken together, these events eventually lead to congestive heart failure (CHF). Figure 2. Illustrates these cardiac structural and functional changes in obese subjects [23].

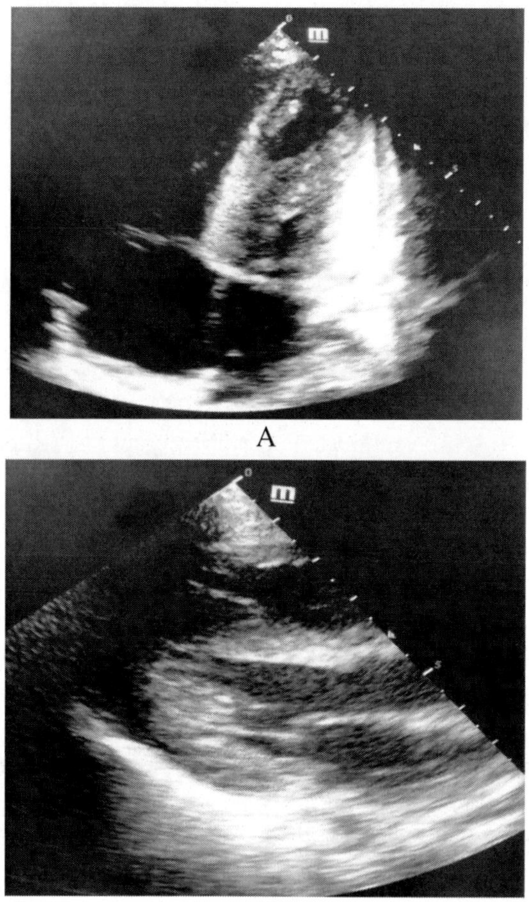

Figure 1. 2D echocardiographic findings indicate left ventricular hypertrophy in a 5 year old boy with hypertension. A: 4 chamber view. B: Long axis view.

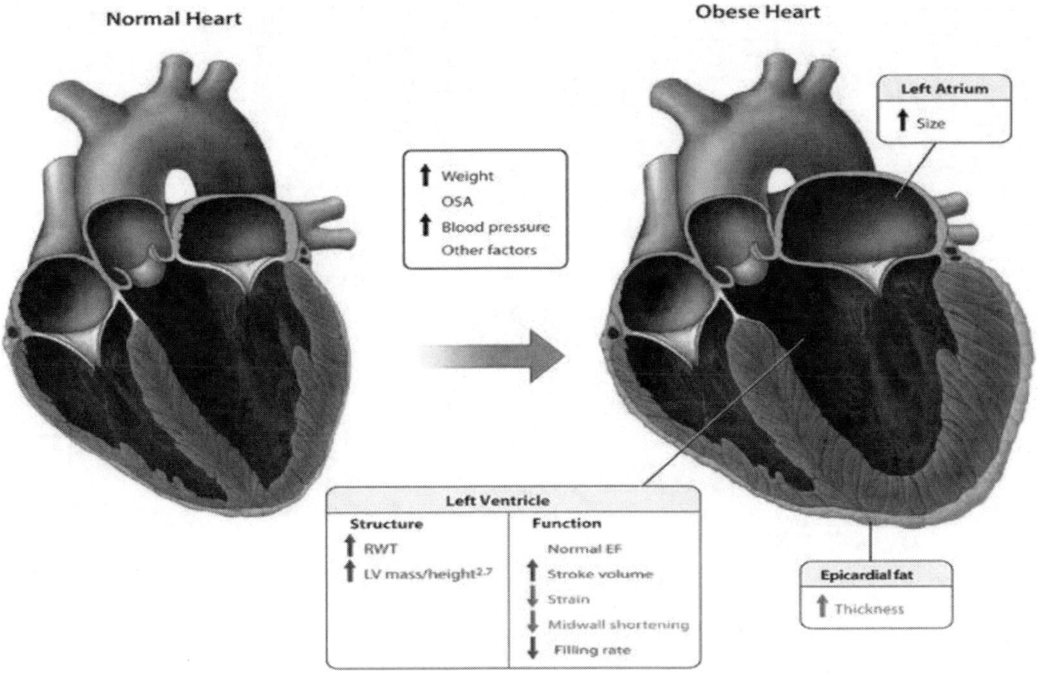

Figure 2. Cardiac structural and functional abnormalities in obesity. EF: ejection fraction; LV: left ventricle; OSA: obstructive sleep apnea; RWT: relative wall thickness. (Courtesy of Dr. Fitzgibbons)

Zhu et al., [24] have shown that left ventricular mass index, cardiac output, overnight sodium excretion, and ambulatory and nocturnal BP measurements are phenotypes that predict CVD threat in over weight and obese youth.

Research in children is ongoing to upgrade identifying predictors of CVD risk by advanced echocardiographic measures. Zhang et al., [25] showed that LV 3D strain is more sensitive than other echocardiographic variables to identify cardiovascular changes in obese children. This variable may detect early subclinical LV myocardial dysfunction in obese normotensive children even sooner than other changes occur such as reduced ejection fraction. Figure 3. Shows these changes on LV global longitudinal strain in an obese child.

However, research demonstrates that these obesity-induced structural and functional cardiac effects will be reversible throughout teenage years with weight reduction. Erbs et al. [26] showed that these improvements occur in LV mass index, left venricular hypertrophy (LVH), LA volume index, global longitudinal LV strain and strain rate. Interestingly, the method of weight reduction is not important. Also, It has been shown that twelve weeks of high intensity interval and moderate intensity continuous trainings are more effective than dietary recommendations alone on improving resting LV systolic dysfunction in obese children [27].

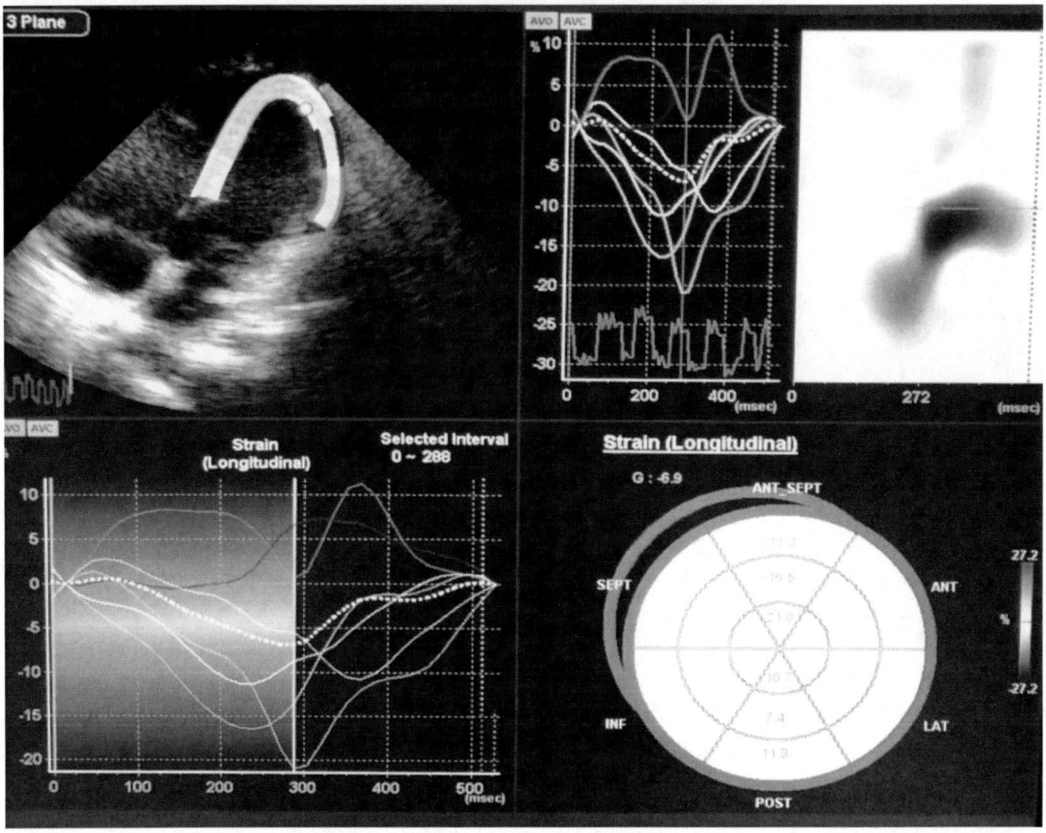

Figure 3. The 2-dimensional global longitudinal strain of the left ventricle in an11 year old obese girl. The color-coded curves in 16 segments indicate diminished myocardial function in different regions in this obese child.

Premature Coronary Artery Disease

Coronary artery disease (CAD) is a multifactorial polygenic disease. It results from damaging effects of different stimuli on arterial wall endothelium by causing inflammation. Inflammation is the principal cause of atherosclerosis as it may disturb lipoprotein metabolism and arterial wall nature [28]. The impact of childhood obesity on future cardiovascular health is well known. Significant morbidities and even deaths from premature ischemic heart disease (before the age of 49) have been proven [21, 29].

Recently scientists have evaluated the genetic relationship among BMI and CAD with study on alleles and demonstrated that there is a causal correlation between BMI and CAD risk. Cole et al., [30] demonstrated that obesity alone is an independent cause of CAD rather than due to the confounding effects on other risk factors such as diabetes mellitus. In addition, new research is identifying biomarkers which may play role in decreasing premature CAD and central obesity such as interleukin 33-rs7044343 T allele [31].

The Importance of Early Life

Several studies [32] have proposed that child and adulthood obesity as risk factors of cardiovascular diseases origin from fetal life. Some environmental stimuli or insults during critical periods in early life affect later health. These early environmental influences are defined by Lucas et al. [8] as "the idea that stimuli or insults during critical or sensitive periods in early life can have lifetime consequences". Three of these critical periods occur during fetal life, the first couple of years of life and at the time of adiposity rebound as early as 5–11 years of age [33].

Dr. David Barker first promoted the idea of fetal origins of adult disease (FOAD). Low birth weight has been known to be associated with coronary artery disease, high blood pressure, insulin resistance, and fatness in future [34]. Calkins et al. [35] have reviewed the consequences of the FOAD further than the low birth weight population. They considered babies exposed to nutritional and non-nutritional insults, during those critical periods of growth, which lead to a chronic adulthood disease. They emphasize that not only maternal starvation and malnutrition influence on neonatal health but also other biological basis (e.g., large for gestational age, stunting, and even rapid weight gain) and environmental factors (high-calorie and high-fat diet, limited active play and excessive media viewing) are associated with coronary artery diseases and hypertension. These unfavorable changes on myocardial function have been detected as early as first trimester both in obese and diabetic mothers [36, 37]. In a study Ingul et al., [38] demonstrated that cardiac function in newborns of obese mothers has decreased compared to normal weight mothers.

Prevention

All data prove the great impact of obesity on cardiovascular system; however, these malicious effects can be prevented from childhood through proper planning and management.

Today, it is properly known that variable stress during growth and developmental periods disturb genetic, structure, and metabolism function resulting in cognitive, behavioral, and body composition which may eventually leading to upcoming disorders [8].

Accordingly, the governments must take measures for community health prevention, medical treatments, and new nutritional/environmental policies to promote population well-being. Pediatricians, obstetricians, perinatalogists, neonatologists, pediatric cardiologists, and everybody who endorse growth during pregnancy, neonatal, infancy, and childhood periods have to be part of these strategies.

Clinicians should monitor the fetus, and later the baby, infant, child and adult when undergoing an adverse pregnancy environment, and understand how these adverse effects can be prohibited or retreated.

REFERENCES

[1] Messiah, SE. Lebron, CN. Arheart, KL. Lipshultz, SE. Miller, TL. (2019). Prevalence of the Metabolic Syndrome in US Youth. Global Perspectives on Childhood Obesity (Second Edition) *Current Status, Consequences and Prevention*, 49-58. https://doi.org/10.1016/B978-0-12-374995-6.10010-6.

[2] Mozaffarian, D. Benjamin, EJ. Go, AS. Arnett, DK. Blaha, MJ, Cushman, M. Das, SR. Ferranti, SD. Després, JP. Fullerton, HJ. Howard, VJ. Huffman, MD. Isasi, CR. Jiménez, MC. Judd,SE. Kissela, BM. Lichtman, JH. Lisabeth, LD. Liu, S. Mackey, RH. Magid, DJ. McGuire, DK. MohlerIII, ER. Moy, CS. Muntner, P. Mussolino, ME. Nasir, Kh. Neumar, RW. Nichol, G. Palaniappan, L. Pandey, DK. Reeves, MJ. Rodriguez, CJ. Rosamond, W. Sorlie, PD. Stein, J. Towfighi, A. Turan, TN. Virani, SS. Woo, D. Yeh, RW. and Turner MB. (2015). Heart disease and stroke statistics-2015 update: a report from the American Heart Association. *Circulation*,131(4):e29-322. doi: 10.1161/ CIR.0000000000000152.

[3] Sarrafzadegan, N. Mohammadifard, N. (2019). Cardiovascular Disease in Iran in the Last 40 Years: Prevalence, Mortality, Morbidity, Challenges and Strategies for Cardiovascular Prevention. *Arch. Iran. Med.*, 22(4):204-210.

[4] Weintraub, WS. Daniels, SR. Burke, LE. Franklin, BA. Goff, DC. Hayman, LL. Lloyd-Jones, D. Pandey, DK. Sanchez, EJ. Schram, AP. Whitsel, LP. (2011). Value of primordial and primary prevention for cardiovascular disease: a policy statement from the American Heart Association. *Circulation,* 124:967–90. doi: 10.1161/CIR.0b013e3182285a81 10.

[5] Expert Panel on Integrated Guidelines for Cardiovascular Health and Risk Reduction in Children and Adolescents; National Heart, Lung, and Blood Institute: summary report. (2011) *Pediatrics,* 128(Suppl 5):S213–56. doi: 10.1542/peds.2009-2107C.

[6] Ferranti, SD. Steinberger, J. Ameduri, R. Baker, A. Gooding, H. Kelly, AS. Snyder, MM. Mitsnefes, MM. Peterson, AL. St-Pierre, J. Urbina, EM. Zachariah, JP. Zaidi, AN. (2019) Cardiovascular Risk Reduction in High-Risk Pediatric Patients. *A Scientific Statement From the American Heart Association.* Circulation, 139 (13): e603-e634. doi: 10.1161/CIR.0000000000000618.

[7] Francis, J. (2018) Coronary Artery Disease in Children. *BMH Med. J.*,5(3):64-66.

[8] Lucas, A. Fewtrell, MS. Cole, TJ. (1999). Fetal origins of adult disease – the hypothesis revisited. *BMJ,* 319:245.

[9] Kwon, EJ. Kim, YJ. (2017). What is fetal programming?: a lifetime health is under the control of in utero health. *Obstet. Gynecol. Sci.*, 60(6):506-519. https://doi.org/10.5468/ogs.2017.60.6.506.

[10] Wirix, AJ. Nauta, J. Groothoff, J W. Rabelink, TJ. Sing, RA. Chinapaw, MJ. Van Holthe, JE. (2016). Is the prevalence of hypertension in overweight children overestimated? *Arch. Dis. Child.*, 101:998–1003. doi: 10.1136/archdischild-2015-309969.

[11] Dadlani, A. Madan, M. Sawhney, JPS. (2019). Ambulatory blood pressure monitoring in clinical practice. *Indian Heart Journal*, 71(1): 91-97.

[12] Pletcher, MJ. Bibbins-Domingo, K. Liu, K. Sidney, S. Lin, F. Vittinghoff, E. Hulley, SB. (2010) Nonoptimal lipids commonly present in young adults and coronary calcium later in life: the CARDIA (Coronary Artery Risk Development in Young Adults) study. *Ann. Intern. Med.*, 153:137–146. doi: 10.7326/0003-4819-153-3-201008030-00004.

[13] Raitakari, OT. Juonala, M. Kahonen, M. Taittonen, L. Laitinen, T. Maki-Torkko, N. Jarvisalo, MJ. Uhari, M. Jokinen, E. Ronnemaa, T. Akerblom, HK. Viikari, JS. (2003). Cardiovascular risk factors in childhood and carotid artery intima-media thickness in adulthood: the Cardiovascular Risk in Young Finns Study. *JAMA*, 290:2277–2283. doi: 10.1001/jama.290.17.2277.

[14] Hartiala, O. Magnussen, CG. Kajander, S. Knuuti, J. Ukkonen, H. Saraste, A. Rinta-Kiikka, I. Kainulainen, S. Kahonen, M. Hutri-Kahonen, N. Laitinen, T. Lehtimaki, T. Viikari, JS. Hartiala, J. Juonala, M. Raitakari, OT. Adolescence risk factors are predictive of coronary artery calcification at middle age: the Cardiovascular Risk in Young Finns study. (2012). *J. Am. Coll. Cardiol.*, 60:1364–1370. doi: 10.1016/j.jacc.2012.05.045.

[15] Magnussen, CG. Koskinen, J. Juonala, M. Chen, W. Srinivasan, SR. Sabin, MA. Thomson, R. Schmidt, MD. Nguyen, QM. Xu, JH. Skilton, MR. Kähönen, M. Laitinen, T. Taittonen, L. Lehtimäki, T. Rönnemaa, T. Viikari, JS. Berenson, GS. Raitakari, OT. (2012). A diagnosis of the metabolic syndrome in youth that resolves by adult life is associated with a normalization of high carotid intima-media thickness and type 2 diabetes mellitus risk: the Bogalusa Heart and Cardiovascular Risk in Young Finns studies. *J. Am. Coll. Cardiol.*. 23;60(17):1631-9. doi: 10.1016/j.jacc.2012.05.056.

[16] Wühl, E. (2019). Hypertension in Childhood Obesity. *Acta Paediatr.* 108(1):37-43. doi: 10.1111/apa.14551.

[17] Kliegman, R. Stanton, B. StGeme, J. Schor, N. Nelson Textbook of Pediatrics. 20nd ed. *The cardiovascular system*. Philadelphia, PA, 2299.

[18] Brady, T. (2016). The Role of Obesity in the Development of Left Ventricular Hypertrophy Among Children and Adolescents. *Current Hypertension Reports,* 18:3

[19] Flynn, J T. Kaelber, D C. Baker-Smith, C M. Blowey, D. Carroll, A E. Daniels, S R. Ferranti, SD. Dionne, JM. Falkner, B. Flinn, SK. Gidding, SS. Goodwin, C. Leu, MG. Powers, ME. Rea, C. Samuels, J. Simasek, M. Thaker, VV. Urbina, EM. (2017). Clinical Practice Guideline for Screening and Management of High Blood Pressure in Children and Adolescents. *Pediatrics,* 140 (3). e20171904; doi: https://doi.org/10.1542/peds.2017-1904.

[20] Jing, L. Binkley, CM. Suever, LD. Umasankar, N. Haggerty, C M. Rich, J. Nevius, CD. Wehner, GJ, Hamlet, SM, Powell, DK. Radulescu, A. Kirchner, HL, Epstein, FH. Fornwalt, BK. (2018). Cardiac remodeling and dysfunction in childhood obesity: a cardiovascular magnetic resonance study. *Journal of Cardiovascular Magnetic Resonance*, 28 doi 10.1186/s12968-016-0247-0.

[21] Raj, M. (2012). Obesity and cardiovascular risk in children and adolescents. *Indian J. Endocrinol. Metab.*,16(1): 13–19.

[22] Chinali, M. Simone, G. Roman, MJ. Lee, ET. Best, LG. Howard, BV. Devereux, RB. (2006). Impact of obesity on cardiac geometry and function in a population of adolescents: The Strong Heart Study. *J. Am. Coll. Cardiol.*, 47:2267–73.

[23] Fitzgibbons, T. Simone, G. Aurigemma, G. (2013). Cardiac Remodeling in Obesity. *Circulation, Cardiovascular Imaging*, 6(1):142-52. doi: 10.1161/CIRCIMAGING.111.964627.

[24] Zhu, H. Yan, W. Ge, D. Treiber, FA. Harshfield, GA. Kapuku, G. Snieder, H. Dong, Y. (2008). Relationships of cardiovascular phenotypes with healthy weight, at risk of overweight, and overweight in US youths. *Pediatrics*, 121:115.

[25] Zhang, C. Deng, Y. Liu, Y. Xu, Y. Liu, Y. Zhang, L. Chen, X. Xie, M. Ge, S. (2018). Preclinical cardiovascular changes in children with obesity: A real-time 3-dimensional speckle tracking imaging study. *Public Library of Science*, 13(10): e0205177

[26] Erbs, S. Broniecki, H. Scheuermann, K. Winzer, E. Adam, J. Spielau, U. Woitek, F. Sandri, M. Zimmer, M. Besler, C. Kiess, W. Linke, A. Körner, A. Mangner, N. (2018). *Impact of Weight Reduction During Adolescence on Parameters of Cardiac Geometry and Function in Obese Children*. JACC: CARDIOVASCULAR IMAGING, 11(12). I SS N 1 9 3 6 - 8 7 8X.

[27] Ingul, CB. Dias, KA. Tjonna, AE. Follestad, T. Hosseini, MS. Timilsina, AS. Hollekim-Strand, MS. Ro, TB. Davies, PS, Cain, PA. Leong, GM. Coombes, JS. (2018). Effect of High Intensity Interval Training on Cardiac Function in Children with Obesity: A Randomised Controlled Trial. *Progress in Cardiovascular Diseases*, 61(2): 214-22.

[28] Moll GX. Inflammatory and Anti-Inflammatory Markers in Acute Coronary Syndromes. Ready for Use in the Clinical Setting? *Rev. Esp. Cardiol.*, 58:615–617. pmid:15970115.

[29] Abderrahma, HA. Al-Abdallat, IM. Idhair, AK. (2018). Age threshold for proper definition of premature coronary artery disease in males. *Journal of Forensic and Legal Medicine*, 58, 45-49.

[30] Cole, C. Nikpay, M. Stewart, A. McPherson, R. (2016). Increased genetic risk for obesity in premature coronary artery disease. *European Journal of Human Genetics*. 24,587–59.

[31] Martínez, AJ. Sánchez, PR. Llorente, L. León, AE. Bello, RJ. Molina, VT. Lima, G. Cardoso-Saldaña, CG. Pérez, RM. Hernández, PN. Fragoso, JM. Romero, PC. Alarcón, VG. (2017). The rs7044343 Polymorphism of the Interleukin 33 Gene Is Associated with Decreased Risk of Developing Premature Coronary Artery Disease and Central Obesity, and Could Be Involved in Regulating the Production of IL-33. *PLoS One*. 3;12(1):e0168828. https://doi.org/10.1371/journal.pone.0168828. e Collection 2017.

[32] Simmons, R. (2006). Developmental origins of adult metabolic disease. *Endo. Metab. Clin.*, 35:193.

[33] Bridger, T. (2009). Childhood obesity and cardiovascular disease. *Paediatr Child Health*, 14(3): 177–182.

[34] Barker, DP. Osmond, C. Kajantie, E. Eriksson, J. (2009). Growth and chronic disease: findings in the Helsinki Birth Cohort. *Ann. Hum. Biol.*, 36:445–58.

[35] Calkins, K. Devaskar, Sh. (2011). Fetal Origins of Adult Disease. *Curr Probl Pediatr Adolesc Health Care*, 41(6): 158–176. doi:10.1016/j.cppeds.2011.01.001.

[36] Kulkarni, A. Li, L. Craft, M. Nnada, M. Lorenzo, JM. Danford, D. Kutty, S. (2017). Fetal myocardial deformation in maternal diabetes mellitus and obesity. *Ultrasound Obstet. Gynecol.*, 49: 630–636. doi: 10.1002/uog.15971.

[37] Ingul, CB. Loras, L. Tegnander, E. Eik-Nes, SH. Brantberg, A. (2016). Maternal obesity affects fetal myocardial function as early as in the first trimester. *Ultrasound Obstet. Gynecol.*; 47: 433–442. doi: 10.1002/uog.14841.

[38] Ingul, CB. Garnaes, K. Moholdt, T. Nyrnes, SA. (2017). Cardiac function in newborns of obese women and the effect of an exercise intervention during pregnancy. *European Heart Journal*, 38(1), ehx501.P651. https://doi.org/10.1093/eurheartj/ehx501.P651.

In: Childhood Obesity
Editor: Roya Kelishadi
ISBN: 978-1-53618-158-6
© 2020 Nova Science Publishers, Inc.

Chapter 10

ASSOCIATIONS OF OVERWEIGHT/OBESITY AND CARDIO METABOLIC RISK FACTORS IN CHILDREN AND ADOLESCENTS PARTICIPATING IN THE PEP FAMILY HEART STUDY

Gerda Maria Haas*[1]*, MPH and Peter Schwandt*[1,2,*]*, MD, PHD
[1]Atherosclerosis Prevention Institute, Munich-Nuremberg, Germany
[2]Ludwig-Maximilians University, Munich, Germany

ABSTRACT

Purpose: Overweight/obesity, hypertension and dyslipidemia are prominent risk factors of cardiovascular diseases (CVD) in children and adolescents. Risk factor profiles of young people should be age-and gender-specific because natural growth influences anthropometric and laboratory components of risk considerably. Therefore, we assessed growth curves of body mass index (BMI), waist circumference (WC), waist-to-hip ratio (WHtR) and body fat distribution (BF) evaluating *overweight/obesity*. Growth curves of high LDL-cholesterol, high triglycerides and low HDL-cholesterol describe *dyslipidemia* and age-specific values of high systolic and/or high diastolic blood pressure (BP) define *hypertension* in 16,036 children (3-11 years old) and 6,015 adolescents (12-18 year old) who participated in the PEP Family Heart Study in the city of Nuremberg.

Methods: We measured body fat from biceps-, triceps- and subscapulary-skinfold thicknesses (SFT). Sum of triceps and subscapulary thicknesses higher than 35 mm defines high body fat. Serum lipids were determined after an overnight fast and auscultatory BP was taken after five minutes sedentary time at home. Age-and gender-adjusted percentile curves were developed using the LMS method.

* Corresponding Author's Email: API.Schwandt.Haas@t-online.de.

Results: Among the main findings are substantial differences between the prevalence of hypertension in different weight groups achieving 24.4% in obese females and 21.9% in obese males with odds ratios of 5.9 (95% CI 5.1- 7.5) respectively 4.3 (95% CI 3.5-5.2). An SFT-sum above 35 mm indicates a fivefold higher risk of hypertension in both genders. Body fat percent above the 85th percentile increased the risk of elevated LDL-Cholesterol twice and of hypertriglyceridemia fourfold.

Conclusions: These and more findings among 22.051 children and adolescents indicate that CVD risk factor profiles should be based on age- and gender-specific percentiles.

INTRODUCTION

Because the risk of cardiovascular diseases (CVD) begins in childhood and adolescents, the purpose of the observational community-based PEP Family Heart Study - performed among 48,667 subjects from 3,370 families living in 94% of the elementary school districts of Nuremberg (Germany) - is to *evaluate associations of cardiovascular risk factors with overweight and obesity.* The first part of this contribution summarizes actual data on body composition and the relation to CVD risk factors. The second part describes major results from the pediatric part of 15-years prospective PEP Family Heart Study among 23,740 children aged 3-18 years.

Body Mass Index and Body Composition

Since 1980, the prevalence of obesity has doubled in more than 70 countries. The prevalence and disease burden of high body mass index (BMI in Kg/m^2) as a measure of overweight and adiposity are increasing globally. In 2015, 107.7 million children were obese corresponding to an overall prevalence of 5.0%. Nearly 70% of the deaths related to high BMI were due to cardiovascular disease (CVD) [1]. In 2-19 y old US youths, overall prevalence of obesity increased from 16.8% to 18.5% between 2007/8 and 2015/6. Among US children aged 2-5 y from 10.1% to 13.9% and in adolescents aged 12-19 y from 18.1% to 20.6% but slightly decreased from 19.6% to 18.4%in the age group 6-11 y whereas severe obesity (BMI at or above 120% of the 95th percentile [2, 3]. Since 2013/14, severe obesity in terms of Class II obesity (BMI $\geq$ 120% of the 95th percentile) and Class III obesity (BMI $\geq$ 140% of the 95th percentile) have significantly increased among children aged 2 to 5 years. The recent WHO study COSI in 6-9y old children from 21 European countries (not including Russia, Germany, France, and the UK) found that the prevalence of severe obesity varied greatly among countries [4, 5]. Among 2-to 19year olds, BMI z-Scores are a poor indicator of body fatness [6]. BMI is an important screening tool, but it must be integrated with other information in the health assessment and body composition like waist circumference (WC), waist-to height ratio (WHtR), skinfold thickness (SFT) and body fat ($BF_{Slaughter}$) based on the sum of triceps skinfold thickness ($SFT_{triceps}$) and subscapulary skinfold thickness ($SFT_{subscapulary}$) that are used to characterize adiposity. Because of physiological growth during youth, they have to be age-related [7-11].

For *German children and adolescents*, we describe a *countrywide Study* and three representative *regional studies* from Heidelberg, Nuremberg and Leipzig. The *nationally representative* KiGGS study from 2003 to 2006 presents BMI percentiles of 17,641 children and adolescents aged 0-17 y from 167 study locations "Compared with the currently used German KH percentiles which are based on pooled data from 17 regional and methodologically heterogeneous German studies [12] smoothed KiGGS BMI percentiles appear more valid for Germany." The cut-offs for overweight and obesity were similar to IOTF from age 18 to 10 y but systematically lower for younger children [13, 14]. Between 1999 and 2008 the prevalence of overweight (>90th percentile) and obesity (>97th percentile) increased among 4-16y old German youths obtained from the CrescNet registry collecting age and gender related height and weight measurements that connects 321 pediatricians in practice from all over Germany and which is considered to be representative of the German population [15, 16]. Age and onset of obesity and the course of BMI over time were analysed in 51,505 children and adolescents from the growth-monitoring database CrescNet. BMI and height were converted to standard-deviation scores by applying German reference data according to current German national guidelines defining overweight as >95th percentile and obesity as >97th percentile of BMI. Among obese adolescents, the most rapid weight gain occurred early in life and persisted into adolescence with the most excessive weight gain between 2 and 6 years, which was the most powerful predictor of adolescent obesity [17].

Among the *regional German studies*, *1989/90* a cross-sectional observational study in *Heidelberg* (Germany) performed among 2,554 schoolchildren aged 6-19 years provides BMI percentiles and skinfold-derived percentage of body fat mass (PFM) demonstrates that the 75th BMI percentile was the most appropriate cut-off value to screen for the 15% most obese patients by PFM. Body fat measured according to Slaughter [10] increased almost steadily with age in girls while boys showed a preadolescent and small increase beyond 16 y. PFM was continuously redistributed across childhood from the extremities to the trunk. [18]. From *1993/4 to 2007/08* the observational community-based longitudinal *PEP Family Heart Study* performed in *Nuremberg* (Germany) described age-and gender-specific percentiles of BMI, WC, WHtR, SFT, percentage body fat, blood pressure (BP) and fasting lipids in 22,051 children and adolescents aged 3-18y living in 3,370 families. For better international comparisons overweight (≥85th- < 85th percentile), obesity (≥95th to < 120% of the 95th percentile) and severe obesity (≥120percentage of the 95th percentile) were defined according to CDC (6-9). In a subpopulation of 2.228 first graders (1.116 boys) from 1994 to 2003 in both genders, mean values of BMI, WC and WHtR remained stable whereas the mean values of blood pressure, high-density cholesterol and serum triglycerides continuously decreased [19-22]. The associations between twelve CVD risk factors and five anthropometric variables in 16,036 children and 6.051 adolescents are shown in the second part of this manuscript. The *Life Child Study* performed in *Leipzig* (Germany) describes age-and sex-related percentiles of SFT, WC, WHtR and hip circumference in 2,363 children and adolescents aged 3-16y from 1,710 families collected as part of the LIFE Child Research Center [23-25].

A meta-analysis of *skinfold thickness* measurements in children and adolescents from 30 developed countries describes nonlinear increases of the ratio $SFT_{triceps}$ to $SFT_{subscapulary}$ indicating increased %BF and a relative shift towards central depots from 1951 to 2004 [26]. Measurements of $SFT_{triceps}$ gave the best results for obesity screening in boys and girls aged 7–17 y [27, 28]. The Amsterdam Growth and Health Longitudinal Study found that adolescent SFT is a better predictor of high body fatness in adults than is BMI [29]. When used in addition to BMI-for-age, SFT can substantially improve the estimation of body fat, though improvement is small among overweight US youths [30-32]. The German PEP Family Heart Study describes age- and gender-specific percentiles for WC, WHR, WHtR, $SFT_{triceps}$ and $SFT_{subscapulary}$ among 3,850 children aged 3-11 years and 3,084 adolescents aged 12-18 years and [33, 34]. A National Health and Nutrition Examination Survey from 2001 to 2006 in 8.216 children aged 6 to 17 years concluded that CVD risk factor screening should be targeted to the most at-risk children, which may involve cholesterol screening of children at the 80th percentile for BMI but diabetes screening only in the very obese category above the 99th percentile [35]. Four German regional populations describe SFT percentiles in Heidelberg [18], Nuremberg [34, 36], Jena [37] and Leipzig [23].

Brambilla and experts [38] from four countries considered *waist circumference* "a good predictor of visceral adipose tissue (VAT) as well as BMI of subcutaneous adipose tissue. The importance of ethnicity and gender on VAT estimation is not negligible:" Fernandez et al. compared 2004 percentiles in nationally representative samples of African-American, European-American, and Mexican-American children and adolescents [39]. We found WC percentiles for children and adolescents from twenty countries including Australia, Brazil, Bulgaria, Canada, China, Cyprus, Germany, Italy, Iran, Japan, Mexico, New Zealand, Netherlands, Nigeria, Poland, Spain, Sweden, Turkey, UK, USA [39-59]. Between 1988–1994 and 1999–2004 mean waist circumference and waist-height ratio and the prevalence of abdominal obesity among US children and adolescents greatly increased [60]. Wang et al. compared WC values at the four commonly used anatomic sites that differ in magnitude depending on sex, are highly reproducible, and correlate with total body and trunk adiposity in a sex-dependent manner. However, there is no universally accepted method of measuring waist circumference [61]. Anthropometric CVD risk factors track from childhood into adulthood [62-65].

Overweight/Obesity Related Cardiovascular Risk Factors

Globally, 41% of BMI-related deaths and 34% of BMI-related disability-adjusted life-years were due to cardiovascular disease among obese persons [1]. In prepubertal children, WC adjusted for age, gender and BMI is independently associated with *cardiovascular risk factors* [66-67]. The Bogalusa Heart Study, the Caspian Study and others confirmed that BMI, WC, SFT and body fat are important predictors of CVD and their risk factors [68-77]. Already in 1980, clustering of risk factors was described [78], adverse WC suggested a simple test for atherogenic disease [79] and central adiposity an indicator of silent CVD risk factors [80]. Using the UK Biobank a Mendelian randomization study described the relation of 14 CVD risk factors to BMI and body composition [81]. Among the CVD risk factors *dyslipoproteinemia* was described in the Bogalusa Heart Study related to WC and SFT in children and adolescents [82], the Taipei Children Heart Study found relationships between anthropometric variables and lipid levels among school children [83] and the PEP Family Heart Study [21, 84]. Among 1721 German children (870 girls, 851 boys) and 2076 Iranian children (1085 girls, 991 boys) aged 6-11 years mean and reference curves of BMI, WC and TG were higher in Iranian than in German children, whereas the mean and reference curves of total and HDL cholesterol were lower in Iranian than in German children [85]. While the prevalence of abdominal adiposity was nearly similar, Iranian and Brazilian youths had considerably higher prevalence of dyslipidemia than German youths [48]. Among 3,850 children (1981 males) aged, 3-11years WHtR > 90th percentile had the strongest association with increased LDL-C (OR:2.0), Non HDL-C (OR:2.1), LDL-C/HDL-C ratio (OR:3.3), TG/HDL-C ratio (OR:2.0) and risk factor clustering (OR:1.7) [86]. A series of growth curves for waist circumference, total cholesterol, LDL cholesterol, triglycerides and HDL cholesterol was created from a combination of two NHANES databases 1988-2006 and cross-sectional data from the Bogalusa Heart Study, the Muscatine Study, the Fels Longitudinal Study and the Princeton Lipid Research Clinics Study [7, 9, 87, 88]. Among 2,720 German child-parent pairs in multivariate models, adjusting for age and gender, child general and abdominal adiposity conferred a significant 2.9-fold and a 2.6-fold enhanced odds among parents of carrying the same risk factors. Similarly, abnormal LDL, HDL, or non-HDL among children conferred a significant 3.0-fold, 2.0-fold, or 2.9-fold increased odds among parents [89]. CVD risk factor clustering was 3–4 times more frequent in 412 adolescents with central obesity than in 2626 adolescents (1639 males) without. Central obesity was the only anthropometric variable that significantly predicted increased risk for all seven non-anthropometric CVD risk factors: hypertension (OR 2.5), elevated triglycerides (OR 4.9), LDL-C (OR 2.0), non-HDL-C (OR 2.1), triglyceride/HDL-C ratio $\geq$3.5 (OR 7.2), low HDL-C (OR 1.6) [90]. In representative samples of Asian and European children, reference curves of anthropometric indices and serum lipid profiles ware presented [91]. The German/Austrian/Swiss registry included 29,711 overweight or obese (based on age- and gender-adjusted BMI-z-scores) children, adolescents and young adults from 162 specialized obesity care centers and described with increasing BMI-category that hypertriglyceridemia and low HDL-cholesterol increased rapidly. Among normal-weight subjects the prevalence was 3.3% for fasting hypertriglyceridemia, 7.2% elevated LDL-C and 3.1% low HDL-C [92]. In obese 12– 14-year-old Swedish children, WC correlates to an atherogenic lipoprotein profile [93].

The epidemic of childhood obesity is associated with an increase in the prevalence of *hypertension* even using the previous percentiles [1]. Obesity hypertension in children and adolescents is a problem of epidemic proportions and the relationship of body mass index and blood pressure is well documented [95, 96]. Elevated BP in children and adolescents is associated with target organ damage and increases the risk of subclinical atherosclerosis [97, 98]. Among 3,850 German children (1981 males) aged 3-11years age- and gender-adjusted hypertension was significantly associated with adiposity (OR:2.8) and high skin-fold thickness (OR:1.7) [71] and among 920 (464 males) 12 y old Chinese children a strong positive relation between BP and BMI and SFT was described [99]. Among 3,038 German adolescents (1639 males), aged 12–18 years the risk of hypertension was 2.5 fold in central obesity and 4.9 fold in adolescents with general adiposity [86]. Seven large nationally representative cross-sectional surveys using certified mercury sphygmomanometers in all seven countries provide BP values from 52 636 non-overweight children and adolescents aged 6 to 19 years that were similar between males and females until the age of 13 years and were higher in males than females thereafter. Systolic BP was lower and diastolic BP were similar at the 90th and 95th percentiles to the widely used US Fourth Report at median height. Oscillometric devices should be clinically validated by the auscultatory method before being widely used because of different types using different manufacturer's proprietary algorithms [99-101]. Rosner et al. described determination of blood pressure percentiles in normal-weight children using the classic auscultatory design excluding overweight and obesity (BMI $\geq$85th percentile).“Whether these norms are also appropriate for oscillometric blood pressure readings remains an open question” [102]. Furthermore, auscultatory BP reference values were published for Northern Europe, China and Germany [103-105] and oscillometric values for Germany and Poland [106, 107]. The German PEP Family Heart Study provides BP percentiles from 18,917 normal-weight, 1,938 overweight and 1,196 obese) aged 3–18 years. Overweight (BMI 85th to < 95th percentile) and obese (BMI $\geq$ 95th percentile) children and adolescents had substantially higher BP percentiles using separate databases for overweight and obesity such as 148/91 vs.136/86 mm Hg for a 17-year-old male and 136/91 vs.123/81 mm Hg for female, respectively, at the 90th percentile [105]. This corresponds with data form Rosner et al. who estimated percentiles using norms based on normalweight children rather than the 7th report which included both normal-weight and overweight children resulting in higher rates of hypertension and prehypertension [106]. Among 8579 children and young adults with a BMI $\geq$85th percentile 46.9% were overweight, 36.4% had class I obesity, 11.9% had class II obesity, and 4.8% had class III obesity. Mean values for some, but not all cardio metabolic variables were higher with greater severity of obesity in both male and female participants, and the values were higher in male participants than in female participants; for HDL cholesterol, the mean values were lower with greater severity of obesity. Multivariable models that controlled for age, race or ethnic group, and sex showed that the greater the severity of obesity, the higher the risks of a low HDL cholesterol level, high systolic and diastolic blood pressures, and high triglyceride levels [108].

RESULTS

The PEP Family Heart Study

Subjects

22,051 youths consisting of 16,036 children aged 3-11y (8,130 boys and 7,906 girls) and 6,015 adolescents aged 12 -18 years (3,198 boys and 2,817 girls) living in 3,370 families participating in the PEP Family Heart Study [21] with complete anthropometric data including including 10,915 children and adolescents with additional laboratory measurements.

Methods

Measurements

At each survey, we measured at home weight and height to the nearest 0.1 cm and 0.1 kg using a calibrated electronic scale SECA (Vogel & Halske, Hamburg, Germany) and a Stadiometer Holtain Ltd (Crymych, UK). We calculated body mass index BMI (kg/m^2), measured waist circumference (WC), waist-to-height ratio (WHtR), skinfold thickness (SFT) triceps ($SFT_{triceps}$) and sub-scapular skinfold thickness ($SFT_{subscapular}$) using a Holtain skinfold calliper (GPM-calliper, Zurich, Switzerland) on the left body side in triplicate to the nearest 0.1 mm calculating %BF using the age-and sex adjusted Slaughter equations [10]. We used IBM SPSS Version 21 calculating p-values < 0.01 for all regression models and bivariate correlations. For regression models, we used univariate regression models for estimating the differences between the single fat patterns and multivariate models for calculating the age-, sex- and bias- adjusted associations between fat patterns and further cardio-vascular risk factors.

Categorization

Non-overweight (normal weight) is defined as BMI < 85th percentile (pctl), overweight as BMI 85th to < 95th pctl, obesity as BMI ≥95th pctl, and severe obesity as ≥120 percentage of the 95th pctl [7]. Estimating percentage of body fat (% BF) we used the original Slaughter formula in terms of triceps skinfold (TSF) in mm and subscapular skinfold (SSF) in mm. The equation for % BF is: %BF = 1.21(TSF + SSF) – 0.008 $(TSF + SSF)^2$ – 1.7 for boys; %BF = 1.33 (TSF + SSF) – 0.013 $(TSF+ SSF)^2$ - 2.5 for girls, when TSF + SSF were ≤35 mm. When the skinfold sum was > 35 mm, the calculation is: % BF = 0.783 (TSF + SSF) + 1.6 for males and 0.546 (TSF + SSF) +9.7 for females. For SFT we used the cut-off point of Slaughter [10] for the sum of TSF plus SSF ≥ 35mm. Cut-offs are described by the expert panel 2012 and CDC growth charts for %body fat the 75th percentile; for WC the 90th percentile [9].

Prehypertension is categorized as the ≥90th to < 95th pctl or ≥120/80 mmHg and hypertension as ≥95th pctl on ≥3 occasions [100]. Elevated values for total Cholesterol (TC), Low Density Cholesterol (LDL-C). Triglycerides (TG) and Non High Density Cholesterol (Non HDL-C) were defined as ≥ 95th percentile analogue to the WHO – cut-offs. High Density Cholesterol (HDL-C) was defined < 40 mg/dl for boys and < 35 mg/dl in girls [9].

Statistical Analysis

We performed all statistical analyses using actual SPSS (Chicago, IL, USA) and conducted bivariate and multivariate analysis and multivariate regression analysis for age and gender adjustments. Using generalized estimating equations to generate adjusted *P* values that accounted for correlation among multiple within-family observations as well as for adjustment for age and gender. We tested all variables for normal distribution. Statistical tests were two-sided, and $P < 0.05$ was considered statistically significant, for correlations with $P < 0.01$ and significances for paired differences and regression coefficients, respectively, odds ratios (ORs), with $P < 0.001$. Smoothed age-, gender-, and height-specific percentiles for children were constructed using the software package LMS Chart Maker Pro (The Institute of Child Health, London), estimating the skewness parameter *L*, the median *M*, and a measure of variation *S* calculating estimated marginal means [11]. We tested the normal distribution of age adjusted exact height and SBP and DBP values by trended and detrended Q-Q diagrams within the age groups. Number of outliers never came close to 5%. We tested the goodness of fit for the final curves by *z*-scores as well as by trended and detrended Q-Q plots and performed age- and sex-adjusted binary logistic regression models defining the crude risk of hypertension (respectively prehypertension) in single weight. For comparison of the three weight groups ($P < 0.001$), we calculated polynomial logistic regression models.

Results

First, we describe the characteristics of the participating 22,051 youths aged 3-18 years. Due to the study-design, far more children (16,036) than adolescents (6,015) took part in the PEP Family Heart Study, whereas the gender distribution in children (8,130 boys and 7,906 girls) and adolescents (3,198 young males and 2,817 young females) was similar. In both genders, all anthropometric variables were higher in adolescents than in children whereas fasting serum lipids were higher in childhood than in adolescence. Table 1 summarizes anthropometric and laboratory variables in 22,051 children and adolescents.

Table 2 describes the prevalence of adverse Cardiovascular Risk Factors (CVD RF) in this cohort.

Next step was testing whether there are significant bivariate correlations between the 5 fat patterns: Body Mass Index (BMI), Waist Circumference (WC), Waist/Height Ratio (WHtR), percentage of Body Fat (% BF), sum of $SFT_{triceps}$ plus $SFT_{subscapular}$ (subtricsum) and the 6 non anthropometric CVD RF: Systolic Blood Pressure SBP, Diastolic Blood Pressure DBP, elevated Total Cholesterol TC, elevated Low Density Cholesterol LDL-C, decreased High Density Cholesterol HDL-C, elevated NonHDL-C, elevated Triglycerides TG. We found significant ones between all factors.

Then we tested the fat patterns for significant linear associations with the 6 non anthropometric CVD and found them confirmed.

Next up it was necessary to find the cut-offs for all RF in children and adolescents using Tim Cole's LMS Percentile Curves. Figures 2.1 to 2.4 show the Curves for BMI. WC WHtR and % BF for both sexes, Figures 3 to 7 the development of the 5 medians for the fat patterns. We did not construct LMS Percentile Curves for the sum of TSF plus SSF as a fixed term $\geq$ 35 mm.

Overweight and obesity have their own section; especially the terms of severe obesity in terms of the 120% and 140% of the 95th percentile of BMI because of the strong association with hypertension.

Next follow the LMS Percentile Curves for TC, LDL-C, HDL-C, NonHDL-C and TG for both gender (Figures 10.1 to 10.5).

At least we calculated the associations between the 5 fat patterns and the 6 non anthropometric CVD RF by multivariate logistic regression analyses including sex and age classes to confirm the hypothesis that all 5 patterns show own relationship with further CVD RF ($p < 0.001$).

Finally we write the summary followed by our conclusion.

Table 1. Characteristics of 22,051 children and adolescents with complete anthropometric measurements including 10,915 youths with additional laboratory measurements

	22,051 youths aged 3-18 years			
	Children (n = 16,036) Adolescents (n = 6,015)			
	3-11 years		12 – 18 years	
	males	females	males	females
N	8130	7906	3198	2817
Mean age, years	7.8(2.0)	7.8(2.0)	14.1(1.8)	14.1(1.9)
Median age, years	8.0	8.0	14.0	14.0
Weight, kg	29.4(9.0)	29.1(9.3)	57.5(14.5)*	53.5(11.1)
Height, cm	131.2(13.3)	130.7(13.7)	167.2(12.0)*	161.9(7.7)
Body mass index (BMI), kg/m²	16.7(2.5)	16.6(2.6)	20.3(3.4)	20.3(3.5)
Waist circumference (WC), cm	60.0(7.4)	58.8(7.2)	73.6(9.6)*	70.7(9.1)
Waist to height ratio (WHtR)	0.458 (0.042)*	0.452(0.045)	0.440(0.042)*	0.437(0.053)
Biceps (BSF) mm	5.29(2.63)	6.20(2.71)*	6,17 (3.38)	7.16(3.36)*
Triceps (TSF) mm	9.01(3.96)	10.54(4.16)*	10,55(5.06)	12.58(5.10)*
Subscapulary (SSF) mm	6.30(3.45)	7.30(3.82)*	8.00(4.70)*	9.71(5.12)*
%Body Fat	15,6(6.0)	16.5(5.6)	17.1(7.1)	21.1(6.3)*
SBP, mm Hg	104.3 (9.0)	103.7(9.2)	114.5 (11.4) *	109.9(9.4)
DBP, mm Hg	67.5 (8.1)	67.3(8.0)	71.5 (8.2) *	69.9(6.0)
Total Cholesterol (TC) mg/dl	170.40(28.93)	173.56(29.54)*	161.48(28.54)	162.52(26.86)
Low Density Cholesterol (LDL-C) mg/dl	99.12(26.21)	103.18(27.05)*	92.50(26.61)	93.21(24.78)
High Density Cholesterol (HDL-C) mg/dl	58.69(12.34)*	56.11(12.54)	55.28(11.83)*	53.78(11.26)
Non HDL-C, mg/dl	111.69(27.28)	117.19(27.81)*	106.25(26.66)	108.74(25.71)
Triglycerides (TG) mg/dl	60.91(24.70)	68.29(28.16)*	65.87(28.72)	74.09(31.59)*

* $p < 0.05$.

All anthropometric values were higher in boys than in girls.

Table 2. Prevalence of Cardiovascular Risk Factors in 22,051 healthy youths (16,036 children and 6,015 adolescents)

Risk Factors	males	females	males	females
	3-11 years	3-11 years	12 – 18 years	12 – 18 years
	%	%	%	%
BMI ≥85th	13.9	14.3	16.3	18.0
WC ≥85th	17.3	13.7	17.1	13.9
WHtR ≥85th	13.1	12.0	12.2	11.2
%Body Fat ≥75th	26.9	24.1	32.0	23.2
(TSF + SSF) ≥35mm	8.0	12.6	16.5	24.8
Prehypertension 90th,-95th	15.0	14.7	15.1	16.1
Hypertension > 95th	7.7	7.7	6.3	7.3
TC ≥ 95th	2.6	1.6	6.0	7.4
LDL-C ≥ 95th	7.4	14.8	4.9	4.0
HDL-C ≤ 95th	2.5	3.3	1.6	1.5
Non HDL-C ≥ 95th	10.6	15.0	8.4	8.1
TG ≥ 95th	0.4	0.9	0.9	1.4

Overweight in terms of BMI above the 85th percentile was higher in females reaching 18% at age 12-18 years. The skinfold-sum ≥35 mm increased more in females than in males of both age groups whereas the prevalence of percentage body fat (% BF) above the 75th percentile was higher in males. 22.7% of the boys, 22.4% of the girls, 21.4% of the male, and 23.4% of the female adolescents had elevated blood pressure values including 7.7% hypertension among children respectively 6.3% in male and 7.3% in female adolescents. 3-11 y old girls had the highest prevalence of elevated LDL-C (14.8) and Non-HDL-C (15.0%) compared with boys and adolescents. The prevalence of combined high TG and low HDL-C was ≥ 3, 3% among youths.

About 25% of more than 22.000 youths had increased body fat in terms of skinfold measurements and 14, 3% had age- and gender-adjusted abdominal obesity in terms of waist circumference respectively general obesity according to increased BMI.

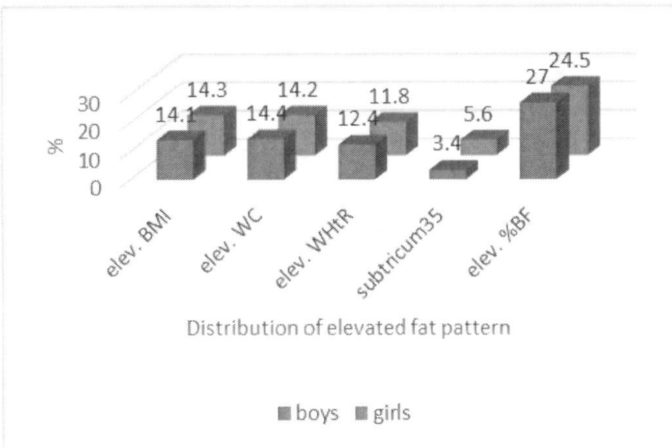

Figure 1. Prevalence of high BMI, WC, WHtR, SFT ratio and % BF in 22,051 children and adolescents aged 3 – 18 years by gender and by age.

Table 3. Bivariate correlations (Pearson) between eight components of fat distribution and seven cardiovascular risk factors in in 22,051 children and adolescents aged 3 – 18 years

WC	BMI	% BF	BSF	TSF	SSF	TSF+SSF	WHtR	
.880**	.687**	.681**	.218**	.267**	.351**	.445**	.510**	SBP
-.153**	-.126**	.020*	.062**	.057**	-0.011	.023*	.075**	TC
-.129**	-.098**	.029**	.062**	.053**	0.006	.033**	.105**	LDL-C
-.207**	-.223**	-.151**	.062**	-.116**	-.194**	-.153**	-.133**	HDL-C
-.071**	-.038**	.087**	.114**	.112**	.072**	.091**	.138**	Non HDL-C
.256**	.268**	.278**	.247**	.273**	.312**	.283**	.197**	TG

**p < 0.05 and ** p < 0.01.

As shown in Table 3, the correlation between these three anthropometric CVD risk factors with systolic hypertension was very strong whereas the correlation was negative between low HDL-C and the anthropometric variables except biceps skinfold.

Correspondingly, the inverse association of BSF and SBP in univariate linear regression models as shown in Table 4 indicate that 1 mm less of biceps skinfold results in 1 mm Hg more of SBP respectively TC, LDL-C and Non HDL-C.

Table 4. Linear associations of BSF, TSF and SSF with further CVDRF in 22,051 children and adolescents aged 3 – 18 years.

SBP	Beta	TC	Beta	LDL-C	Beta	HDL-C	Beta	Non HDL-C	Beta	TG	Beta
BSF	-0.158	BSF	0.101	BSF	0.097	BSF	0.053	BSF	0.087	BSF	-0.029
TSF	0.088	TSF	0.101	TSF	0.061	TSF	0.055	TSF	0.085	TSF	0.095
SSF	0.402	SSSF	-0.166	SSSF	-0.114	SSSF	-0.276	SSSF	-0.06	SSSF	0.26

$P < 0.001$.

For all 22,051 children and adolescents we constructed LMS percentile curves using LMS Pro, Version 2.3 by Tim Cole corresponding to the curves and measurement of NCBLI and NHANES [8, 9, 11]. The 11 curves at the 3rd, 5th 10th, 25th, 50th (median), 75th, 85th, 90th, 95th, 97th and 99th percentiles for cut-off values are shown in Figures 2.1-2.5 for BMI, WC, WHtR, %BF, SFT- sum. They indicate the utmost importance of age-dependency of these anthropometric measures and allow exact graduations and cut-offs.

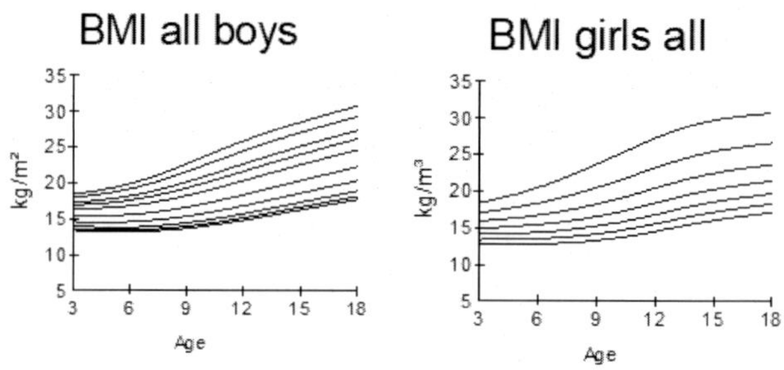

Figure 2.1. BMI.

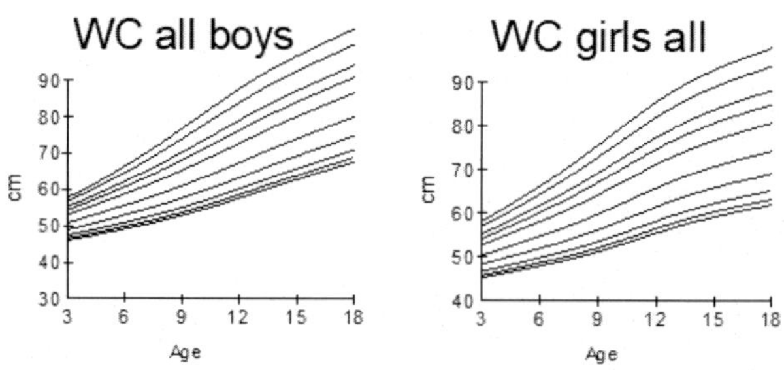

Figure 2.2. WC.

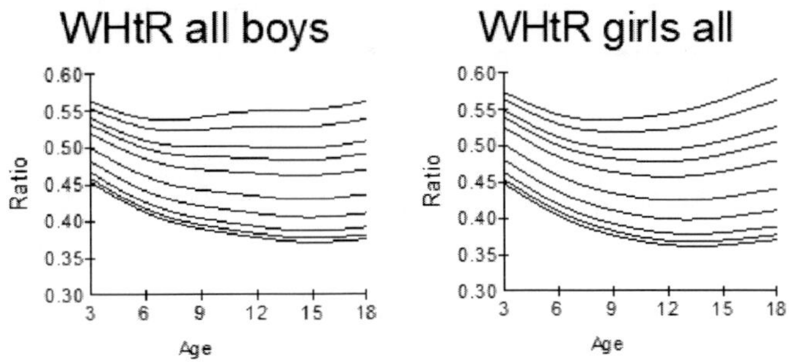

Figure 2.3. WHtR.

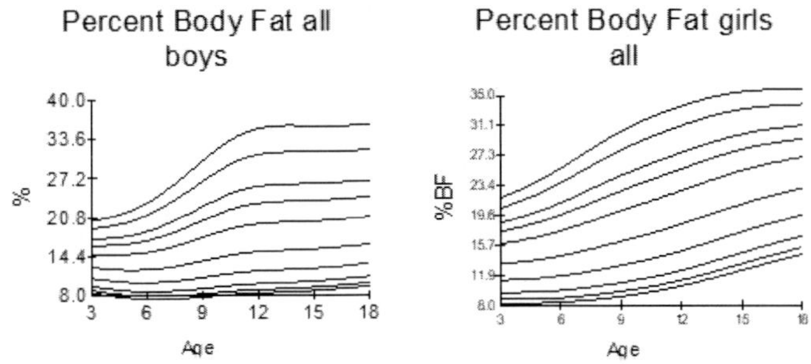

Figure 2.4. %BF Boys %BF Girls.

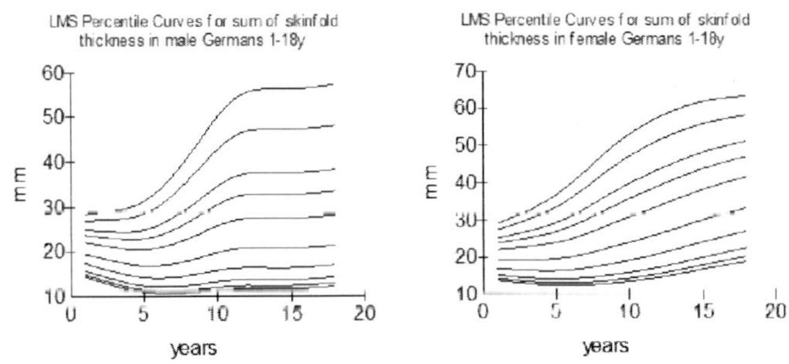

Figure 2.5. Sum of TSF plus SSF $\geq$ 35mm.

Curves depicting BMI, WC, %BF and the sum of TSF plus SSF $\geq$35mm increase more steeply in children and tend plateauing in adolescents while WHtR first decrease and then increase between ages 3-18 years.

In late adolescence WC medians increase slightly but continuously above 12 years in males but flatten in females whereas BMI medians are not different between males and females a stronger increase of abdominal adiposity in adolescents.

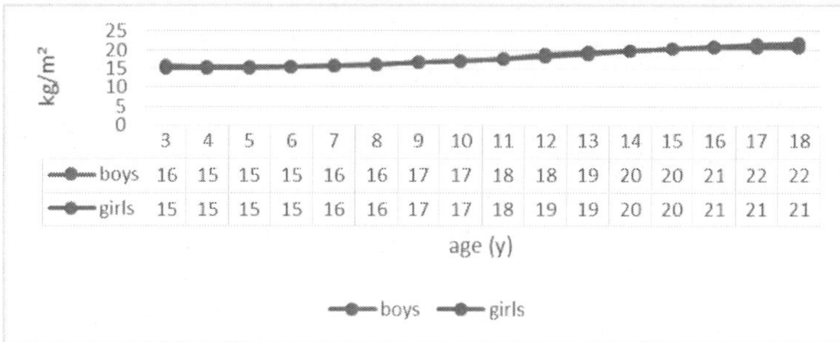
kg/m²
25
20
15
10
5
0
3 4 5 6 7 8 9 10 11 12 13 14 15 16 17 18
boys 16 15 15 15 16 16 17 17 18 18 19 20 20 21 22 22
girls 15 15 15 15 16 16 17 17 18 19 19 20 20 21 21 21
age (y)
boys girls

Figure 3. BMI medians in 11.328 males and 10.723 females aged 3-18 years.

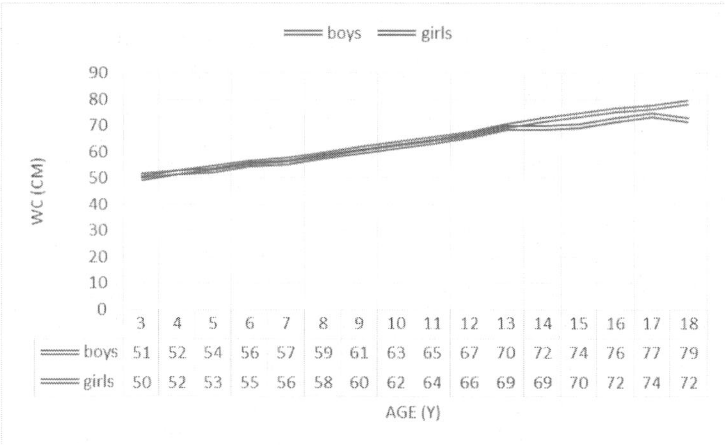

Figure 4. WC medians in 11.328 males and 10.723 females aged 3-18 years.

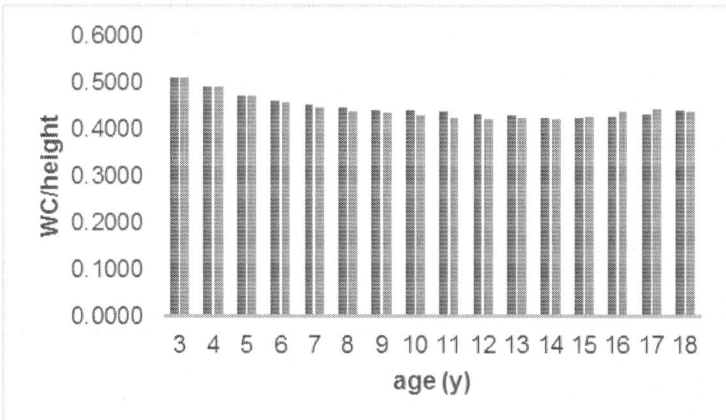

Figure 5. Development of WHtR in 16,036 children and 6,015 adolescents aged 3 -18 years.

In both genders WHtR decreases throughout childhood and increases slightly in adolescence.

Compared with % BF the median curves of the SFT-sum are higher in boys than in girls whereas the increase of the SFT-sum is stronger in female adolescents.

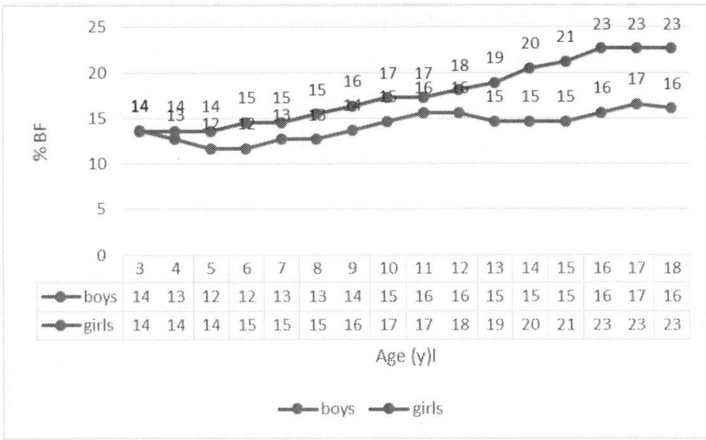

Figure 6. Medians of percentage body fat in 16,036 children and 6,015 adolescents aged 3 – 18 years. The % body fat median increases more in girls than in boys, whereas the male curves are plateauing at 16% compared with 23% in girls in adolescence.

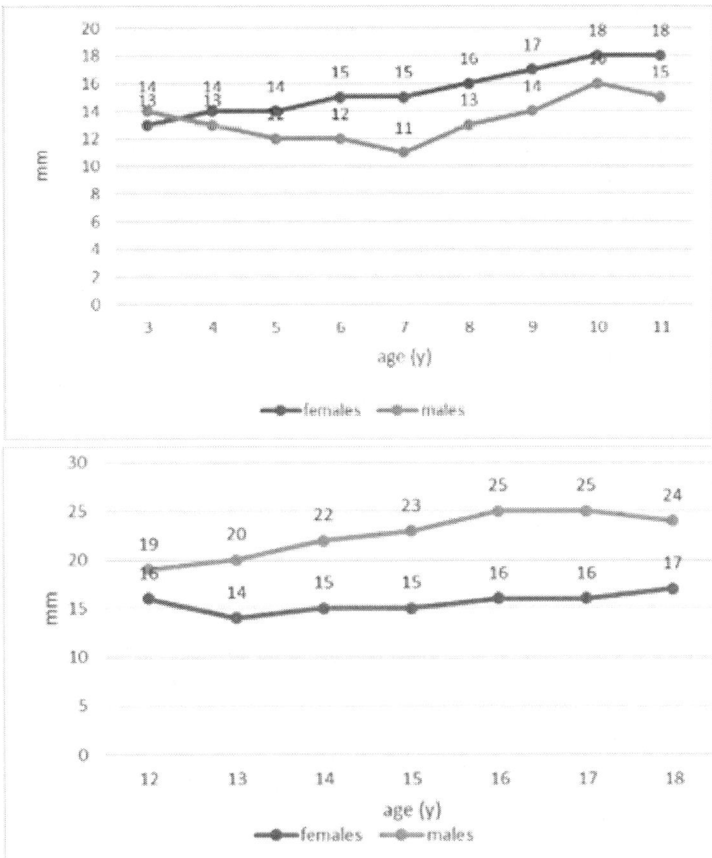

Figures 7. Development of the sum of triceps plus subscapular skinfold (mm) medians in 16,036 children and 6,015 adolescents of both genders.

Overweight and Obesity

Table 5. Percentage of overweight, obesity I and severe obesity II and III over 15y among 16,036 children and 6,015 adolescents participating in the PEP Study

children	1994	95	96	97	98	99	2000	2001	2002	2003	2004	2005	2006	2007	Mean
overw.	3.6	4.2	3.9	4.7	4.2	4.2	4	4.7	4.6	5.3	4.8	5.2	4.7	4.4	4.5
obese	2.5	3.4	3.9	4.2	4.6	3.7	4.8	4.2	4.2	5.1	6	4.5	5.4	3.9	4.3
obese II	1.5	1.5	1.8	1.5	1.3	2.2	2.2	2.1	2.6	2	2	1.9	1.9	1.9	1.9
obese III	2.8	2.5	2.7	2.2	3.7	4.5	4.3	3.2	4.1	3.6	3.7	3.8	3.5	3.2	3.4

adolesc	1994	95	96	97	98	99	2000	2001	2002	2003	2004	2005	2006	2007	Mean
overw.	8.1	4.7	2.7	6	4.8	4.1	4.5	5.5	4.5	3.7	3.5	4.3	4.8	3.6	4.6
Obese II	1.6	3.4	4.8	3	2.6	3.4	4.7	3.8	3.8	4.2	4.5	4.5	5.8	5.4	4.0
obese III	3.2	2	3.2	2.3	3.2	2.2	2.6	1.2	2.4	2.3	2.6	2.7	1.9	2.5	2.5
obese III	4.8	6.8	4.3	6	4.2	3	3.1	2.8	2.6	2.7	3.5	3.3	4.1	2.7	3.9

Legend: Overweight ≥ 85th percentile BMI, obesity I BMI ≥ 95th percentile, obesity II 120% of the 95th percentile and obesity III 140% of the 95th percentile.

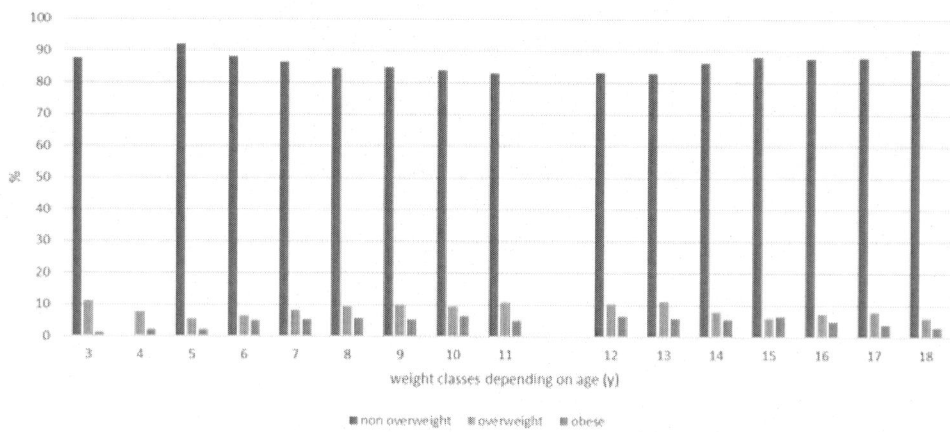

Figure 8. Prevalence of non-overweight, overweight and obesity in youths.

Whereas the prevalence of overweight in childhood remains stable around 10%, it decreases to around 6% in adolescence, the prevalence of obesity in children increases from 1.3% to 6.6% and decreases in adolescents to 3.3%.

We performed multivariate regression analysis of the risk of CVD risk factors comparing overweight and obese youths in terms of BMI (Figure 9).

Defining overweight/obesity either by BMI or by % BF results in different degrees of risk: OR for hypertension is either 2.2 or 3.7 times higher respectively for low HDL-C 2.6 and 2.0, but much more different for hypertriglyceridemia as OR 1.5 and 4.7.

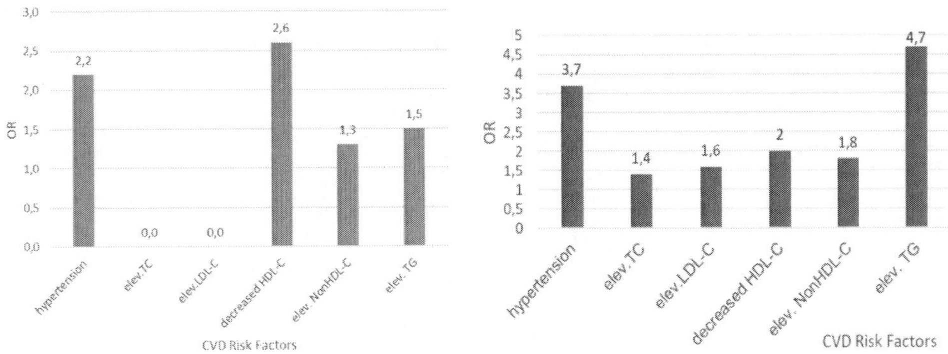

Figure 9. Probability for six CVD risk factors comparing overweight and obese children and adolescents in terms of BMI (left) and %BF (right).

Serum Lipids

Most of our 10.915 children and adolescents aged 3-18 years who had fasting lipid analyses were non-overweight. Figures 9.1-9.5 show the percentile curves for Total-Cholesterol, LDL-C, HDL-C Non HDL-C and triglycerides. The 11 curves represents the 3$^{rd.}$, 5th 10th, 25th, 50th (median), 75th, 85th, 90th, 95th, 97th and 99th percentile.

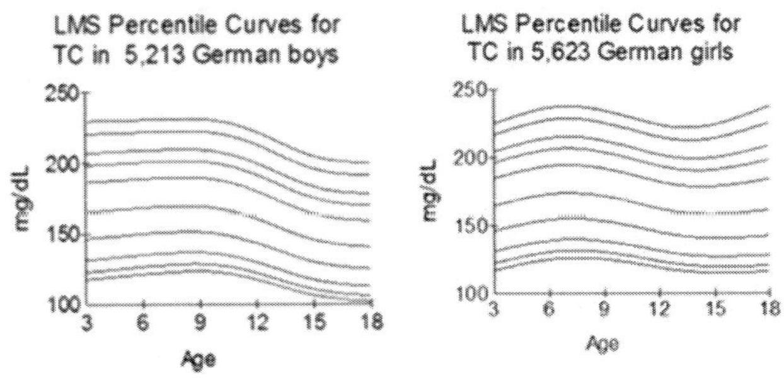

Figure 9.1. Total Cholesterol.

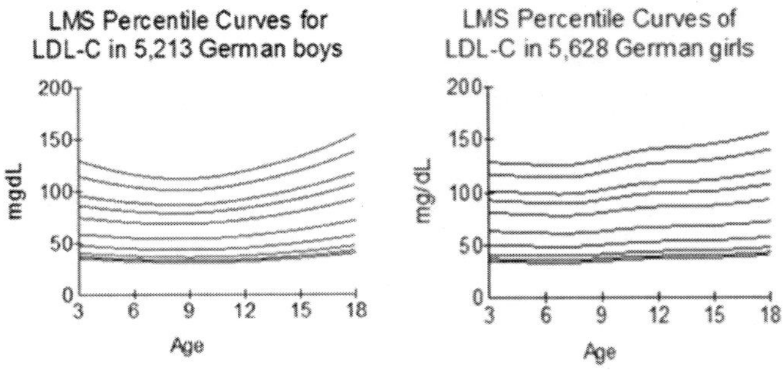

Figure 9.2. LDL-Cholesterol.

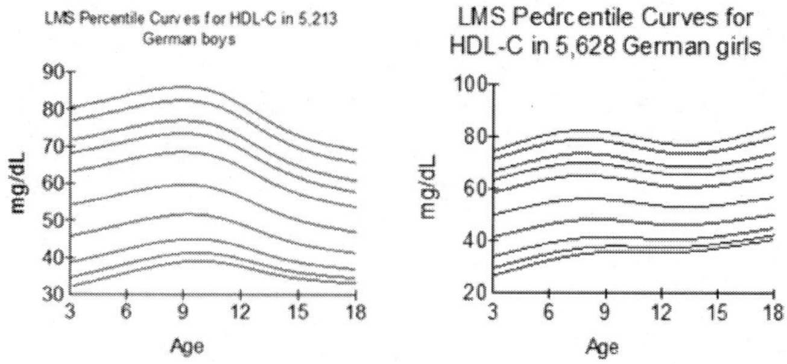

Figure 9.3. HDL-Cholesterol.

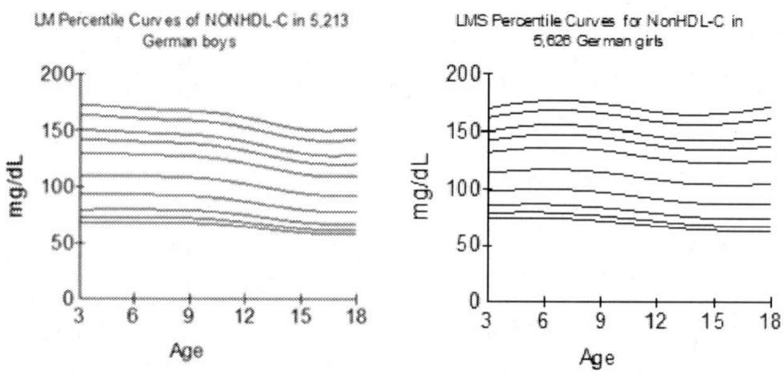

Figure 9.4. Non-HDL-Cholesterol.

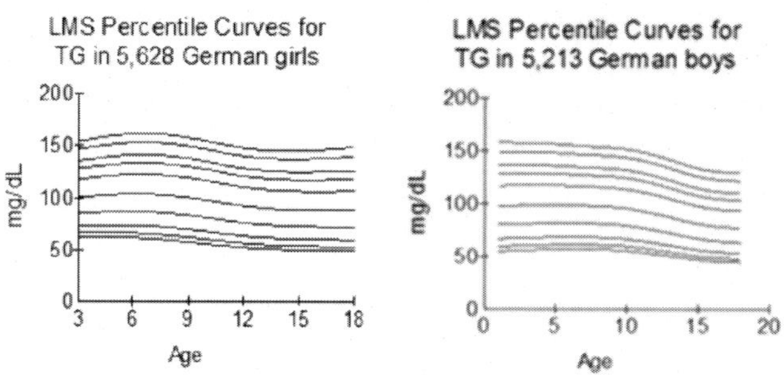

Figure 9.5. Triglycerides.

The growth curves of Non HDL-C and TG are similar, decreasing slightly more in male than in female adolescents.

Among children, total cholesterol is nearly stable until age 10 y, decreases in adolescents but re-increases after 13 years in females.

In both genders, the LDL-C median is stable throughout childhood and adolescence, which means that the cut-off remains constant in youths. However, the HDL-C median decreases in male adolescents but increases in females after puberty. This affects the age-dependent cut-off of the LDL/HDL-C ratio that decreases considerably in females (from 2.09 to 1.52 at the 50th percentile).

BLOOD PRESSURE

Among 22,051 youths, the mean prevalence of hypertension and obesity was 7.3% and 5.2% in children respectively 7.2% and 5.8% in adolescents. Here we present only the growth curves for systolic blood pressure (SBP) among normalweight, overweight and obese youths.

Figure 11. Ten age-, gender-, and height-adjusted LMS percentile curves for systolic blood pressure at the 3rd, 5th, 10th, 25th, 50th, 85th, 90th, 95th, and 97th percentile in 18,917 normalweight (BMI < 85th), 1,938 overweight (BMI 85th to < 95th) and 1,196 obese (≥95th) 3-18 years old males and females.

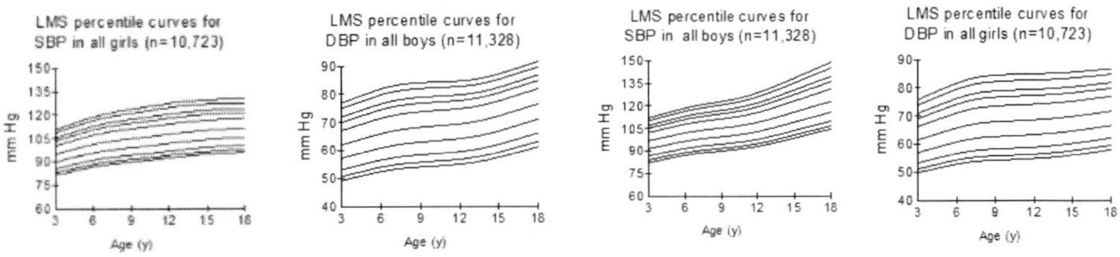

Figure 11. LMS Percentile Curves for SBP and DBP in 22,051 youths.

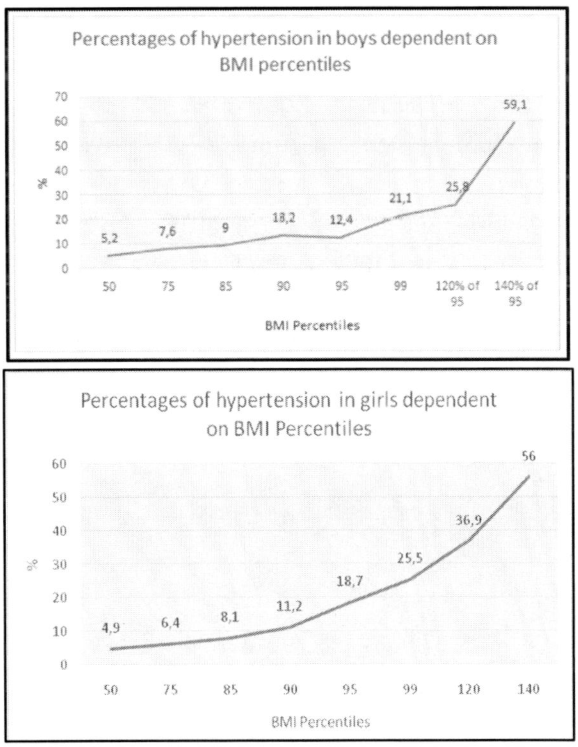

Figure 12 depicts a steep increase of the prevalence of hypertension beyond the 99th percentile of BMI, reaching 59% in males and 56% in females at very severe obesity.

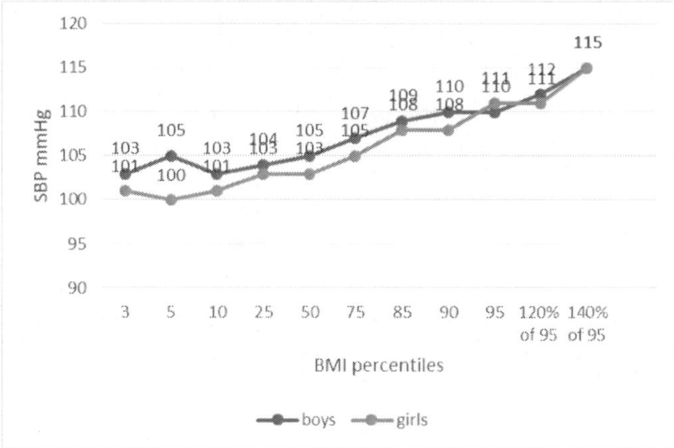

Figure 13. The higher BMI is the higher increase Systolic Blood Pressure means.

The shapes of the SBP percentile curves are different between genders independently from weight groups. In males at younger age, they increase continuously by 1 mm Hg/year and steeper by 2 mm Hg/year from age 13 years upward, whereas in females, the curves increase by 2 mm Hg/year until age 7 years thereafter plateauing until age 14 years with increasing tendency. These changes by age are stronger in overweight and obese youths.

As complained that BMI does not consider (9) whether the children have lean or strong body fat mass we calculated the multivariate models for two further variations namely for children and adolescents with combined overweight from BMI and % Body Fat and combined BMI, %BF and WC. The results for overweight (BMI combined with overBF) demonstrates a probability for hypertension from 5.3 vs. 3.7 for BMI-overweight alone, for elevated TC 1.2 for both, no difference OR 1.3 for LDL-C in both, for low HDL-C a small difference for BMBF-combined OR 2.1 vs. 23, no difference for NonHDL-C with an OR 1.6 as well as for elevated TG the OR 4.9. The combination of elevated BMI, elevated %BF and elevated WC resulted in hypertension 5.3 vs. 3.7 for BMI alone, no significant association for TC or LDL-C with BMBFWC, for HDL-C 2.4 vs. 2.1, no difference for NonHDL-C and for elevated TG 5.4 vs. 4.9.

What Are the Risk Factors Besides Hypertension Associated with Different Adverse CVD RF?

The associations have been analyzed by multivariate logistic models including sex and age classes (children, adolescents).

We found WHtR ≥ 90th percentile as highest risk at all.

Impressive differences are observed when the cohort is divided for sex and age-classes.

Table 6. Attributable Risk for children and adolescents depending on sex and age compared for all fat patterns

Risk Factors	hypertension	TC ≥95th p'tile	LDL-C≥95th p'tile	HDL-C≤5th/10=th p'tile	NonHDL-C ≥95th p'tile	TG≥95th p'tile
sex(1)	0,9 (0,8-1,0)	1,3 (1,1-1,5)	1,3 (1,2 -1,5)	n.s.	1,4 (1,2 -1,6)	1,7 (1,2 -2,5)
agegr(1)	n.s.	2,5 (2,1-3,0)	2,7 (2,2 -3,2)	n.s.	2,2 (1,9-2,7)	0,5 (0,3 - 0,7)
BMI ≥85th p'tile	1,5 (1,2- 2,0)	n.s.	n.s.	n.s.	n.s.	2,9 (1,5 - 5,3)
WC≥90th p'tile	n.s.	0,6 (0,4-0,9)	0,6 (0,4-9,0)	0,3 (0,1 -0,7)	n.s.	n.s.
WHtR≥90th p'tile	1,4(1,1-1,8)	1,5 (1,1 -2,2)	1,5 (1.0 -2,5)	3,6 (1,9 - 6,8)	n.s.	3,0 (1,5 -6,1)
%BF≥85th p'tile	1,5 (1,2-1,8)	n.s.	n.s.	n.s.	n.s.	n.s.
subtricsum>35mm	n.s.	n.s.	n.s.	n.s.	n.s.	n.s.
constant	0,1	0,1	0	0	0,1	0

Legend: sex (1) means girls compared with boys; agegr(1) means adolescents (12-18Y) compared with children (3-11y).

Table 7. Comparison between boys and girls and younger and older children

			boys		girls
			OR (CI 95%)		OR (CI85%)
hypertension	children	BMI> = 85th	1,5(1,1-2,0)	BMI> = 85th	1,7(1,3-2,3)
		WHtR≥90th	1,5(1,1-2,0)		
		BF> = 85th	1,6(1,3-2,0)	BF> = 85th	2,0(1,6-2,6)
		tricplussub35	1,7(1,1-2,4)	tricplussub35	2,3(1,7-3,2)
	adolescents	WHtR≥90th	1,8(1,0-3,3)	BMI> = 85th	4,0(2,4-6,5)
elev. TC	children	BF> = 85th	1,5 (1,1-2,0)	BMI> = 85th	1,5(1,0-2,1)
	adolescents	BF> = 85th	1,7(1,0-2,6)	tricplussub35	2,3(1,1-4,6)
elev. LDL-C	children	WHtR≥90th	1,7(1,0-2,6)	no pattern	
		BF> = 85th	1,4(1,1-2,0)	no pattern	
	adolescents	BF> = 85th	2,2(1,3-3,5)	BF> = 85th	2,6(1,2-5,6)
decr. HDL-C	children	no pattern		BMI> = 85th	2,1 (1,0-2,9)
		no pattern		WHtR≥90th	2,9(1,5-5,6)
	adolescents	no pattern			
elev. NonHDL-C	children	WHtR≥90th	1,6(1,0-2,5)	BMI> = 85th	1,8(1,2-2,5)
		BF> = 85th	1,4(1,0-1,8)	no pattern	
	adolescents	BF> = 85th	1,9(1,2-3,0)	no pattern	
		tricplussub35	2,3(1,1-5,1)	tricplussub35	2,3(1,2-4.4)
elev. TG	children	no pattern		BMI> = 85th	2,8(1,3-5,9)
		no pattern		BF> = 85th	2,2(1,1-4,2)
	adolescents	tricplussub35	4,5(1,5-13,2)	BMI> = 85th	3,4(1,4-8,0)

The risk for adverse CVD RF besides unhealthy fat patterns is higher for girls than in boys and higher for adolescents than in children.

CONCLUSION

The risk for hypertension is for obese youths twofold higher than in non overweights,and the risk for low HDL-C 2,5-fold higher. For TC and LDL-C is no association and no difference between overweights and obese. The results for hypertriglyceridemia and elevated NonHDL-C are nearly the same for overweight and obese children and adolescents. Higher differences are demonstrated for"obese-fat" versus "over"- fat". The risk for all adverse lipids and TG increases. For hypertension the probabilty is 2-fold higher and for hypertriglyceridemia nearly 3-fold higher than in "overfats".

Overweight defined by WHtR showed a 1.5- fold higher risk for elevated LDL-C whereas overweight defined by BMI showed the 1.3-fold risk. Significant probability for elevated Total Cholesterol was only shown for WHtR $\geq 90^{th}$ percentile. No raw association for elevated NonHDL-Cholesterol with adverse fat patterns were found calculating univariate logistic regression.

Demonstrated were in linear associations yet that with each increasing unit of fat pattern the risk of for each unit of hypertension as well as for lipids and TG increases, too.

6,555 youths (601%) had no CVD Risk factor at all. The tables and figures in this chapter establish that "overweight" not always is BMI $\geq 85^{th}$ percentile. As demonstrated with figures and tables out of the percentile tables overweight is not only a fixed definition based on weight and height. Depending on age and sex relationships are observed between waist circumference and adverse lipids or TG as well as for blood pressure. Weight-to Height ratio is an independent indicator, the fat composition of the body is another one (% body fat as well as the sum of triceps and subscapular skinfold thickness), too. The less or more strong associations with further CVD risk factors prove the importance of them all for the definition of overweight, too.

Each of the five possibilities to define "over" the "normal" body composition has its own justification to examine children and adolescents. Sometimes it is sufficient to measure two skinfolds (triceps plus subscapular skinfold) to detect CVD risk factors in children and adolescents.

REFERENCES

[1] Afshin A, Forouzanfar MH, Reitsma MB et al. Health effects of overweight and obesity in 195 countries over 25 years. *N Engl J Med* 2017; 377: 13–27.

[2] Ogden CL, Carroll MD, Lawman HG, et al. Trends in obesity prevalence among Children and adolescents in the United States, 1988-1994 through 2013-2014. *JAMA*. 2016; 315(21):2292-2299.

[3] Hales CM, Fryar CD, Carroll MD, Freedman DS, Ogden CL. Trends in obesity and severe obesity prevalence in US youth and adults by sex and age, 2007-2008 to 2015-2016. *JAMA* 2018; 319: 1723-5.

[4] Skinner AC, Ravanbakht SN, Skelton JA, et al. Prevalence of Obesity and Severe Obesity in US Children, 1999–2016. *Pediatrics*. 2018;141(3):e20173459

[5] Spinelli A, Buoncristiano M, Kovacs CA, Yngv A, Spiroski I, Obreja G et al. Prevalence of severe obesity among primary school children in 21 European countries, *Obes Facts* 2019 doi:10.1159/000500436

[6] Freedman DS, Butte BF, Taveras EM, Lundeen EA, Blanck HM, Goodman AB, Ogden CL BMI z-Scores are a Poor Indicator of Adiposity Among 2- to 19-Year-Olds with Very High BMIs, NHANES 1999-2000 to 2013-2014. *Obesity* 2017 25, 739-746.

[7] Barlow SE and the Expert Committee. Expert committee recommendations regarding the prevention, assessment, and treatment of child and adolescent overweight and obesity: Summary Report. *Pediatrics* 2007; 120 (Suppl 4): S164 – 192

[8] Ogden CL, Kuczmarski RJ, Flegal KM, Mei Z, Guo S, Wei R, Grummer-Strawn LM, Curtin LR, Roche AF & Johnson CL. Centers for Disease Control and Prevention 2000 growth charts for the United States: improvements to the 1977 National Center for Health Statistics version. *Pediatrics*. 2002; 109, 45–60.

[9] Daniels SE et al. Expert Panel on integrated guidelines for cardiovascular health and risk reduction in children and adolescents: Summary Report. *Clinical Practice guidelines NLHBI*, access 2 .April 2020

[10] Slaughter MH, Lohman TG, Boileau RA, Horswill CA, Stillman RJ, van Loan MD, et al. Skin fold equations for estimation of body fatness in children and youth. *Hum Biol*. 1988; 60:709–23.

[11] Cole TJ, Green PJ (1992). Smoothing reference centile curves: the LMS method and penalized likelihood. *Stat Med* 11, 1305–1319.

[12] Kurth BM, Kamtsiuris P, Holling H, Schlaud M, Dolle R, Ellert U, Kahl H, Knopf H, Lange M, Mensink GB, Neuhauser H, Rosario AS, Scheidt-Nave C, Schenk L, Schlack R, Stolzenberg H, Thamm M, Thierfelder W, Wolf U: The challenge of comprehensively mapping children's health in a nation-wide health survey: design of the German KiGGS-study. *BMC Public Health* 2008; 8: 196

[13] Schaffrath Rosario AS, Kurth BM, Stolzenberg H, Ellert U, Neuhauser H. Body mass index percentiles for children and adolescents in Germany based on a nationally representative sample (KiGGS 2003-2006). *Eur J Clin Nutr* 2010; 64: 341-9

[14] Kromeyer-Hauschild K, Wabitsch M, Kunze D, Geller F, Geiß HC, Hesse V, et al. Perzentile für den Body-Mass-Index für das Kindes- und Jugendalter unter Heranziehung verschiedener deutscher Stichproben [Percentiles for the body mass index for children and adolescents using various German samples]. *Monatsschr Kinderheilkunde*. 2001; 149(8): 807–18

[15] Blüher S, Molz E, Wiegand S, Otto KP, Sergeyev E, Tuschy S, et al.; Adiposity Patients Registry Initiative and German Competence Net Obesity. Body mass index, waist circumference, and waist-to-height ratio as predictors of cardiometabolic risk

in childhood obesity depending on pubertal development. *J Clin Endocrinol Metab.* 2013; Aug; 98(8): 3384–93.

[16] Keller E, Gausche R, Meigen C, Keller A, Burmeister J, Kiess W. Auxological computer based network for early detection of disorders of growth and weight attainment. *J Pediatr Endocrinol Metab* 2002; 15: 149-56

[17] Geserick M, Vogel M, Gausche R, et al. Acceleration of BMI in early childhood and risk of sustained obesity. *N Engl J Med* 2018; 379: 1303-12.

[18] Schaefer F, Geordi M, Wühl E, Schärer K. Body mass index and percentage fat mass in healthy German schoolchildren and adolescents. *Int J Obes* 1998; 22:461–9

[19] Schwandt P, Geiss HC, Ritter MM, Üblacker C, Parhofer KG, Otto C, Laubach E, Donner MG, Haas GM, Richter WO. The Prevention Education Program (PEP). A prospective study of the efficacy of family oriented life style modification in the reduction of cardiovascular risk and disease: Design and baseline data. *J Clin Epidemiol* 1999; 52:791 800.

[20] Öhrig E, Geiss HC, Haas GM, Schwandt P. The Prevention Education Program (PEP) Nuremberg: design and baseline data of a family oriented intervention study. *Int J Obes*. 2001; Suppl 1: 89 – 92

[21] Schwandt P, Haas GM. What do we learn from the Prevention Education Program Family Heart Study about Lifestyle change, Blood Pressure, and Lipids in Children and Parents? *Int J Prev Med* 2018; 9:107-.

[22] Schwandt P, Haas GM. Family based prevention of cardiovascular disease risk factors in children by lifestyle change: The PEP Family Heart Study. In: *Primordial Prevention of Noncommunicable Disease*, R. Kelishadi (Ed.), Springer Nature Switzerland AG 2019.

[23] Rönnecke E, Vogel M, Bussler S, Grafe N, Jurkutat A, Schlingmann M, et al. Age- and sex related percentiles of skinfold thickness, waist and hip circumference, waist-to-height ratio: Results from a population-based pediatric cohort in Germany (Life Child) *Obesity Facts* 2019;12:25-39

[24] Quante M, Hesse M, Döhnert M, Fuchs M, Hirsch C, Sergeyev E, et al.; LIFE Child Study Investigators. The LIFE child study: a life course approach to disease and health. *BMC Public Health*. 2012 Nov; 12(1): 1021.

[25] Poulain T, Baber R, Vogel M, Pietzner D, Kirsten T, Jurkutat A, et al.; LIFE Child study team. The LIFE Child study: a population-based perinatal and pediatric cohort in Germany. *Eur J Epidemiol*. 2017 Feb; 32(2): 145–58.

[26] Olds TS. One million skinfolds: secular trends in the fatness of young people 1951-2004. *Eur J Clin Nutr* 2009; 63:934–46.

[27] Sarria A, Garcia Llop LA, Moreno LA, Fleta J, Morellón MP, Bueno M. Skin fold thickness measurements are better predictors of body fat percentage than body mass index in male Spanish children and adolescents. *Eur J Clin Nutr*.1998; 52:573-6

[28] Bedogni G, Iughetti L, Ferrari M, Malavolti M, Poli M, Bernasconi S et al. Sensitivity and specificity of body mass index and skin fold thickness in detecting excess adiposity in children aged 8-12 years. *Ann Hum Biol.* 2003; 30:132–9-

[29] Nooyens AC, Koppes LL, Visscher TL, Twisk JW, Kemper HC, Schuit AJ, et al. Adolescent skinfold thickness is a better predictor of high body fatness in adults than is body mass index: the Amsterdam Growth and Health Longitudinal Study. *Am J Clin Nutr.* 2007 Jun; 85(6): 1533–9.

[30] Freedman DS, Wang J, Ogden C, Thornton JC, Mei Z, Pierson RN, Dietz WH, Horlick M. The prediction of body fatness by BMI and skinfold thickness among children and adolescents. *Annals Human Biology* 2007; 34(2): 183-194

[31] Ogden CL, Li Y, Freedman DS, Borrud LG, Flegal KM. National health statistic reports; no 43. Hyattsville, MD: National Center for Health Statistics; 2011. *Smoothed percentage body fat percentiles for U.S. children and adolescents*, 1999-2004.

[32] Laurson KR, Eisenmann JC, Welk GJ. Body fat percentile curves for U.S. children and adolescents. *Am J Prev Med.* 2011; 41 (4 Suppl 2):S87–92.

[33] Schwandt P, Kelishadi R, Haas GM. First reference curves of waist circumference for German children in comparison to international values: the PEP Family Heart Study. *World J Pediatr.* 2008 Nov; 4(4): 259–66.

[34] Haas GM, Liepold E, Schwandt P. Percentile curves for fat pattering in German adolescents. *World J Pediatr* 2011; 7:16-23.

[35] Skinner AC, Ravanbakht SN, Skelton JA, Perrin EM, Armstrong SC. Prevalence of Obesity and Severe Obesity in US Children, 1999-2016. *Pediatrics* 2018; 141(3): e20173459

[36] Schwandt P, von Eckardstein A, Haas GM. Percentiles of percentage body fat in German children and adolescents: An international comparison. *Int J Prev Med* 2012; 3:846-52

[37] Kromeyer-Hauschild K, Gläser N, Zellner K. Percentile curves for skinfold thickness in 7- to 14-year-old children and adolescents from Jena, Germany. *Eur J Clin Nutr* 2012, 66:615-21

[38] Brambilla P, Bedogni G, Moreno LA, Goran MI, Gutin B, KR Fox KR, Peters DM, P Barbeau P, De Simone M, Pietrobelli A. Crossvalidation of anthropometry against magnetic resonance imaging for the assessment of visceral and subcutaneous adipose tissue in children. *International Journal of Obesity* (2006) 30, 23–30

[39] Fernandez JR, Redden DT, Pietrobelli A, Allison DB. Waist circumference percentiles in nationally representative samples of African-American, European-American, and Mexican-American children and adolescents. *J Pediatr.* 2004; 145:439–44.

[40] McCarthy HD, Jarrett KV, Crawley HF.The development of waist circumference percentiles in British children aged 5.0–16.9 y. *Eur J Clin Nutr.* 2001; 55:902–907

[41] Savva SC, Kourides Y, Tornaritis M, Epiphanious-Savva M, Tafouna P & Kafatos A. Reference growth curves for Cypriot children 6-17 years of age. *Obes Res* 2001; 9: 754 -762

[42] Katzmarzyk PT. Waist circumference percentiles for Canadian youth 11-18y of age. *Eur J Clin Nutr* 2004; 58: 1011-1015

[43] Gómez-Diaz RA, Martinez-Hernández AJ, Aguilar-Salinas CA, Violante R, López-Alarcó M, Jiménez-Viallarruel M, Wacher-Rodarte.N, & Solozano-Santos F. Percentile distribution of the waist circumference among Mexican preadolescents of a primary school in Mexico City. *Diabetes Obes Metab*; 2005; 7: 716 - 721

[44] Eisenmann JC..Waist circumference percentiles for 7-to 15-year-old Australian children. *Acta Paediatr* 2005, 94:, 1182 - 1185

[45] Hatipoglu N, Ozturk A, Mazicioglu MM, Kurtoglu S, Seyhan S & Lokoglu F. Waist circumference percentiles for 7-17-year-old Turkish children and adolescents. *Eur J Pediatr* 2007; published online 9 May

[46] Inokuchi M, Matsuo N, Anzo M, Takayama JI & Hasegawa T. Age dependent percentile for waist circumference for Japanese children based on the 1992-1994 cross-sectional national survey data. *Eur J Pediatr* 2007; 166: 655-661

[47] Galcheva SV, Iotova VM, Yotov YT, et al. Waist circumference percentile curves for Bulgarian children and adolescents aged 6-18 years. *Intern J Pediatr Obesity* 2009; 4:381-388

[48] Schwandt P, Kelishadi R, Ribeiro RQ, Haas GM, Poursafa P. A three country study on the components of the metabolic syndrome in youths: The BIG study. *Int J Pediatr Obes* 2010; 5:334 41.

[49] Nawarycz T, Haas GM, Krzyżaniak A, Schwandt P, Ostrowska Nawarycz L. Waist circumference and waist-to-height ratio distributions in polish and German schoolchildren: Comparative analysis. *Int J Prev Med* 2013; 4:786-96.

[50] Janssen I, Katzmarzyk PT, Ross R. Waist circumference and not body mass index explains obesity-related health risk. *Am J Clin Nutr*. 2004 Mar; 79(3): 379–84.

[51] Taylor SA, Hergenroeder AC. Waist circumference predicts increased cardiometabolic risk in normal weight adolescent males. *Int J Pediatr Obes*. 2011 Jun; 6(2-2):e307–11.

[52] Fredriks AM, van Buuren S, Fekkes M, Verloove-Vanhorick SP, Wit JM. Are age references for waist circumference, hip circumference and waist-hip ratio in Dutch children useful in clinical practice? *Eur J Pediatr*. 2005; 164:216–22.

[53] Kelishadi R, Gouya MM, Ardalan G, Hosseini M, Mtaghian M, Delavari A et al. First reference curves of waist and hip circumferences in an Asian population of youth: CASPIAN study. *J Tropical Pediatr*. 2007; 53:158–64.

[54] Sung RYT, So HK, Choi KC, Nelson EAS, Li AM, Yin JA, Kwok CWL, Ng PC, Fok TF. Waist circumference and waist-to-height ratio of Hong Kong Chinese children. *BMC Public Health*. 2008;8:324. doi:10.1186/1471-2458/8/324 .

[55] Senbanjo IO, Njokanma OF, Oshikoya KA. Waist circumference values of Nigerian children and adolescents. *Ann Nutr Metab*. 2009;54:145–50.

[56] Moreno LA, Fleta J, Mur L, Rodríquez G, Sarría A, Bueno M. Waist circumference values in Spanish children – gender related differences. *Eur J Clin Nutr*. 1999; 53:429–33.

[57] McCarthy HD, Jarrett KV, Crawley HF. The development of waist circumference percentiles in British children aged 5.0–16.9 y. *Eur J Clin Nutr*. 2001;55:902–7.

[58] McCarthy HD, Ellis SM, Cole TJ. Central overweight and obesity in British youth aged 11–16 years: cross sectional surveys of waist circumference. *BMJ* 2003; 326:624–6.

[59] Schwandt P, Haas GM. Reference Curves of Waist Circumference in Children and Adolescents. 2012, Part 13: 1405 -1412. DOI: 10.1007/978-1-1788-1_85 in: *Handbook of Anthropometry*, Preedy Victor R. (Ed.)

[60] Li C, Ford ES, Mokdad AH, Cook S. Recent trends in waist circumference and waist-to height ratio among US children and adolescents. *Pediatrics*. 2006; 118:e1390–98.

[61] Wang J, Thornton, Bari S, Williamson B, Gallagher D, Heymsfi eld SB et al. Comparisons of waist circumference measured at 4 sites. *Am J Clin Nutr*. 2003; 77:379–84.

[62] Katzmarzyk PT, Perusse L, Malina RM, Bergeron J, Despres JP, Bouchard C. Stability of indicators of the metabolic syndrome from childhood and adolescence to young adulthood: the Quebec Family Study. *J Clin Epidemiol*. 2001; 54:190–195

[62a.]Chen X, Wang Y. Tracking of blood pressure from childhood to adulthood: a systematic review and meta-regression analysis. *Circulation*. 2008; 117:3171–3180

[63] Singh AS, Mulder C, Twisk JW, van Mechelen W, Chinapaw MJ. Tracking of childhood overweight into adulthood: a systematic review of the literature. *Obes Rev*. 2008; 9(5):474-488

[64] Ward ZJ, Long MW, Resch SC, Giles CM, Cradock AE, Gortmaker SL. Simulation of growth trajectories of childhood obesity into adulthood. *N England J Med* 2017, 377: 2440-50

[65] Ogden CL, Freedman DS, Craig M, Hales CM. BMI Trajectories in youth and adulthood. *Pediatrics* 2018;141(1):e20343317

[66] Maffeis C, Grezzani A, Pietrobelli A, Provera S, Tatò L. Waist circumference and cardiovascular risk factors in prepubertal children. *Obes Res*. 2001; 9:179–87

[67] Geiss HC, Parhofer KG, Schwandt P. Parameters of childhood obesity and their relationship to cardiovascular risk factors in healthy prepubescent children. 2001 *Int J Obes Relat Metab Disord* 25: 830-837

[68] Sung RYT, Yu CCW, Choi KC, McManus A, Li AMC, Xu SLY, Chan D, Lo AFC, Chan JCN, Fok TF. Waist circumference and body mass index in Chinese children: cut off values for predicting cardiovascular risk factors. *Intern J Obesity*. 2007; 31:550–558

[69] Savva SC, Tornaritis M, Savva ME. Waist circumference and waist to height ratio are better predictors of cardiovascular disease risk factors in children then body mass index. *Int J Obesity Relat Metab Disord.* 2000;24(11):1453–8.

[70] Freedman DS, Katzmarzyk PT, Dietz WH, Srinivasan SR, Berenson GS. Relation of body mass index and skinfold thicknesses to cardiovascular disease risk factors in children: the Bogalusa Heart Study. *Am J Clin Nutr.* 2009; 90:210–6.

[71] Haas GM, Liepold E, Schwandt P. Predicting cardiovascular risk factors by different body fat patterns in 3850 German children: The PEP Family Heart Study. *Int J Prev Med* 2011; 2:15

[72] Daniels SR, Morrison JA, Sprecher DL, Khoury P, Kimball TR. Association of body fat distribution and cardiovascular risk factors in children and adolescents. *Circulation* 1999; 99: 541-545

[73] Morrison JA, Sprecher DL, Barton BA, Waclawiw MA, Daniels SR. Overweight, fat patterning, and cardiovascular disease risk factors in black and white girls: the National Heart, Lung, and Blood Institute Growth and Health Study. *J Pediatr.* 1999; 135:458–464

[74] Kelishadi R, Gheiratmand R, Ardalan G, Adeli K, Mehdi Gouya M, et al. Association of anthropometric indices with cardiovascular disease risk factors among children and adolescents: CASPIAN Study. *Int J Cardiol* 2007117: 340-348.

[75] Matsushita Y, Tomita K, Yokoyama T, Mizoue T. Optimal measurement site of waist circumference for assessing the metabolic syndrome. *Diabetes Care.* 2009; 32:e70.

[76] Moreno LA, Pineda I, Rodriguez G, Fleta J, Sarria A, Bueno M. Waist circumference for the screening of the metabolic syndrome in children. *Acta Paediatr.* 2002; 91:1307–1312

[77] Freedman DS, Ogden CL, Brian K. Kit BK. Interrelationships between BMI, skinfold thicknesses, percent body fat, and cardiovascular disease risk factors among U.S. children and adolescents. *BMC Pediatrics* 2015, 15:188

[78] Khoury P, Morrison JA, Kelly K, Mellies M, Horvitz R, Glueck CJ. Clustering and interrelationships of coronary heart disease risk factors in schoolchildren, ages 6–19. *Am J Epidemiol.* 1980; 112:524–538

[79] Zannolli R, Morgese G. Waist percentiles: a simple test for atherogenic disease? *Acta Paediatr.* 1996; 85:1368–1369

[80] Haas GM, Schwandt P. Age- and gender-specific silent cardiovascular risk factors in children and adolescents. *Trends in Research* 2018 doi: 10.15761/TR.1000107

[81] Larsson SC, Bäck M, Rees JMB, Mason AM, Burgess S. Body mass index and body composition in relation to 14 cardiovascular conditions in UK Biobank: a Mendelian randomization study. *European Heart Journal* 2020; 41:221-226

[82] Freedman DS, Serdula MK, Srinivasan SR, Berenson GS. Relation of circumferences and skinfold thicknesses to lipid and insulin concentrations in

children and adolescents: the Bogalusa Heart Study. *Am J Clin Nutr.* 1999; 69:308–317

[83] Chu N-F, Rimm EB, Wang D-J, Liou H-S, Shieh S-M. Relationship between anthropometric variables and lipid levels among schoolchildren: the Taipei Children Heart Study. *Int J Obes Relat Metab Disord.* 1998; 22:66–72

[84] Schwandt P, Haas GM.Waist Circumference in Children and Adolescents from Different Ethnicities. Chapter 4, p. 79 -94 in: Childhood Obesity Sevil An Yuca (Ed.) ISBM 978-953-51-0374-5 e-book www.intechopen.com / articles/show/title/ waist-circumference-in-children-and-adolescents-from-different-ethnicities

[85] Kelishadi R, Schwandt P, Haas GM, Hosseini M, Mirmoghtadaee P. Reference curves of anthropometric indices and serum lipid profiles in representative samples of Asian and European children. *Arch Med Sci* 2008; 4: 329 – 335

[86] Haas GM, Liepold E, Schwandt P. Predicting Cardiovascular Risk Factors by Different Body Fat Patterns in 3850 German Children: the PEP Family Heart Study. *Int J Prev Med* 2011; Jan. 2(1): 15 -19

[87] Daniels SR, Greer FR. the Committee on Nutrition. Lipid Screening and Cardiovascular Health in Childhood. *Pediatrics* 2008; 122(1):198–208.

[88] Cook S, Auinger P, Huang TTK. Growth Curves for Cardio-Metabolic Risk Factors in Children and Adolescents J Pediatr. 2009 September; 155(3): S6.e15–S6.e26. doi: 10.1016/j.jpeds.2009.04.051

[89] Schwandt P, Bischoff -Ferrari HA, Staehelin HB, Haas GM. Cardiovascular risk screening in schoolchildren predicts risk in parents. *Atherosclerosis* 2009: 250: 626 – 631

[90] Schwandt P, Bertsch T, Haas GM. Anthropometric screening for silent cardiovascular risk factors in adolescents: The PEP Family Heart Study. *Atherosclerosis* 2010; 211:667-71.

[91] Mirmoghtadaee P. (2008) Reference curves of anthropometric indices and serum lipid profiles in representative samples of Asian and European children. *Arch Med Sci*; 4: 329-335

[92] Holl RW, Hoffmeister U, Thamm M et al. Does obesity lead to a specific lipid disorder? Analysis from the German/Austrian/Swiss APV registry. *Int J Pediatr Obes* 2011 Suppl 1:53-58.

[93] Flodmark CE, Sveger T, Nilsson-Ehle P. Waist measurement correlates to a potentially atherogenic lipoprotein profile in obese 12–14-year-old children. *Acta Paediatr.* 1994; 83:941 945

[94] Sorof J, Daniels S. Obesity hypertension in children: a problem of epidemic proportions. *Hypertension* 2002:40(4): 441-447.

[95] Falkner ML, Gidding SS, Ramirez-Garnica G, Wiltrout SA, West D, Rappaport EB. The relationship of body mass index and blood pressure in primary care pediatric patients. *J Pediatr* 2006; 148(2):195-200

[96] Kollias A, Dafni M, Poulidakis E, Ntineri A, Stergiou GS. Out-of-office blood pressure and target organ damage in children and adolescents: a systematic review and meta-analysis. *J Hypertens*. 2014; 32:2315–2331;

[97] Juhola J, Magnussen CG, Berenson GS, Venn A, Burns TL, Sabin MA, Srinivasan SR, Daniels SR, Davis PH, Chen W, Kahonen M, Taittonen L, Urbina E, Viikari JS, Dwyer T, Raitakari OT, Juonala M. Combined effects of child and adult elevated blood pressure on subclinical atherosclerosis: the International Childhood Cardiovascular Cohort Consortium. *Circulation*.2013; 128: 217–224

[98] Ying-xiu Z, Zhan-xia W, Ling Y, Ghun-bo G, Guo-lin G. Association between body mass index, skinfold thickness and blood pressure in 12-year-old children. *Eur J Pediatr* doi 10.1007/s00431-013-2014-7

[99] Bo Xi, PhD*; Xin'nan Zong, Kelishadi R. Establishing International Blood Pressure References Among Nonoverweight Children and Adolescents Aged 6 to 17 Years. *Circulation*. 2016; 133:398-408

[100] National High Blood Pressure Education Program Working Group on High Blood Pressure in Children and Adolescents. The fourth report on the diagnosis, evaluation, and treatment of high blood pressure in children and adolescents. *Pediatrics* 2004; 114 (Suppl):555–76.

[101] Lurbe E, Cifkova R, Cruickshank JK, Dillon MJ, Ferreira I, Invitti C, Kuznetsova T, Laurent S, Mancia G, Morales-Olivas F, Rascher W, Redon J, Schaefer F, Seeman T, Stergiou G, Wuhl E, Zanchetti A; European Society of Hypertension. Management of high blood pressure in children and adolescents: recommendations of the European Society of Hypertension. *J Hypertens*. 2009; 27:1719–1742.

[102] Rosner B, Cook N, Portman R, Daniels S, Falkner B. Determination of blood pressure percentiles in normal-weight children: some methodological issues. *Am J Epidemiol*. 2008; 167:653–666.

[103] Munkhaugen J, Lydersen S, Wideroe TE, Hallan S. Blood pressure reference values in adolescents: methodological aspects and suggestions for Northern Europe tables based on the Nord-Trondelag Health Study II. *J Hypertens*. 2008; 26:1912–1918.

[104] Yan W, Liu F, Li X, Wu L, Zhang Y, Cheng Y, Zhou W, Huang G. Blood pressure percentiles by age and height for non-overweight Chinese children and adolescents: analysis of the China Health and Nutrition Surveys 1991-2009. *BMC Pediatr*. 2013; 13:195.

[105] Schwandt P, Scholze JE, Bertsch T, Liepold E, Haas GM. Blood pressure percentiles in 22,051 German children and adolescents: the PEP Family Heart Study. *Am J Hypertens*. 2015; 28:672–679.

[106] Neuhauser HK, Thamm M, Ellert U, Hense HW, Rosario AS. Blood pressure percentiles by age and height from nonoverweight children and adolescents in Germany. *Pediatrics*. 2011; 127: e978–e988.

[107] Kułaga Z, Litwin M, Grajda A, Kułaga K, Gurzkowska B, Góźdź M, Pan H; OLAF Study Group. Oscillometric blood pressure percentiles for Polish normal-weight school-aged children and adolescents. *J Hypertens*. 2012; 30:1942–1954.

[108] Skinner AC, Perrin EM, Moss LA, Skelton JA. Cardiometabolic risks and severity of obesity in children and young adults. *N Engl J Med*. 2015; 373 (14):1307-1317.

In: Childhood Obesity
Editor: Roya Kelishadi

ISBN: 978-1-53618-158-6
© 2020 Nova Science Publishers, Inc.

Chapter 11

METABOLICALLY HEALTHY OBESITY IN THE CHILDHOOD: A PATTERN OR A TRANSIENT STATE?

Cézane Priscila Reuter[1,*], PhD, Éboni Marília Reuter[2], PhD, Leticia Borfe[3], Letícia Welser[4], Letícia de Borba Schneiders[4], Elza Daniel de Mello[3], MD, Jane Dagmar Pollo Renner[5], PhD and Roya Kelishadi[6], MD

[1]Department of Health Sciences and Graduate Program in Health Promotion, University of Santa Cruz do Sul, Santa Cruz do Sul, Rio Grande do Sul, Brazil
[2]Department of Health Sciences, University of Santa Cruz do Sul, Santa Cruz do Sul, Rio Grande do Sul, Brazil
[3]Graduate Program in Human Movement Sciences, Federal University of Rio Grande do Sul, Porto Alegre, Rio Grande do Sul, Brazil
[4]Graduate Program in Health Promotion, University of Santa Cruz do Sul, Santa Cruz do Sul, Rio Grande do Sul, Brazil
[5]Department of Life Sciences and Graduate Program in Health Promotion, University of Santa Cruz do Sul, Santa Cruz do Sul, Rio Grande do Sul, Brazil
[6]Child Growth and Development Research Center, Research Institute for Primordial Prevention of Non-Communicable Disease, Isfahan University of Medical Sciences, Isfahan, Iran

ABSTRACT

The high frequency of childhood obesity, as well as its association with cardiometabolic alterations are evidenced worldwide. However, many studies have

[*] Corresponding Author's Email: cezanereuter@unisc.br.

focused on assessing metabolically healthy obesity (MHO) in childhood, which consists of the presence of adiposity without metabolic disorders. In contrast, little is known about childhood MHO and there is no standardized definition of this phenotype in this population, with diverse information in the literature. In addition, the mechanisms involved in this obesity pattern are still unknown, suggesting the possibility of differentiation of visceral fat accumulation, birth weight, fat cell size, inflammatory action, and genetic factors. Moreover, several authors have discussed this terminology to assess how healthy is an obese individual? Controversial evidence exists about evidences suggesting if MHO is a pattern of obesity or a transient state to metabolically unhealthy obesity (MUO). The clinical implications for both groups were also reviewed since obesity alone is a major risk factor for cardiovascular disease from childhood. A better understanding of MHO and MUO phenotypes is important for the development of strategies for the prevention, management, and treatment of obesity and metabolic disorders in childhood. Thus, this chapter aims to review the literature on MHO in the pediatric age group, exploring the mechanisms proposed to understand this phenotype, as well as discussing the use of terminology in the literature.

Keywords: obesity, Metabolically Healthy Obesity, prevention, management, children

INTRODUCTION

Obesity is a highly prevalent disorder that presents itself as a physiopathological complex disease. It results from the interaction of behavioral, environmental, metabolic and genetic factors (Hoebel, Malan, and Ridder 2012; Rey-López et al. 2014). However, some obese individuals have a normal metabolic profile, with lower risk of developing metabolic changes, such as type 2 diabetes mellitus (DM), dyslipidemia, and hypertension, even for a not determined period of time (Jung, Lee, and Song 2017; Martínez-Larrad et al. 2014). This condition was termed as Metabolically Healthy Obesity (MHO), characterized by a normal metabolic profile and low levels of inflammatory responses, although with excess weight of fat. Therefore, even with the presence of the pathology, these individuals demonstrate to have less amount of visceral fat (Yaghootkar et al. 2014) when compared to individuals that present altered metabolic profile, the denominated Metabolically Unhealthy Obesity (MUO) (Jung, Lee, and Song 2017; Seo and Rhee 2014).

Although obesity can be characterized as an independent risk factor for the development of metabolic changes (Galić et al. 2016), the prevalence of MHO individuals is different between populations, ranging from 6 to 75% of some studied populations (Rey-López et al. 2014; Jung, Lee, and Song 2017; Martínez-Larrad et al. 2014; Seo and Rhee 2014; Eckel et al. 2015; M. Blüher 2010). Differences in prevalence are due to their definition being based on different metabolic evaluation criteria, and there is still no consistent criterion as a diagnostic standard. Among variations found, are the definition of the study population - whether only obese or overweight -, as well as which items compose MHO and how many factors are considered to be at risk (Jung, Lee, and Song 2017). As a consequence, there is a difficulty in comparing the findings which are reflected in the mechanisms that determine metabolic disorders or control metabolic changes in obese individuals that have not yet been totally understood and its long-term behavior.

Thus, this chapter aims to review the literature on MHO in the pediatric age group, exploring the mechanisms proposed to better understand this phenotype, as well as discussing the use of terminology in the literature - if MHO is a pattern of obesity or a transient state to MUO.

METABOLICALLY HEALTHY OBESITY CRITERIA

The lack of standardization of the MHO criteria, including the markers to be considered, their cutoff points, and the number of risk factors, makes it difficult to compare outcomes, understand the phenotype and prognosis. The literature has diverged on the existence of a "healthy obesity," and the conclusion has not yet been reached for the adoption of a single criterion that meets children and adolescents, regardless of sex or pubertal stage, which would facilitate conclusions on the subject (Stefan et al. 2008; Cadenas-Sanchez et al. 2017; Jung, Lee, and Song 2017; Damanhoury et al. 2018).

One of the decisive elements for the study of MHO is what is considered obesity. This is because part of the studies includes overweight subjects in the sample, and body mass index (BMI) is usually used as a marker of nutritional status (Ortega et al. 2015; Damanhoury et al. 2018). Thus, variants of the acronym MHO are found in the literature, which can mean Metabolically Healthy Obese or Metabolically Healthy Overweight, in addition to related terms.

As for risk factors, changes in blood pressure (BP) (systolic and diastolic), triglycerides (TG), glucose and high-density lipoprotein (HDL-C) levels are commonly considered. The use of insulin sensitivity markers, metabolic syndrome and absence of fatty liver is also described (Damanhoury et al. 2018; S. Blüher and Schwarz 2014). Ortega et al. (2015) proposed a definition of MHO criteria for adolescents, considering that in this age group the literature is more restricted and there is less frequency of changes in the metabolic profile. They emphasize the importance of cut-off points specific to sex and age, for the physiological changes that occur during the development phase. They recommend linking MHO with the metabolic syndrome criteria, except for waist circumference (WC), since BMI and WC are strongly associated and would hardly provide different answers (Stefan et al. 2013). However, there are criteria for metabolic syndrome that are not applicable in children. In addition, there is low agreement between criteria for the metabolic syndrome in the pediatric population, indicating that new criteria should be established for its diagnosis (Reuter et al. 2018).

Table 1. International prevalence of MHO in children and adolescents

Author (year)	Local	n; age range(yr)	Prevalence of MHO
Nasreddine et al. 2018	Saudi-Arabia	1,047; 1-19	20.9% (IDF) and 23.8% (RC) 12.8% (both of criteria)
Remor et al. 2019	South America	340;10-18	49.4% (IDF) and 55.9% (IR)
Heshmat et al. 2018	Iran	3843; 7-18	Boys 10.35% and Girls 7.74% (ATP III)
Reinehr et al. 2015	Germany	2,017;	49.3% at baseline (CMRF)
Prince et al. 2014	Canada	181; 8–17	31.5% (IR) and 21.5% (CR)
Bervoets and Massa 2016	Belgium	156; 10–18	11.6% (both of criteria)
Stenzel et al. 2018	Brazil	60;10-19	18.6% (IDF), 19.2% (HOMA-IR) 6.4% (both of criteria)
Mangge et al. 2013	Austria	299;8-17	23.3% (ATP III)
Zhao et al. 2019	Brazil, China, Greece, Italy, and Spain	3,497;6-17	36% (MS) 4.5% (NCEP) and 8.2% (IDF)
Yoon et al. 2017	Korea	530; 10-19	36.8% (CMRF) and 68.8% (IR)
Arenaza et al. 2019	Europe	137;12-17	32.8% (Jolliffe and Janssen criteria)

Note: IDF/ATP III/CR/MS/NCEP/CMRF/Jolliffe and Janssen Criteria refer to MHO = being obese but not having other components of Metabolic Syndrome; HOMA-IR/IR Criteria refer to MHO = absence of insulin resistance.

Despite the heterogeneity of the methods, common points are perceived by those who represent metabolically favorable profiles, such as high insulin sensitivity, blood pressure levels and preserved lipid profile (S. Blüher and Schwarz 2014; Cadenas-Sanchez et al. 2017). Thus, in consultation with experts in the field, consensus was defined as: a) the HDL-C, TG, systolic and diastolic BP markers and a blood glucose measurement, without agreement on which glycemic indicator is most appropriate; b) as in most publications (Table 1), those who do not have changes in risk markers should be considered metabolically healthy; c) finally, the BMI measurement must be maintained to assess nutritional status, using the World Health Organization cutoff points (Damanhoury et al. 2018).

Pathophysiological Mechanisms

It is not clear yet which mechanisms interact for the expression of the MHO phenotype, with limited data on the key points of protection. However, there are theories that aim to contribute to its understanding. The amount and distribution of body fat have been described as important in this process, rather than the isolated value of BMI, to determine a healthy or unhealthy metabolic profile. A smaller amount of visceral adipose tissue contributes to the favorable profile of MHO (Jung, Lee, and Song 2017; Gonçalves, Glade, and Meguid 2016).

Regarding fat storage, it is indicated that lipids can accumulate in visceral fat deposits, which have a low capacity when compared to subcutaneous tissue, being distributed to the liver, muscle (including the heart muscle) and β cells. This distribution contributes to metabolic damages. In MHO phenotype, on the other hand, the subcutaneous adipose tissue would expand, preserving insulin sensitivity. The size of adipocytes (visceral or subcutaneous) has also been associated with the metabolic profile. There are indications that genetic factors may contribute to the pattern of distribution of central or peripheral fat. However, the contribution of both genetic and environmental factors to the expansion of subcutaneous fat remains under discussion (Denis and Obin 2013; Jung, Lee, and Song 2017).

Visceral fat in higher concentrations is accompanied by a set of changes that characterize the metabolic syndrome: insulin resistance, type 2 DM, systemic arterial hypertension, dyslipidemia, systemic inflammation, and cardiovascular diseases. Insulin resistance, in turn, is accompanied by higher levels of low-density lipoprotein cholesterol (LDL-C), TG, fasting glucose, low concentrations of HDL-C, changes in epithelial tissue and microalbuminuria. Both visceral fat and insulin resistance are related to an increased concentration of free fatty acids in the portal circulation, which stimulate changes in the lipid profile (Gonçalves, Glade, and Meguid 2016). Furthermore, the accumulation of liver fat may be more relevant than visceral deposits in determining a metabolically healthy phenotype, since obese with insulin sensitivity showed a 54% lower accumulation of liver fat compared to obese with insulin resistance (Stefan et al. 2008).

The activity of liver enzymes can also contribute to the metabolic profile. Reduced levels of some enzymes, especially alanine aminotransferase (ALT), may reflect lower insulin resistance and lower hepatic fat content. Thus, the higher oxidation rate of free fatty acids could result in a lower amount of fat in the liver Messier et al. 2010. In addition, increased levels of visceral fat have been associated with pro-inflammatory markers such as interleukin-6 (IL-6), tumor necrosis factor-α (TNF-α) and chemokines. As a consequence of inflammation, there is the occurrence of insulin resistance, which determines an increased risk for the development of diabetes mellitus, cardiovascular diseases and fatty liver (Gonçalves, Glade, and Meguid 2016). One of these biomarkers is C-reactive protein (CRP), which is positively associated with anthropometric parameters (S. Blüher and Schwarz 2014). On the other hand, MHO has a reduced inflammatory profile (Denis and Obin 2013; DeBoer 2013). In this sense, the homeostasis of adipose tissue inflammation has been shown to be an important element for metabolic health, with MHO presenting inflammatory markers in low concentrations and adiponectin in the normal range, in addition to less visceral fat and smaller size of adipocyte cells (S. Blüher and Schwarz 2014; Cadenas-Sanchez et al. 2017). Therefore, it is notable that the unfavorable metabolic profile is a sum of factors that culminate in insulin resistance, such as visceral obesity, increased levels of free fatty acids, systemic inflammation, low levels of adiponectin and genetic factors (DeBoer 2013).

Clinical Implications of Metabolically Healthy Obesity

In general, despite the presence of excessive fat mass, MHO phenotype is considered as a subset of characteristics that reduce cardiometabolic risk factors (Gonçalves, Glade, and Meguid 2016). The risks of type 2 DM, cardiovascular diseases, and mortality for all causes are higher in MUO than MHO. Nevertheless, the risks are higher in the MHO phenotype if compare to nonobese and metabolically healthy (MHNO) individuals (Zheng, Zhou, and Zhu 2016; Mongraw-Chaffin et al. 2018; Bell, Kivimaki, and Hamer 2014; Hamer and Stamatakis 2012).

Presently, there are no consensus criteria for the definition of MHO. However, the lipid profile, the glycemic index, and the blood pressure have shown relation with MHO. In this aspect, studies show that MHO individuals exhibit a lipid and enzyme hepatic profile more favorable than MUO individuals (Karelis et al. 2005; Aguilar-Salinas et al. 2008; Marini et al. 2007; Succurro et al. 2008).

Another clinic characteristics of MHO individuals include more favorable levels of LDL-C (Shin et al. 2006) and free fatty acids (Stefan et al. 2008; Succurro et al. 2008). However, blood pressure results differ than those find for the blood lipids, whilst some studies noticed lower blood pressure in MHO individuals (Marini et al. 2007; Genelhu et al. 2009; Succurro et al. 2008) while others do not (Brochu et al. 2001; Karelis et al. 2005).

The risk of developing type 2 DM is lower in MHO than MUO, although it is still about four times higher than MHNO (Bell, Kivimaki, and Hamer 2014). Also, there is a direct relation with the risk of developing type 2 DM and cardiovascular events with the number of metabolic abnormalities in the baseline (Twig et al. 2014; Caleyachetty et al. 2017). Studies report that, in MHO individuals, greater sensitivity to insulin was accompanied by lower levels of fasting glucose and insulin (Brochu et al. 2001; Stefan et al. 2008; Marini et al. 2007).

The risk of cardiovascular events in MHO individuals is also lower than in MUO individuals, but it is still higher compared to individuals with MHNO (Caleyachetty et al. 2017; Eckel et al. 2015). Also, MHO individuals have fewer mortality risks for all causes than those with MUO (Hamer and Stamatakis 2012). However, in relation to those are MHNO, depends on the number of metabolic abnormalities and its gravity, as well the metabolic health stability (Hamer, Johnson, and Bell 2017; Kuk et al. 2018).

Lifestyle and Associated Factors to Metabolically Healthy Obesity in Childhood

It is known that behavioral risk factors, sedentarism, and abdominal obesity are associated with metabolic syndrome in childhood (Wang et al. 2013). A study realized in the Czech Republic identified that metabolic health had been related to the total of sleep hours, time to sleep, time of the last meal, regular consumption of meals, and protein ingest (Aldhoon-Hainerová, Hainer, and Zamrazilová 2017).

The MHO condition may be due by the genetic predisposition, lifestyle or the combination of both of them (Gonçalves, Glade, and Meguid 2016). A study by Li et al. (2016) confirms that both genetic predispositions than the environmental factors and their interaction contributes to MHO prevision status, suggesting the existence of a partial genetic-environmental base in this phenotype. The same study also identified in addition to the current lifestyle and the socio economics factors, such as walking until the school and the soda consume, the early nutritional intrauterine environmental can predict the MHO for independent way as well.

The literature did not still report enough evidence that explains why some obese children developing associated metabolic complications and others do not. However, it is speculated that this condition can be due to specific factors of the lifestyle such as physical activity (Damanhoury et al. 2018). In a study realized with Canadian children and adolescents, Prince et al. (2014) showed that moderate and vigorous physical activity were independently associated with MHO.

Thus, Arenaza et al. (2019) highlight that cardiorespiratory fitness can play a key role in the MHO phenotype of European adolescents. Although, other research realizes with American, Canadian, and Arabs adolescents did not report association with physical activity and MHO (Camhi et al. 2013; Heinzle, Ball, and Kuk 2016; Nasreddine et al. 2018).

So that the metabolic health situation of obese children and adolescents does not worsen, actions are necessary in order to encourage the control of a more balanced and healthy diet, and an increase in the practice of physical exercises (Li et al. 2016; Lin et al. 2017) with the purpose to increase the cardiorespiratory fitness in this population, contributing to the comorbidities prevention related to obesity more late in life (Arenaza et al. 2019).

Metabolically Healthy Obesity as a Pattern of Obesity or a Transient State to Metabolically Unhealthy Obesity?

Since the term was proposed, many studies have been published, describing the prevalence (Kelishadi et al. 2008; Nasreddine et al. 2018; Remor et al. 2019) and factors associated with MHO in children and adolescents (Payab et al. 2019; Remor et al. 2019; Zhao et al. 2019). However, a new debate has been conducted in the literature: is an obese really healthy? Or is this pattern a transient state for MUO?

In fact, the metabolically healthy status can be changed to metabolically unhealthy and vice versa. In this sense, MHO has not considered a static condition (Jung, Lee, and Song 2017), due to the fact that it is not clear whether these individuals continue with this pattern throughout life. It has been suggested, however, that visceral obesity is one of the predictive factors for the progression from MHO to MUO (Kang et al. 2017; Hwang et al. 2015). Therefore, MHO can be considered as a syndrome that presents a relevant prognosis implication (Denis and Obin 2013).

In this context, some studies demonstrate the transient effect from MHO to MUO, especially in adults. In a 10 years-cohort study with a representative sample of adults, 64.7% converted to MUO. Dyslipidemia, higher insulin resistance, greater abdominal visceral area, and subcutaneous fat were the univariate predictors to MUO conversion (Hwang et al. 2015). Also, another cohort study showed that for one-third MHO subjects were a transient state, that turned MHO cases in MUO during the follow-up (Appleton et al. 2013). In children, the transient effect appears to be less evident. In a longitudinal study conducted with 1,002 children classified as MHO in the baseline, 68% maintained this pattern of obesity after a 1-year follow-up (Reinehr et al. 2015). Therefore, more longitudinal studies are essential to better understand this pattern of obesity and the transitory effect for MUO (Damanhoury et al. 2018).

An important point that we must consider is the prevention of progression from MHO to MUO phenotype, through the preservation of the individual's metabolic health, including increased levels of aerobic fitness, circulating levels of adiponectin and incretin responses to the meal, for example. On the other hand, it is important to reduce visceral adiposity, liver lipids, and inflammatory activity. Through an active and healthy lifestyle, it is possible to promote these metabolic actions (Jung, Lee, and Song 2017). Also, if the transition from MHO to MUO occurs, modifiable predictors of this change should be the key to intervention programs to maintain the healthy metabolic profile of children throughout their lives (Damanhoury et al. 2018).

Conclusion

It is suggested that MHO individuals have a lower risk of developing cardiometabolic diseases than the MUO individuals. Based on this review, it is believed the terminology MHO in use for the literature seems to be a transient state with a limited and variable period of time until they would become MUO. It depends on the time the individual has the extra amount of the fat deposited in its body, the healthy lifestyle including physical activity and dietary habits, as well as genetics aspects.

Given its transitory effect from healthy to unhealthy obesity profile, it should be considered by health care providers and public intervention and prevention programs. Knowledge about the predictors of this transition is the key to intervention programs focused on aspects of lifestyle, with the aim of maintaining a healthy metabolic profile throughout life. It is also suggested that it is necessary to standardize the classification of MHO in children and adolescents, which would facilitate the international actions for this condition.

REFERENCES

Aguilar-Salinas, C. A., Eduardo García García, Lorena Robles, Daniela Riaño, Doris Georgina Ruiz-Gomez, Ana Cristina García-Ulloa, Marco A. Melgarejo, et al. 2008. "High Adiponectin Concentrations Are Associated with the Metabolically Healthy Obese Phenotype." *The Journal of Clinical Endocrinology & Metabolism* 93 (10): 4075–79. https://doi.org/10.1210/jc.2007-2724.

Aldhoon-Hainerová, I., V. Hainer, and H. Zamrazilová. 2017. "Impact of Dietary Intake, Lifestyle and Biochemical Factors on Metabolic Health in Obese Adolescents." *Nutrition, Metabolism and Cardiovascular Diseases* 27 (8): 703–10. https://doi.org/10.1016/j.numecd.2017.05.002.

Appleton, Sarah L., Christopher J. Seaborn, Renuka Visvanathan, Catherine L. Hill, Tiffany K. Gill, Anne W. Taylor, and Robert J. Adams. 2013. "Diabetes and Cardiovascular Disease Outcomes in the Metabolically Healthy Obese Phenotype: A Cohort Study." *Diabetes Care* 36 (8): 2388–94. https://doi.org/10.2337/dc12-1971.

Arenaza, Lide, Inge Huybrechts, Francisco B. Ortega, Jonatan R. Ruiz, Stefaan De Henauw, Yannis Manios, Ascensión Marcos, et al. 2019. "Adherence to the Mediterranean Diet in Metabolically Healthy and Unhealthy Overweight and Obese European Adolescents: The HELENA Study." *European Journal of Nutrition* 58 (7): 2615–23. https://doi.org/10.1007/s00394-018-1809-8.

Bell, J. A., M. Kivimaki, and M. Hamer. 2014. "Metabolically Healthy Obesity and Risk of Incident Type 2 Diabetes: A Meta-Analysis of Prospective Cohort Studies." *Obesity Reviews* 15 (6): 504–15. https://doi.org/10.1111/obr.12157.

Bervoets, Liene, and Guy Massa. 2016. "Classification and Clinical Characterization of Metabolically 'Healthy' Obese Children and Adolescents." *Journal of Pediatric Endocrinology and Metabolism* 29 (5): 553–60. https://doi.org/10.1515/jpem-2015-0395.

Blüher, Matthias. 2010. "The Distinction of Metabolically 'healthy' from 'Unhealthy' Obese Individuals." *Current Opinion in Lipidology* 21 (1): 38–43. https://doi.org/10.1097/MOL.0b013e3283346ccc.

Blüher, Susann, and Peter Schwarz. 2014. "Metabolically Healthy Obesity from Childhood to Adulthood - Does Weight Status Alone Matter?" *Metabolism: Clinical and Experimental* 63 (9): 1084–92. https://doi.org/10.1016/j.metabol.2014.06.009.

Brochu, Martin, André Tchernof, Isabelle J. Dionne, Cynthia K. Sites, Georgia H. Eltabbakh, Ethan A. H. Sims, and Eric T. Poehlman. 2001. " What Are the Physical Characteristics Associated with a Normal Metabolic Profile Despite a High Level of Obesity in Postmenopausal Women? 1 ." *The Journal of Clinical Endocrinology & Metabolism* 86 (3): 1020–25. https://doi.org/10.1210/jcem.86.3.7365.

Cadenas-Sanchez, Cristina, Jonatan R. Ruiz, Idoia Labayen, Inge Huybrechts, Yannis Manios, Marcela González-Gross, Christina Breidenassel, et al. 2017. "Prevalence of Metabolically Healthy but Overweight/Obese Phenotype and Its Association With Sedentary Time, Physical Activity, and Fitness." *Journal of Adolescent Health* 61 (1): 107–14. https://doi.org/10.1016/j.jadohealth.2017.01.018.

Caleyachetty, Rishi, G. Neil Thomas, Konstantinos A. Toulis, Nuredin Mohammed, Krishna M. Gokhale, Kumarendran Balachandran, and Krishnarajah Nirantharakumar. 2017. "Metabolically Healthy Obese and Incident Cardiovascular Disease Events Among 3.5 Million Men and Women." *Journal of the American College of Cardiology* 70 (12): 1429–37. https://doi.org/10.1016/j.jacc.2017.07.763.

Camhi, Sarah M., Molly E. Waring, Susan B. Sisson, Laura L. Hayman, and Aviva Must. 2013. "Physical Activity and Screen Time in Metabolically Healthy Obese Phenotypes in Adolescents and Adults." *Journal of Obesity* 2013 (s/n): 1–10. https://doi.org/10.1155/2013/984613.

Damanhoury, S., A. S. Newton, M. Rashid, L. Hartling, J. L.S. Byrne, and G. D.C. Ball. 2018. "Defining Metabolically Healthy Obesity in Children: A Scoping Review." *Obesity Reviews* 19 (11): 1476–91. https://doi.org/10.1111/obr.12721.

DeBoer, Mark D. 2013. "Obesity, Systemic Inflammation, and Increased Risk for Cardiovascular Disease and Diabetes among Adolescents: A Need for Screening Tools to Target Interventions." *Nutrition* 29 (2): 379–86. https://doi.org/10.1016/j.nut.2012.07.003.

Denis, Gerald V., and Martin S. Obin. 2013. "'Metabolically Healthy Obesity': Origins and Implications." *Molecular Aspects of Medicine* 34 (1): 59–70. https://doi.org/10.1016/j.mam.2012.10.004.

Eckel, Nathalie, Karina Meidtner, Tamara Kalle-Uhlmann, Norbert Stefan, and Matthias B. Schulze. 2015. "Metabolically Healthy Obesity and Cardiovascular Events: A Systematic Review and Meta-Analysis." *European Journal of Preventive Cardiology* 23 (9): 956–66. https://doi.org/10.1177/2047487315623884.

Galić, Biljana Srdić, Tatjana Pavlica, Mirjana Udicki, Edita Stokić, Milena Mikalački, Darinka Korovljev, Nebojša Čokorilo, Zorka Drvendžija, and Dragan Adamović. 2016. "Somatotype Characteristics of Normal-Weight and Obese Women among Different Metabolic Subtypes." *Archives of Endocrinology and Metabolism* 60 (1): 60–65. https://doi.org/10.1590/2359-3997000000159.

Genelhu, Virginia A., Bruno M.J. Celoria, Stenio Fernando Pimentel Duarte, Pedro H. Cabello, and Emilio A. Francischetti. 2009. "Not All Obese Subjects of Multiethnic

Origin Are at Similar Risk for Developing Hypertension and Type 2 Diabetes." *European Journal of Internal Medicine* 20 (3): 289–95. https://doi.org/10.1016/j.ejim.2008.09.009.

Gonçalves, Carolina G., Michael J. Glade, and Michael M. Meguid. 2016. "Metabolically Healthy Obese Individuals: Key Protective Factors." *Nutrition* 32 (1): 14–20. https://doi.org/10.1016/j.nut.2015.07.010.

Hamer, Mark, William Johnson, and Joshua A. Bell. 2017. "Improving Risk Estimates for Metabolically Healthy Obesity and Mortality Using a Refined Healthy Reference Group." *European Journal of Endocrinology* 177 (2): 169–74. https://doi.org/10.1530/EJE-17-0217.

Hamer, Mark, and Emmanuel Stamatakis. 2012. "Metabolically Healthy Obesity and Risk of All-Cause and Cardiovascular Disease Mortality." *Journal of Clinical Endocrinology and Metabolism* 97 (7): 2482–88. https://doi.org/10.1210/jc.2011-3475.

Heinzle, S., G. D. C. Ball, and J. L. Kuk. 2016. "Variations in the Prevalence and Predictors of Prevalent Metabolically Healthy Obesity in Adolescents." *Pediatric Obesity* 11 (5): 425–33. https://doi.org/10.1111/ijpo.12083.

Heshmat, Ramin, Zeinab Hemati, Moloud Payab, Shirin Seyed Hamzeh, Mohammad Esmaeil Motlagh, Gita Shafiee, Majzoubeh Taheri, Hasan Ziaodini, Mostafa Qorbani, and Roya Kelishadi. 2018. "Prevalence of Different Metabolic Phenotypes of Obesity in Iranian Children and Adolescents: The CASPIAN V Study." *Journal of Diabetes and Metabolic Disorders* 17 (2): 211–21. https://doi.org/10.1007/s40200-018-0363-5.

Hoebel, S., L. Malan, and J. H. Ridder. 2012. "Determining Cut-off Values for Neck Circumference as a Measure of the Metabolic Syndrome amongst a South African Cohort: The SABPA Study." *Endocrine* 42 (2): 335–42. https://doi.org/10.1007/s12020-012-9642-y.

Hwang, Y. C., T. Hayashi, W. Y. Fujimoto, S. E. Kahn, D. L. Leonetti, M. J. McNeely, and E. J. Boyko. 2015. "Visceral Abdominal Fat Accumulation Predicts the Conversion of Metabolically Healthy Obese Subjects to an Unhealthy Phenotype." *International Journal of Obesity* 39 (9): 1365–70. https://doi.org/10.1038/ijo. 2015.75.

Jung, Chang Hee, Woo Je Lee, and Kee Ho Song. 2017. "Metabolically Healthy Obesity: A Friend or Foe?" *Korean Journal of Internal Medicine* 32 (4): 611–21. https://doi.org/10.3904/kjim.2016.259.

Kang, Yu Mi, Chang Hee Jung, Yun Kyung Cho, Jung Eun Jang, Jenie Yoonoo Hwang, Eun Hee Kim, Woo Je Lee, Joong Yeol Park, and Hong Kyu Kim. 2017. "Visceral Adiposity Index Predicts the Conversion of Metabolically Healthy Obesity to an Unhealthy Phenotype." *PLoS ONE* 12 (6): e0179635. https://doi.org/10.1371/journal.pone.0179635.

Karelis, Antony D., May Faraj, Jean Philippe Bastard, David H. St-Pierre, Martin Brochu, Denis Prud'homme, and Remi Rabasa-Lhoret. 2005. "The Metabolically Healthy but

Obese Individual Presents a Favorable Inflammation Profile." *Journal of Clinical Endocrinology and Metabolism* 90 (7): 4145–50. https://doi.org/10.1210/jc.2005-0482.

Kelishadi, Roya, Stephen R. Cook, Mohammad Esmaeil Motlagh, Mohammad Mehdi Gouya, Gelayol Ardalan, Molouk Motaghian, Reza Majdzadeh, and Mohammad A. Ramezani. 2008. "Metabolically Obese Normal Weight and Phenotypically Obese Metabolically Normal Youths: The CASPIAN Study." *Journal of the American Dietetic Association* 108 (1): 82–90. https://doi.org/10.1016/j.jada.2007.10.013.

Kuk, J. L., M. Rotondi, X. Sui, S. N. Blair, and C. I. Ardern. 2018. "Individuals with Obesity but No Other Metabolic Risk Factors Are Not at Significantly Elevated All-Cause Mortality Risk in Men and Women." *Clinical Obesity* 8 (5): 305–12. https://doi.org/10.1111/cob.12263.

Li, Lujiao, Jinhua Yin, Hong Cheng, Ying Wang, Shan Gao, Mingyao Li, Struan F. A. Grant, Changhong Li, Jie Mi, and Ming Li. 2016. "Identification of Genetic and Environmental Factors Predicting Metabolically Healthy Obesity in Children: Data From the BCAMS Study." *The Journal of Clinical Endocrinology & Metabolism* 101 (4): 1816–25. https://doi.org/10.1210/jc.2015-3760.

Lin, Hanli, Liqun Zhang, Ruizhi Zheng, and Yishan Zheng. 2017. "The Prevalence, Metabolic Risk and Effects of Lifestyle Intervention for Metabolically Healthy Obesity: A Systematic Review and Meta-Analysis." *Medicine (United States)* 96 (47): e8838. https://doi.org/10.1097/MD.0000000000008838.

Mangge, Harald, Sieglinde Zelzer, Peter Puerstner, Wolfgang J. Schnedl, Gloria Reeves, Teodor T. Postolache, and Daniel Weghuber. 2013. "Uric Acid Best Predicts Metabolically Unhealthy Obesity with Increased Cardiovascular Risk in Youth and Adults." *Obesity* 21 (1): 71–77. https://doi.org/10.1002/oby.20061.

Marini, Maria Adelaide, Elena Succurro, Simona Frontoni, Marta Letizia Hribal, Francesco Andreozzi, Renato Lauro, Francesco Perticone, and Giorgio Sesti. 2007. "Metabolically Healthy but Obese Women Have an Intermediate Cardiovascular Risk Profile between Healthy Nonobese Women and Obese Insulin-Resistant Women." *Diabetes Care* 30 (8): 2145–47. https://doi.org/10.2337/dc07-0419.

Martínez-Larrad, María Teresa, Arturo Corbató N. Anchuelo, Ná Yade Del Prado, José María Ibarra Rueda, Rafael Gabriel, and Manuel Serrano-Ríos. 2014. "Profile of Individuals Who Are Metabolically Healthy Obese Using Different Definition Criteria. a Population-Based Analysis in the Spanish Population." *PLoS ONE* 9 (9): e106641. https://doi.org/10.1371/journal.pone.0106641.

Messier, Virginie, Antony D. Karelis, Marie Ève Robillard, Philippe Bellefeuille, Martin Brochu, Jean Marc Lavoie, and Rémi Rabasa-Lhoret. 2010. "Metabolically Healthy but Obese Individuals: Relationship with Hepatic Enzymes." *Metabolism: Clinical and Experimental* 59 (1): 20–24. https://doi.org/10.1016/j.metabol.2009.06.020.

Mongraw-Chaffin, Morgana, Meredith C. Foster, Cheryl A.M. Anderson, Gregory L. Burke, Nowreen Haq, Rita R. Kalyani, Pamela Ouyang, et al. 2018. "Metabolically Healthy Obesity, Transition to Metabolic Syndrome, and Cardiovascular Risk." *Journal of the American College of Cardiology* 71 (17): 1857–65. https://doi.org/10.1016/j.jacc.2018.02.055.

Nasreddine, Lara, Hani Tamim, Aurelie Mailhac, and Fadia S. AlBuhairan. 2018. "Prevalence and Predictors of Metabolically Healthy Obesity in Adolescents: Findings from the National 'Jeeluna' Study in Saudi-Arabia." *BMC Pediatrics* 18 (1): 281. https://doi.org/10.1186/s12887-018-1247-z.

Ortega, Francisco B., Cristina Cadenas-Sánchez, Xuemei Sui, Steven N. Blair, and Carl J. Lavie. 2015. "Role of Fitness in the Metabolically Healthy but Obese Phenotype: A Review and Update." *Progress in Cardiovascular Diseases* 58 (1): 76–86. https://doi.org/10.1016/j.pcad.2015.05.001.

Payab, Moloud, Mostafa Qorbani, Nazila Shahbal, Mohammad Esmaeil Motlagh, Shirin Hasani-Ranjbar, Hoda Zahedi, Gita Shafiee, et al. 2019. "Association of Anthropometric Indices With Metabolic Phenotypes of Obesity in Children and Adolescents: The CASPIAN-V Study." *Frontiers in Endocrinology* 10 (786): 1–10. https://doi.org/10.3389/fendo.2019.00786.

Prince, Rhiannon L., Jennifer L. Kuk, Kathryn A. Ambler, Jasmine Dhaliwal, and Geoff D. C. Ball. 2014. "Predictors of Metabolically Healthy Obesity in Children." *Diabetes Care* 37 (5): 1462–68. https://doi.org/10.2337/dc13-1697.

Reinehr, Thomas, Barbara Wolters, Caroline Knop, Nina Lass, and Reinhard W. Holl. 2015. "Strong Effect of Pubertal Status on Metabolic Health in Obese Children: A Longitudinal Study." *Journal of Clinical Endocrinology and Metabolism* 100 (1): 301–8. https://doi.org/10.1210/jc.2014-2674.

Remor, Jane Maria, Wendell Arthur Lopes, João Carlos Locateli, Ronano Pereira Oliveira, Caroline Ferraz Simões, Carlos Andrés Lopera Barrero, and Nelson Nardo. 2019. "Prevalence of Metabolically Healthy Obese Phenotype and Associated Factors in South American Overweight Adolescents: A Cross-Sectional Study." *Nutrition* 60 (s/n): 19–24. https://doi.org/10.1016/j.nut.2018.08.017.

Reuter, Cézane Priscila, Miria Suzana Burgos, Cláudia Daniela Barbian, Jane Dagmar Pollo Renner, Silvia Isabel Rech Franke, and Elza Daniel de Mello. 2018. "Comparison between Different Criteria for Metabolic Syndrome in Schoolchildren from Southern Brazil." *European Journal of Pediatrics* 177 (10): 1471–77. https://doi.org/10.1007/s00431-018-3202-2.

Rey-López, J. P., L. F. de Rezende, M. Pastor-Valero, and B. H. Tess. 2014. "The Prevalence of Metabolically Healthy Obesity: A Systematic Review and Critical Evaluation of the Definitions Used." *Obesity Reviews* 15 (10): 781–90. https://doi.org/10.1111/obr.12198.

Seo, Mi Hae, and Eun Jung Rhee. 2014. "Metabolic and Cardiovascular Implications of a Metabolically Healthy Obesity Phenotype." *Endocrinology and Metabolism* 29 (4): 427–34. https://doi.org/10.3803/EnM.2014.29.4.427.

Shin, M. J., Y. J. Hyun, O. Y. Kim, J. Y. Kim, Y. Jang, and J. H. Lee. 2006. "Weight Loss Effect on Inflammation and LDL Oxidation in Metabolically Healthy but Obese (MHO) Individuals: Low Inflammation and LDL Oxidation in MHO Women." *International Journal of Obesity* 30 (10): 1529–34. https://doi.org/10.1038/sj.ijo.0803304.

Stefan, Norbert, Hans Ulrich Häring, Frank B. Hu, and Matthias B. Schulze. 2013. "Metabolically Healthy Obesity: Epidemiology, Mechanisms, and Clinical Implications." *The Lancet Diabetes and Endocrinology.* https://doi.org/10.1016/S2213-8587(13)70062-7.

Stefan, Norbert, Konstantinos Kantartzis, Jürgen Machann, Fritz Schick, Claus Thamer, Kilian Rittig, Bernd Balletshofer, Fausto Machicao, Andreas Fritsche, and Hans Ulrich Häring. 2008. "Identification and Characterization of Metabolically Benign Obesity in Humans." *Archives of Internal Medicine* 168 (15): 1609–16. https://doi.org/10.1001/archinte.168.15.1609.

Stenzel, Ana Paula, Roberta Carvalho, Patricia Jesus, Aline Bull, Silvia Pereira, Carlos Saboya, and Andrea Ramalho. 2018. "Serum Antioxidant Associations with Metabolic Characteristics in Metabolically Healthy and Unhealthy Adolescents with Severe Obesity: An Observational Study." *Nutrients* 10 (2). https://doi.org/10.3390/nu10020150.

Succurro, Elena, Maria A. Marini, Simona Frontoni, Marta L. Hribal, Francesco Andreozzi, Renato Lauro, Francesco Perticone, and Giorgio Sesti. 2008. "Insulin Secretion in Metabolically Obese, but Normal Weight, and in Metabolically Healthy but Obese Individuals." *Obesity* 16 (8): 1881–86. https://doi.org/10.1038/oby.2008.308.

Twig, Gilad, Arnon Afek, Estela Derazne, Dorit Tzur, Tali Cukierman-Yaffe, Hertzel C. Gerstein, and Amir Tirosh. 2014. "Diabetes Risk among Overweight and Obese Metabolically Healthy Young Adults." *Diabetes Care* 37 (11): 2989–95. https://doi.org/10.2337/dc14-0869.

Wang, Qiaoxuan, Jinhua Yin, Lu Xu, Hong Cheng, Xiaoyuan Zhao, Hongding Xiang, Hugh Simon Lam, Jie Mi, and Ming Li. 2013. "Prevalence of Metabolic Syndrome in a Cohort of Chinese Schoolchildren: Comparison of Two Definitions and Assessment of Adipokines as Components by Factor Analysis." *BMC Public Health* 13 (1): 249. https://doi.org/10.1186/1471-2458-13-249.

Yaghootkar, Hanieh, Robert A. Scott, Charles C. White, Weihua Zhang, Elizabeth Speliotes, Patricia B. Munroe, Georg B. Ehret, et al. 2014. "Genetic Evidence for a Normal-Weight 'Metabolically Obese' Phenotype Linking Insulin Resistance,

Hypertension, Coronary Artery Disease, and Type 2 Diabetes." *Diabetes* 63 (12): 4369–77. https://doi.org/10.2337/db14-0318.

Yoon, Da Young, Young Ah Lee, Jieun Lee, Jae Hyun Kim, Choong Ho Shin, and Sei Won Yang. 2017. "Prevalence and Clinical Characteristics of Metabolically Healthy Obesity in Korean Children and Adolescents: Data from the Korea National Health and Nutrition Examination Survey." *Journal of Korean Medical Science* 32 (11): 1840–47. https://doi.org/10.3346/jkms.2017.32.11.1840.

Zhao, Min, Abel López-Bermejo, Carmelo A. Caserta, Carla Campos Muniz Medeiros, Anastasios Kollias, Judit Bassols, Elisabetta L. Romeo, et al. 2019. "Metabolically Healthy Obesity and High Carotid Intima-Media Thickness in Children and Adolescents: International Childhood Vascular Structure Evaluation Consortium." *Diabetes Care* 42 (1): 119–25. https://doi.org/10.2337/dc18-1536.

Zheng, Ruizhi, Dan Zhou, and Yimin Zhu. 2016. "The Long-Term Prognosis of Cardiovascular Disease and All-Cause Mortality for Metabolically Healthy Obesity: A Systematic Review and Meta-Analysis." *Journal of Epidemiology and Community Health* 70 (10): 1024–31. https://doi.org/10.1136/jech-2015-206948.

In: Childhood Obesity
Editor: Roya Kelishadi
ISBN: 978-1-53618-158-6
© 2020 Nova Science Publishers, Inc.

Chapter 12

PROTECTING CHILDREN FROM UNFAVORABLE FOOD MARKETING

***Behnaz Abiri*[1]*, PhD and Mohammadreza Vafa*[2,*]**
[1]Nutritional Sciences, Department of Nutrition, Faculty of Paramedicine, Ahvaz Jundishapur University of Medical Sciences, Ahvaz, Iran
[2]Professor of Nutritional Sciences, Department of Nutrition, School of Public Health, Iran University of Medical Sciences, Tehran, Iran

ABSTRACT

The increasing prevalence of childhood obesity worldwide imposes a major burden on society in health care system costs and children's physical and mental health; thus, early intervention is necessary. Food marketing is often discriminated as the leading cause of the obesity epidemic. The food industry spends massive amounts of money marketing calorie-dense, nutrient-poor foods, and its marketing particularly targets children. Today's children use multiple types of media and spend more time in front of computer, television, and game screens than any other activity in their lives except for sleeping. Research has found strong relationships between increases in advertising for non-nutritious foods and rates of obesity in children. Exposure to the marketing of unhealthy foods and beverages is a widely established risk factor for the development of childhood obesity and non-communicable diseases. Food marketing includes the use of various persuasive techniques to affect children's food attitudes, preferences and consumption. Obesity is probably a natural response to the modern food environment, where the marketing and advertising of inexpensive, highly palatable, energy-dense and nutrient poor foods and beverages is prevalent. Children are specifically susceptible to persuasive messages used in marketing communications, because their cognitive development is relatively limited. Acute and accumulative exposures to food marketing affects children's thoughts and behaviors, particularly, their attitudes, preferences and consumption of unhealthy products. Thus, the

* Corresponding Author's Email: vafa.m@iums.ac.ir.

obesity crisis cannot be solved without notable alterations in the obesogenic marketing environment that encloses children. The present review examines evidence that how this marketing negatively influences children's food intake and elevates children's risk for obesity. Then, we will highlight potentially practical local policy options to limit the marketing of obesogenic food to children.

Keywords: childhood obesity, marketing, food

INTRODUCTION

The prevalence of overweight and obesity has risen dramatically among children, worldwide [1]. Obesity, a disease in itself, is also a modifiable behavioral risk factor for long-term non-communicable diseases, such as cardiovascular diseases and some cancers [2, 3]; hence, early intervention is crucial.

Obesity is a public health concern that has taken the attention of a broad set of citizens and institutions, and calls for action are becoming increasingly strong. However, it is a complex issue. Obesity is the result of numerous behaviors that occur through time, and many factors help form children's food preferences, eating behaviors, and physical activity levels. Some of these are specific to individuals (genetics, taste predispositions), and others are specific to families (parent food intake, household food availability, family meals), communities (schools, food retail outlets), and macro systems (culture, food production and distribution systems, advertising, governmental regulations) [4]. In attempting to remove angle potential contributors to obesity, particular attention has been focused on the influences of food marketing.

Obesity is possibly a natural response to the modern food environment, where the marketing and advertising of low-priced, highly palatable, energy-dense foods and beverages is ubiquitous [5, 6]. The techniques used to market unhealthy foods to children are substantial, sophisticated and convincing [7, 8] and target different vehicles of promotion (such as television) via various marketing methods (such as product placement). Analysis of children's environments shows convincing marketing has an especially strong presence on television [9], websites [10] and games [11] and expands its promotion to supermarkets [12] and outside schools [13], leading to minimal un-commercialised space.

Children are specifically susceptible to convincing messages used in marketing communications, as their cognitive development (cognition that allows one to recognize the selling and convincing aim of marketing communications) is somewhat limited [14] Children are more likely to interpret marketing as truthful [15]. Younger children are established to understand advertising as assistive information to make sure they are up-to-date with what is available in the shops [15].

Acute and accumulative exposures to food advertising affect children's thoughts and behaviors, in particular, their attitudes, preferences and consumption of unhealthy products

[16-18]. These factors are key components of a cascade of impacts of marketing that may result in childhood weight gain [19].

Therefore, this chapter aimed to investigate the impact of food marketing on children's food attitudes, preferences and consumption. We describe ways in which food companies market calorie- dense, nutrient-poor foods directly to children in national media and local communities. In addition, we present evidence that this marketing negatively affects children's diets, elevates children's risk for obesity and obesity-associated illness, and takes benefit of youths' unique vulnerabilities.

Marketing Channels

Children initiate to watch television quite early, and do it for several hours each time. The report published by the Institute of Medicine (IOM) found that "for younger and older children, the evidence obviously supports the finding that television advertising affects their food and beverage purchase requests" [20]. Even though television remains a primary promotional medium to reach large numbers of children, increasingly, children are the target of marketing communications programs, which may consist of product placements, sales promotions, special packaging, and in-school and Internet marketing, as well as television and print media [21].

Internet marketing is playing an ever increasing role between children and adolescents. Indeed, in a business context, the Internet has become a main marketing channel [22]. The number of hours that young people spend on the Internet also appears to be elevating [23].

Sponsorship is another channel utilized. Fast-food chains usually sponsor activities including sporting competitions, television programmes and music shows [24].

Promotions are another marketing tool, and direct to encourage the purchase of products directly at the points of sale. The most routinely used promotions by fast-food chains consist of giving prizes, or discounts on products [25].

Children's Vulnerability

Children have long been identified as a vulnerable group. Children, especially up to 8 years old, have not yet attained a sufficient level of cognitive and psychological development to become aware of the nature and intentions of marketing and advertising and are, thus, defenceless regarding them [26].

Therefore, some authors have focused on children's fragility in the face of marketing and advertising, as they often still cannot distinguish, for example, television advertising from the programming itself [27]. It is determined that children begin to make this distinction between the ages of 4 and 7 years of age, becoming aware of the intention of persuading at 8 years old. However, it is only around the age of 11 or 12 that they can formulate critical thinking about advertising itself [28]. Although older children and adolescents comprehend the intent of advertising, they do not regularly act on that knowledge nor do they try to counteract its influence.

Unfavorable Impacts of Food Marketing

Food companies have traditionally claimed that their advertising simply encourages children to prefer one brand over another and hence does not lead to childhood obesity [29]. Most evaluations on the impacts of television food advertising to children affirms that it elevates children's preferences for advertised brands, choices of specific foods after advertisement exposure, and requests to parents for advertised food products [30]. Another research has indicated, however, that food marketing also has potentially great impacts on children's overall diet and health. For example, television food advertising elevates consumption of any available snack foods through and immediately after exposure, and exposure to commercial television is related to elevated overall calorie consumption, higher body mass index, and decreased fruit and vegetable consumption 5 years later [31]. Research has also reported a relationship between exposure to soft drink advertising and consumption of all sugar-sweetened beverages [32].

Because of its omnipresence, food marketing likely affects children's normative beliefs about the kinds of foods that are acceptable to eat routinely without adverse side effects, may affect how much children like the taste of advertised foods, and may automatically prime other unrelated aims and behaviors, such as children's motivation to engage in unhealthful behaviors.

The Impact of Food Marketing on Child's Behavior

Several studies carried out since 1970 have concentrated on the role of television on childhood obesity. These studies led to the conclusion that children who were most exposed to television commercials were more likely to prefer food advertised in them. An association between the number of hours of television viewing and the number of requests that children make to their parents to buy specific products from certain brands has also been shown. It was also found that the number of hours children watch television is associated with a higher consumption of high energy density foods rich in calories, fat, sugar and salt. Likewise, the relationship between the number of hours of television viewing and the prevalence and incidence of obesity has also been demonstrated [25, 33].

Children between the ages of 2 and 11 years are the most vulnerable group to the impacts of advertising on food consumption [34]. Considering that most advertised foods are unhealthy, the WHO believes television advertising to be an important contributor in weight gain and childhood obesity [35].

Government's Role in Promoting Public Health

Because the food marketing environment leads to the health problems facing our nation's children and since members of the food industry seem unlikely to voluntarily make the notable alterations needed to improve this environment, government at all levels has an obligation to involve oneself where it can. In fact, a core responsibility of government is to protect and promote public health - specifically among vulnerable populations, such as children. Public health is essential in society because it provides the general population with basic security and welfare that can be achieved only via collective action [36].

Public health advocates have recognized several policy proposals that localities can consider to decrease marketing of unhealthful food to children in stores, restaurants, schools, and elsewhere in the community.

Protecting children from the unfavorable impacts of food marketing needs a range of policy interventions at all levels of government, and finally an alteration in social norms of acceptable behavior.

Food Marketing and Childhood Overweight/Obesity

Food marketing is often identified as the leading cause of the childhood obesity epidemic. Many of today's children routinely consume more calories than they expend in physical activity, but this imbalance leads from many alterations in home, school, and neighborhood environments. According to the IOM, food marketing intentionally targets children who are too young to recognize advertising from truth and induces them to eat high-calorie, low-nutrient "junk" foods; companies succeed so well in this effort that business-as-usual cannot be allowed to continue.

Childhood obesity has become an epidemic around the world [37]; the related risks to children's health and wellbeing are considerable. Marketing's role as both a contributor to the problem and a force in its alleviation is complex. Marketing strongly influences children's food preferences, requests, and consumption. The IOM mentioned the idea that some forms of marketing elevate the risk of obesity "cannot be ignored."

But the most insidious purpose of marketing is to convince children to eat foods made "just for them" and not what adults are eating. Some campaigns aim to persuade children that they know more about what they are "supposed to" eat than their parents do. Marketers clearly try to undermine family decisions about food choices through convincing children that they, not adults, should control those choices [38]. In fact, children now routinely report that they, and not their parents, decide what to eat.

Nowadays, the food industry spends large amounts of money for marketing calorie-dense, nutrient-poor foods, and this marketing specifically targets children [39]. The obesity epidemic cannot be solved without notable alterations in the obesogenic marketing environment that surrounds children [29].

The White House Task Force on Childhood Obesity has called for immediate action: "Key actors - from food and beverage companies, to restaurants, food retailers, the media, government and others - all have an important role to play in founding a food marketing environment that supports, rather than undermines, the attempts of parents and other caregivers to encourage healthy eating among children and prevent obesity" [40].

Exposure to the advertising and marketing of unhealthy foods and beverages is a broad established risk factor for the development of childhood obesity and non-communicable diseases. Food marketing involves the use of several convincing techniques to affect children's food attitudes, preferences and consumption.

Acute and accumulative exposures to food marketing affect children's thoughts and behaviors, especially, their attitudes, preferences and consumption of unhealthy products [16-18]. These factors are key elements of a cascade of impacts of marketing that may result to childhood weight gain [19].

Altogether, the identified studies present a strong, comprehensive body of evidence reporting the powerful influence of food marketing exposure. The studies also recognize the impacts on children's attitudes, preferences and consumption of the vehicles of promotion and related techniques, especially with regard to television commercials, and the marketing techniques utilized in packaging of commodities.

The IOM concluded that television advertising affects key dietary patterns, including children's food and beverage preferences, purchase requests, and short-term consumption in 2-11 years old children. Correlational evidence also connected exposure to television advertising to adiposity in children and youth. A key conclusion of that report [4] was that "food and beverage marketing practices geared to children and youth are out of balance with healthy diets and lead to an environment that puts their health at risk" [4].

As might be anticipated, perspectives differ notably with regard to the most effective courses of action for addressing marketing's effect in decreasing childhood obesity. Some critics claimed that limits should be exerted on marketing activities targeted children. For example, in 2003, the Center for Science in the Public Interest published a position paper that discussed for restrictions on the advertising of high-calorie, low-nutrient foods for children. The American Psychological Association has also called for restrictions but has adopted a more extensive approach in recommending that all television advertising to children (ages 7 and younger) be terminated [41]. This is according to the premise that advertising is inherently undeserved because of young children's limited understanding of the nature and purpose of advertising. The American Academy of Pediatrics [42] has called for a prohibition on advertisements for "junk food" in television programs that are viewed mainly by children.

In 2007, the Office of Communications, the media regulatory agency in the United Kingdom, established new rules inhibiting advertisements for high-fat, -salt, and -sugared foods in and around television programs that are either designed for or appeal to children less than the age of 16 years old.

The impact and potentials of the self-regulatory system, particularly the Children's Advertising Review Unit (CARU), were also hotly discussed. For many years, CARU has served a critically important role for protecting children from misleading or deceptive advertising.

Although television advertising remains a primary medium to reach children, other media, such as the Internet, have significantly extended advertising's reach and offer novel opportunities to target a young audience. For example, new technics of marketing, such as "advergames," have become a growing common feature of Web sites designed for children. These advertiser-sponsored video games include brand messages in fast-paced, animated adventures and are made by a firm for the aim of elevating one or more of its brands. Brand exposures in this medium are basically different from those in traditional media, prompting calls for a review of online marketing technics from policy makers, consumer advocates, and industry groups. In "The Online Marketing of Food to Children: Is It Just Fun and Games?" [43] it was reported the results of a detailed content analysis of food marketers' Web sites for children and its implications for public policy. Findings are debated in regards of 11 marketing technics that the authors recognize as relevant and potentially of concern to policy makers. Their study provides insights into the nature and area of these marketing activities, to the challenges this new environment presents to young children, and to the areas in which protections may be required.

The final article in the specific section expands the empirical analysis beyond marketing communications to product utilization. In "Fast-Food Marketing and Children's Fast-Food Consumption: Exploring Parents' Influences in an Ethnically Diverse Sample," it was evaluated how marketing to parents may influence their children's food intake. Particularly, they ask whether fast-food marketing directed at parents has an impact on children's eating behavior throughout parents' attitudes and beliefs about the social norms for consuming fast food. To examine this issue, the authors evaluated caregivers of children ages 2–12 years old in medically underserved communities. The evidence-based findings are interesting and help recognize some of the key mechanisms by which parents may mediate marketing effects. The study sample was ethnically diverse, which also enabled an informative exploration of variations across groups. Because rates of childhood obesity differ considerably by ethnicity, empirical research is required to understand the drivers of these variations and the steps that might be taken to reach various groups. A one-size-fits-all manner to the problem may mask important variations, rendering some manners more or less effective, depending on how specific attempts are targeted. One of the key contributions of this study is that it demonstrates how marketing to parents can be a pathway to childhood overweight/obesity. To this point, when researchers and others have evaluated marketing effects, the focus has been squarely on communications targeted children. Grier et al. propose that a broader perspective is required.

Hobin et al's [44] findings among Canadian children, who also displayed an overall preference for unhealthy foods. Such findings may be due to children's inherent preference for sweet and salty foods [45] which is probably exacerbated by their prior exposure to a 'real world' food marketing environment that is heavily distorted towards the promotion of such foods, and established to affect children's food predilection [46, 47].

Commercial marketing of energy-dense, nutrition-poor foods and beverages (unhealthy foods) has been recognized as contributing to population levels of overweight and obesity and poor diet worldwide [47]. Systematic reviews have reported that food promotions have a direct impact on children's nutrition knowledge, predilections, purchase behavior, consumption patterns and diet-associated health [46, 47].

In addition, the World Health Organization [48], the IOM (20), and the British Food Commission [49] carried out reviews of academic research pointing to a connection between child-targeted marketing and childhood overweight/obesity. The 2006 report published by the IOM concluded that "for younger and older children, the evidence obviously supports the report that television advertising affects their food and beverage purchase requests" [20]. The WHO, which reported that "the heavy marketing of high-calorie and low-nutrient foods and fast food channels represents a possible elevated risk for childhood obesity" [20].

As a result of elevating evidence that advertising persuades children to eat too much of the wrong types of food [50], food marketing has emerged as a clear target for action.

The findings of this review support more restriction on food marketing to children as a key solution for the management of childhood obesity [18].

Conclusion

This chapter found a strong body of evidence that exposure to food marketing affects children's attitudes, predilection and consumption of unhealthy foods, with harmful consequences to health such as obesity. The health problems caused by childhood obesity need strategies to impede it. Childhood obesity has become an epidemic all over the world; the associated risks to children's health and wellbeing are considerable. Marketing's effect as both a contributor to the issue and a force in its alleviation is complex. Present studies provide valuable insights and provide convincing evidence to support the restriction of food marketing to children. Future research to evaluate contemporaneous marketing techniques, using a wider range of methodologies, could more strengthen this evidence. Many important questions are yet to be addressed. Further research in this special section is required.

REFERENCES

[1] Abarca-Gómez, L.; Abdeen, Z. A.; Hamid, Z. A.; Abu-Rmeileh, N. M.; Acosta-Cazares, B.; Acuin, C.; Adams, R. J.; Aekplakorn,W.; Afsana, K.; Aguilar-Salinas, C. A.; et al. Worldwide trends in body-mass index, underweight, overweight, and obesity from 1975 to 2016: A pooled analysis of 2416 population-based measurement studies in 128_9 million children, adolescents, and adults. *Lancet* 2017, 390, 2627–2642.

[2] World Health Organization. *Noncommunicable Diseases: Progress Monitor 2017*; Report No.: 9241513020; World Health Organization: Geneva, Switzerland, 2017.

[3] World Health Organization. *Obesity and Overweight*; World Health Organization: Geneva, Switzerland, 6 November 2018.

[4] IOM (2006), *Food Marketing to Children and Youth: Threat or Opportunity?* Washington, DC: National Academies Press.

[5] Swinburn, B. A.; Sacks, G.; Hall, K. D.; McPherson, K.; Finegood, D. T.; Moodie, M. L.; Gortmaker, S. L. The global obesity pandemic: Shaped by global drivers and local environments. *Lancet* 2011, 378, 804–814.

[6] Boyland, E. J.; Whalen, R. Food advertising to children and its e_ects on diet: A review of recent prevalence and impact data. *Pediatr. Diabetes* 2015, 16, 331–337.

[7] Boyland, E. J.; Halford, J. C. Television advertising and branding. E_ects on eating behaviour and food preferences in children. *Appetite* 2013, 62, 236–241.

[8] Boyland, E.; Harrold, J.; Kirkham, T.; Halford, J. Persuasive techniques used in television advertisements to market foods to UK children. *Appetite* 2012, 58, 1170.

[9] Kelly, B.; Smith, B.; King, L.; Flood, V.; Bauman, A.; Smith, B. Television food advertising to children: The extent and nature of exposure. *Public Health Nutr.* 2007, 10, 1234–1240.

[10] Potvin Kent, M.; Pauzé, E. The frequency and healthfulness of food and beverages advertised on adolescents' preferred web sites in Canada. *J. Adolesc. Health* 2018, 63, 102–107.

[11] Lee, M.; Choi, Y.; Quilliam, E. T.; Cole, R. T. Playing With Food: Content Analysis of Food Advergames. *J. Consum. A* 2009, 43, 129–154.

[12] Harris, J. L.; Schwartz, M. B.; Brownell, K. D. Marketing foods to children and adolescents: Licensed characters and other promotions on packaged foods in the supermarket. *Public Health Nutr.* 2010, 13, 409–417.

[13] Kelly, B.; Cretikos, M.; Rogers, K.; King, L. The commercial food landscape: Outdoor food advertising around primary schools in Australia. *Aust. N. Z. J. Public Health* 2008, 32, 522–528.

[14] Rozendaal, E.; Buijzen, M.; Valkenburg, P. Comparing Children's and Adults' Cognitive Advertising Competences in the Netherlands. *J. Child Media* 2010, 4, 77–89.

[15] Ludvigsen, A.; Scott, S. Real kids don't eat quiche: What food means to children. *Food Cult. Soc.* 2009, 12, 417–436.

[16] Obesity Policy Coalition and the Global Obesity Centre. *Tipping the Scales: Australian Obesity Prevention Consensus; Obesity Policy Coalition and the Global Obesity Centre*: Melbourne, Australia, 2017.

[17] Boyland, E. J.; Nolan, S.; Kelly, B.; Tudur-Smith, C.; Jones, A.; Halford, J. C.; Robinson, E. Advertising as a cue to consume: A systematic review and meta-analysis of the effects of acute exposure to unhealthy food and nonalcoholic beverage advertising on intake in children and adults. *Am. J. Clin. Nutr.* 2016, 103, 519–533.

[18] World Health Organization. *Report on the Commission on Ending Childhood Obesity*; World Health Organization: Geneva, Switzerland, 2016.

[19] Kelly, B.; King, M. L.; Chapman, M. K.; Boyland, E.; Bauman, A. E.; Baur, L. A. A Hierarchy of Unhealthy Food Promotion E_ects: Identifying Methodological Approaches and Knowledge Gaps. *Am. J. Public Health* 2015, 105, e86–e95.

[20] McGinnis, J. Michael, Jennifer Gootman, and Vivica I. Kraak, eds. 2006. *Food marketing to children and youth: Threat or opportunity?* Washington, DC: Institute of Medicine of the National Academies.

[21] Moore, Elizabeth S. (2004), "Children and the Changing World of Advertising," *Journal of Business Ethics,* 52 (June), 161–67.

[22] Cardoso, P. J. R and Cardoso, A. (2012). Adolescents' attitudes toward internet advertising. *Revista Portuguesa de Mark*eting. 14(27): 20-31.

[23] Herédia A., Hipólito J., Nunes O., Ribeiro L, Moura T., Laneiro T. (2017). Fast-Food Marketing Strategies and Their Impact on Childhood Obesity. *Journal of Spatial and Organizational Dynamics,* CIEO-Research Centre for Spatial and Organizational Dynamics, University of Algarve, vol. 5(3), pages 296-315.

[24] World Health Organization (2013b). *Marketing of foods high in fat, salt and sugar to children: update 2012 2013.* Copenhagen, Denmark. WHO Regional Office for Europe.

[25] Boulos, R., Vikre, E. K., Oppenheimer, S., Chang, H., Kanarek, R. B. (2012). ObesiTV: how television is influencing the obesity epidemic. *Physiology & Behavior.* 107(1): 146-53. doi: 10.1016/j.physbeh.2012.05.022. Epub 2012 Jun 4.

[26] Swinburn, B., Sacks, G., Lobstein, T., Rigby, N., Baur, L. A., Brownell, K. G., Gill, T., Seidell, J. and Kumanyika, S. (2008). The 'Sydney Principles' for reducing the

commercial promotion of foods and beverages to children. *Public Health Nutrition*. 11: 881–886.

[27] World Health Organization (2013a). Lax marketing regulations contribute to obesity crisis in children. Retrieved from: http://www.euro.who.int/en/media-centre/sections/pressreleases/2013/06/lax-marketing-regulations-contribute-to-obesity-crisis-in-children.

[28] Iglesias, F., Caldas, L. S. and Lemos, S. M. S. (2013). Advertising to children: an analysis of persuasive tactics on a free channel. *Psicologia & Sociedade*. 25(1): 134-141. https://dx.doi. org/10.1590/S0102-71822013000100015.

[29] Harris JL, Pomeranz JL, Lobstein T, Brownell KD. 2009. 30 211 225 A crisis in the marketplace: how food marketing contributes to childhood obesity and what can be done *Annu Rev Public Health* Harris J. L., Pomeranz J. L., Lobstein T., Brownell KD. A crisis in the marketplace: how food marketing contributes.

[30] Institute of Medicine, Committee on Food Marketing and the Diets of Children and Youth. *Food marketing to children and youth: threat or opportunity?* Washington (DC): National Academies Press; 2006.

[31] Harris J. L., Brownell KD, Bargh J. A. The food marketing defense model: integrating psychological research to protect youth and inform public policy. *Soc Issues Policy Rev*. 2009;3(1):211–271.

[32] Andreyeva T., Kelly I. R., Harris J. L. Exposure to food advertising on television: associations with children's fast food and soft drink consumption and obesity. *Econ Hum Biol*. 2011;9(3):221–233.

[33] Bingham, D. D., Varela-Silva, M. I., Ferrão, M. M., Gama, A., Mourão, I., Nogueira, H., Marques, V. R. and Padez, C. (2013). Socio-Demographic and Behavioral Risk Factors Associated with the High. Prevalence of Overweight and Obesity in Portuguese Children. *American Journal of Human Biology*. 25: 733-742.

[34] Rodrigues, A. S., Carmo, I., Breda, J. and Rito, A. I. (2011). Associação entre o marketing de produtos alimentares de elevada densidade energética e a obesidade infantil. *Revista Portuguesa de Saúde Pública*. 29(2): 180-187. doi: http://dx.doi.org/10.1016/S0870- 9025(11)70022-0.

[35] World Health Organization (2013b). *Marketing of foods high in fat, salt and sugar to children: update 2012–2013*. Copenhagen, Denmark. WHO Regional Office for Europe.

[36] Gostin L. O. *Public health law: power, duty, restraint*. 2nd edition. Berkeley (CA): University of California Press; 2010.

[37] World Health Organization (2003), *"Obesity and Overweight,"* Global Strategy on Diet, Physical Activity and Health, (accessed July 12, 2007), [available at http://www.who.int/ dietphysicalactivity/publications/facts/obesity/en/].

[38] *Pestering parents: how food companies market obesity to children*. Washington, D.C.: Center for Science in the Public Interest, November 2003.

[39] Marketing food to children and adolescents: A review of industry expenditures, activities, and self-regulation. A report to Congress. Federal Trade Commission; 2008. [Accessed October 4, 2010]. http://www.ftc.gov/os/2008/07/P064504 foodmktingreport. pdf.

[40] White House Task Force on Childhood Obesity. Report to the President: solving the problem of childhood obesity within a generation. *Executive Office of the President of the United States;* 2010. [Accessed October 4, 2010]. p. 28. http://www. letsmove.gov/sites/letsmove.gov/files/TaskForce_on_Childhood_Obesity_May201 0_ FullReport.pdf.

[41] Kunkel, Dale, Brian L. Wilcox, Joanne Cantor, Edward Palmer, Susan Linn, and Peter Dowrick (2004), *Report of the Task Force on Advertising and Children.* Washington, DC: American Psychological Association.

[42] American Academy of Pediatrics (2006), "Policy Statement: Children, Adolescents, and Advertising," *Pediatrics*, 118 (December), 2563–69.

[43] Grier, Sonya A., Janell Mensinger, Shirley H. Huang, Shiriki K. Kumanyika, and Nicolas Stettler (2007), "Fast-Food Marketing and Children's Fast-Food Consumption: Exploring Parents' Influences in an Ethnically Diverse Sample," *Journal of Public Policy & Marketing*, 26 (Fall), 221–35.

[44] Hobin, E. P., Hammond, D. G., Daniel, S., Hanning, R. M., & Manske, S. (2012). The happy meal® effect: the impact of toy premiums on healthy eating among children in Ontario, Canada. *Canadian Journal of Public Health* = Revue Canadienne De Santé Publique, 103, e244-e248.

[45] Mennella, J. A. (2014). Ontogeny of taste preferences: basic biology and implications for health. *Am J Clin Nutr*, 99, 704S-711S.

[46] Cairns, G., Angus, K., Hastings, G., & Caraher, M. (2013). Systematic reviews of the evidence on the nature, extent and effects of food marketing to children. A retrospective summary. *Appetite,* 62, 209-215.

[47] World Health Organization. (2010). *Set of recommendations on the marketing of foods and non-alcoholic beverages to children.* Geneva, Switzerland: World Health Organization.

[48] World Health Organization (WHO). 2003. *Diet, nutrition, and the prevention of chronic diseases.* Geneva, Switzerland: WHO. http://whqlibdoc.who.int/trs/WHO_ TRS_916.pdf.

[49] Dalmeny, Kathy, Elizabeth Hanna, and Tim Lobstein. 2004. *Broadcasting bad health: Why food marketing to children needs to be controlled.* London: International Association of Consumer Food Organizations for the World Health Organization Consultation on a Global Strategy for Diet and Health. http://www. foodcomm.org.uk/Broadcasting_bad_health.pdf (accessed September 29, 2006).

[50] Institute of Medicine. *Food Marketing to Children and Youth: Threat or Opportunity?.* Washington, DC: National Academies Press; 2005.

In: Childhood Obesity
Editor: Roya Kelishadi
ISBN: 978-1-53618-158-6
© 2020 Nova Science Publishers, Inc.

Chapter 13

ACTIONS TO PROMOTE THE INTAKE OF HEALTHY FOODS BY CHILDREN

Cintia Chaves Curioni**, PhD,
Evelyn Kowalczyk dos Santos,
Ana Carolina Felderheimer da Silva, PhD,
Evelyne Florido Lobato Cavalcante
and Jorginete de Jesus Damião, PhD
Institute of Nutrition, State University of Rio de Janeiro,
Rio de Janeiro, Brazil

ABSTRACT

Childhood obesity is a public health problem that has raised concern worldwide, specially, because it is a complex, multidisciplinary issue, with many drivers, including behavior, environment, genetics, and culture. To be successful in managing childhood obesity, it is necessary coordinated and multisectoral pool of actions including not only the children, but also their families and communities. These actions should involve different sectors, including health - responsible for the growth monitoring and the guarantee of access to care and obesity treatment, education (food meals programs, health promotion, nutrition literacy), justice (implementation of laws and marketing restriction), and others. Regarding healthy eating initiatives, the combination of actions taken by a country or region should be able to promote the intake of healthy foods and/or inhibit the intake of unhealthy foods for children at the individual, household, and/or community levels. Accordingly, this chapter review will discuss the strengths, limitations, uncertainties, and recommendations of the following actions that may influence healthy food choices: dietary

* Corresponding Author's Email: cintiacurioni@gmail.com.

guidelines, taxes on unhealthy food and beverages, food labeling and food advertising and regulatory controls on the marketing of unhealthy foods and beverages to children.

Keywords: child, obesity, nutrition policy, government regulation

Introduction

Childhood obesity is a public health problem that has raised concern worldwide, especially because it is a complex, multidisciplinary issue, with many drivers, including behavior, environment, genetics and culture.

Similarly to other lifestyle-related chronic diseases, overweight and obesity are largely preventable, although the global prevalence of childhood overweight and obesity has increased in recent decades (Lobstein et al. 2015). In 2018, an estimated 40 million of the children under the age of 5 were overweight, which represents 5.9% of the children in this age group around the world (UN/WHO 2019), and it is estimated that the majority of overweight or obese children live in developing countries, where the rates are increasing faster than in developed countries, with trends no longer correlated to those observed in adults (Abarca-Gómez et al. 2017).

Overweight and obese children are likely to maintain their status into adulthood and are at higher risks for developing chronic diseases such as hypertension, dyslipidemia, type 2 diabetes, heart disease, stroke, gallbladder disease, osteoarthritis, sleep apnea, orthopedic and respiratory problems, and certain cancers (Kumar and Kelly 2017; Lobstein, Baur, and Uauy 2004; Perry et al. 2017; Shore et al. 2018; Styne et al. 2017; Chen et al. 2019; Simmonds et al. 2016).

This epidemic situation calls for effective approaches to face its challenges. To be successful in managing childhood obesity, it is necessary coordinated and multisectoral pool of actions including not only the children, but also their families and communities. These actions should involve different sectors, including health - responsible for the growth monitoring and the guarantee of access to care and obesity treatment, education (food meals programs, health promotion, nutrition literacy), justice (implementation of laws and marketing restriction), and others.

Governments play an important role in ensuring their citizens have a healthy start in life. The prevention of childhood obesity will require inputs of different governmental sectors and institutions contributing to policy development and implementation (WHO 2017a).

Regarding healthy eating initiatives, the combination of actions taken by a country or region should be able to promote the intake of healthy foods and/or inhibit the intake of unhealthy foods for children at the individual, household and/or community levels.

This chapter review will discuss the strengths, limitations, uncertainties, and recommendations of the following actions that may influence healthy food choices: dietary guidelines, taxes on unhealthy food and beverages, food labelling and food advertising, and regulatory controls on the marketing of unhealthy foods and beverages to children.

DIETARY GUIDELINES

Obesity is a significant health and social problem. To reverse this scenario, it needs to be implemented public policies and population-based strategies aimed to tackle the influence of "obesogenic" environments. These responses must be allied to actions to reduce differences in socioeconomic conditions since the poor and less-educated people are most vulnerable to environmental impacts (Swinburn 2002).

Global actions are essential. However, they should be associated with actions target on individuals, aiming to increase access to information and the empowerment of families to choose healthy food and develop healthier eating practices (Onis 2015).

To support these actions, several countries developed dietary guidelines (DG) as a tool to be used directly to the general population and to assist health professionals. Furthermore, beyond the health sector, dietary guidelines are also an important source to guide other public policies and regulations, such as food production, food labeling, restrictions on food advertising and marketing regulation of unhealthy foods (FAO 2014). The sectors must work in a synergic way focusing the incorporation of recommendations presented by dietary guidelines transversely to sectoral objectives.

Since 1992, at the 1st International Nutrition Conference and later, World Health Organization (WHO) documents encouraged the countries to develop dietary guidelines for different age groups, considering factors as culture and national food and nutrition status (Barbosa, Colares and Soares 2008). In this chapter, dietary guidelines are treated generically, as not all countries have child-specific guidelines, and when they do, they are only for children under 2 years old.

Many countries have mobilized efforts to develop DG, but only 83 countries have national guidelines. Among the guidelines, most of them did not incorporate the promotion of healthy food aligned with economic and social aspects related to sustainability and health (Fischer and Garnett 2016). This approach involves components of sustainable food systems, from production to consumption. It becomes essential considering that the population's eating practices interfere with food production and sales. Besides it, the consumption of ultra-processed foods interferes with the environment, food cultures and, increases the obesity epidemic.

The effectiveness of DG depends on how many different aspects are presented and discussed. The first concerns about the adequacy of its content to the epidemiological, nutritional, and food profile of each region. The messages delivered in each guideline should be appropriate to the reality of its population. As well, the cultural aspects of eating should be valued, based on the rescue and strengthening of local and family eating practices. Thus, scientific knowledge must be combined with folk wisdom and not opposed to it.

A key influence on the infant diet is the quality of the family diet and should be strongly considered in DG for young children. The aim is to encourage healthy eating habits for the whole family, and not just for children (Robinson et al. 2007).

Home cooking is an essential issue, mainly in low-and-middle-income countries. They experienced the process of nutritional transition (traditional diets replaced by diets based on ultra-processed food - UPF) while they face challenges, health problems and sustainability questions also present in high-income countries (Fischer and Garnett 2016). UPF is ready to eat and, sometimes, just need to be heated. Losing the habit of cooking had an impact on the increased consumption of UPF. People who do not know how to cook food are more dependent on UPF. Thus, guidelines for healthy eating should stimulate and support the improvement of families' cooking skills (Oliveira 2018).

Historically, the labor division between men and women implies an overload of female work. Women are used to be inserted in the formal and informal market summed to domestic work, which involves the care of the house, food, and family (Damião and Rotenberg 2019). Thus, approaches that stimulate the division of responsibility for the tasks related to eating: cook, planning the menu, buying food, organizing and cleaning the kitchen must be a guideline topic. Guidelines focused on children under 2 years must also discuss the sharing of the childcare.

Another necessary issue is their perceptibility by the population. The texts must be written in plain language, easily understandable by the population, and by their capacity to disseminate information. These two aspects are challenges, especially in low-and-middle-income countries, where a great part of the population has poor access to health and education policies, and where the know-how and resources for building guidelines may be insufficient (Fischer and Garnett 2016). Moreover, it is common that guidelines were written using technical language, focusing on health professionals. However, the technical language is frequently not understood by the population.

In addition to the appropriateness of language, the translation of the recommendations on the guidelines to deal with the challenges of everyday life promotes and facilitates understanding and the adherence to the messages.

Most of the dietary guidelines are based on the food portion of food groups that hinder the assessment and identification of ultra-processed foods, which have been linked to negative health consequences (FAO 2014; Fischer and Garnett 2016). The classification elaborated by Monteiro et al. (2010) divides the foods into three groups according to their level of processing: "in natura" or minimally processed foods, processed foods used as ingredients in culinary preparations or by the food industry and ultra-processed foods. The Brazilian food guide (Brazil 2014) and the food guide for Brazilian children below 2 years (Brazil 2019) adopted this classification, which facilitates understanding and application in everyday life. This approach was presented by the Food and Agriculture Organization as a differential of the Brazilian food guide (Fischer and Garnett 2016).

The production of educational materials and strategic investment to facilitate access to the messages contained in dietary guidelines have been neglected by countries (FAO 2014). For dietary guidelines for young children, training of multipliers, including training of health professionals, is even more strategic for the dissemination, since this is a priority target of the public health agenda, and consequently, more frequent in health services.

Monitoring children's growth and development is primordial on the children's health agenda. This action becomes more important due to the actual scenario of the rise of obesity. The weight monitoring and the precocious identification of excess of weight is an important issue and a public health concern (Onis 2015).

Dietary guidelines are an important strategy for influencing healthy food choices but they need to be linked to policies and actions such as taxation of unhealthy food and beverage, food labeling and regulation of advertising and marketing of unhealthy food.

Sugar-sweetened Beverages Taxes

> "Sugar, rum, and tobacco are commodities which are nowhere necessaries of life, which are become objects of almost universal consumption, and which are therefore extremely proper subjects of taxation."
>
> Adam Smith, 1776, An Inquiry into the Nature and Causes of The Wealth of Nations

The World Health Organization (WHO) recommends that both adults and children restrict consumption of free sugars to less than 10% of total daily energy intake – and preferably less than 5%, based on the assumption that free sugars contribute to dental caries and the overall energy density of diets (WHO 2015). Therefore, could be positively associated with or has an effect on obesity indices in children, an important noncommunicable disease (NCDs) with high prevalence and rising trends among children's worldwide (Martin-Calvo et al. 2014; Bucher Della Torre et al. 2016; Abarca-Gómez et al. 2017; Frantsve-Hawley et al. 2017; Perry et al. 2017; Luger et al. 2018; Charvet and Huffman 2019).

In recent studies, a large proportion of children, within all age groups, exceeded the WHO recommended cut-off for free sugars (Lei et al. 2016; Bailey et al. 2018; Crowe et al. 2019). Additionally, some lifestyle and diet patterns also play a role in the free sugars' intake (Farajian et al. 2016). The excess consumption of added sugars, especially from sugary drinks, disproportionately affects children of minority and low-income communities (Muth et al. 2019). Nonetheless, reducing the overconsumption of sugary foods and drinks with low nutrient density may help improve diet quality among children (Gibson et al. 2016). Studies also found that children might not make up the missing calories from other sources of beverages when they're substituted, providing a background to recommend water intake rather than sugar sweetened beverages consumption as a strategy to address childhood obesity (de Ruyter et al. 2013; Gombi-Vaca, Sichieri, and Verly 2016).

Accordingly, sugar-sweetened beverage taxation can be considered as an effective intervention to reduce sugar consumption and help address NCDs in all age groups, and WHO cited an average cost-effectiveness ratio of ≤ 100 international dollars (I$) per Disability-Adjusted Life Year (DALY) averted in low- and lower-middle-income countries (WHO 2017b).

In this scenario, it is also important to recognize the "corporate" or "commercial" determinants of health – strategies, approaches, and influences from such manufacturers that are detrimental to health (Maani Hessari et al. 2019). The corporate political activity of the food industry could include reframing policy debates, build opposing constituencies, and lobby politicians to avert public health policies that could undermine their profits (Mialon et al. 2015). In addition, the social and cultural norms related to sugar-sweetened beverages, and the subsequent level of trust in health expert messages or food and beverage industry can impact the support and affect the perceived effectiveness of taxes (Pell et al. 2019). These conditions need to be carefully evaluated in every context, as they can facilitate or hinder the implementation of sugar-sweetened beverages taxes.

The World Health Organization also supported a commission on "Ending Childhood Obesity" (ECHO). The report of the Commission presented a comprehensive, integrated package of recommendations to guide countries to address childhood obesity. The implementation of an effective tax on sugar-sweetened beverages is highlighted as a recommendation among one of the six key areas of action, entitled "comprehensive programs that promote the intake of healthy foods and reduce the intake of unhealthy foods and sugar-sweetened beverages by children and adolescents" (WHO 2017a).

Globally, taxation of sugar-sweetened beverage was first implemented in 1981, in Norway, and is gaining strength worldwide as a public health concern in the last decade. Thereafter, nearly 40 countries and many cities already implemented sugar-sweetened beverage taxes (WCRF 2018a), with compelling evidence of an association with decreased sales, purchasing, and dietary intake of taxed beverages (Teng et al. 2019).

Table 1. Common steps in sugar-sweetened beverages tax design

Steps of the tax design and implementation	Important questions to be explored	Aspects to consider
Policy objectives	Are they health related, revenue related, or both?	Choices must be supported by independent and robust evidence.
Monitoring and evaluation	– Indicators framework are be specific, measurable, achievable, relevant and time-bound? – How to identify whether the implementation is on course and performing as expected? – - It is necessary to refine the tax design to avoid some loophole that manufacturers have exploited?	It is not appropriate to solely evaluate the effectiveness of the tax based on obesity rates. Implemented policies can have unintended impacts
Types of products to be taxed	What products are subject to the tax? A threshold or level of tax according to sugar content will be adopted? If the tax has thresholds or levels, how and who will analyze the sugar content within products? Imported products are subject to the same tax conditions?	Different beverages that can be taxed: soft drinks, juices, milk, yoghurts, energy drinks and waters. The rationale for the distinction between taxed beverages must be clear and relevant to the context
Types of tax	The types of tax can be combined	Building on existent tax infrastructure is important to ensure effective implementation
	Specific excise taxes: they can be content-based (e.g., per gram of sugar) or volumetric (per volume)	Jurisdictions with strong tax administrations are encouraged to implement content-based excise taxes Content-based tax can encourage industry to reformulate products
	Ad valorem tax: charge according to the product price, usually pre-tax price	These taxes have the advantage of being easily adjusted for inflation In countries and local jurisdictions with limited tax infrastructure or resources, they are more easily applied
	Sales tax: collected from consumers at point of purchase by retailers	

Table 1. (Continued)

Steps of the tax design and implementation	Important questions to be explored	Aspects to consider
	Value added tax: each stage of production supply chain is charged	
	Custom/import duty tax: taxes levied on imported products	International trade law says that countries cannot tax international products differently from similar domestic ones, making taxes susceptible to challenge
How high should the tax be?	Enough to impact purchase behavior	Understand how price elastic sugar sweetened beverages are is important to set the value of the tax Effective results can be achieved through taxes with values from 10% to 20% Align tax with inflation and economic growth in order to maintain its effect
Who should the tax be levied on?	Excise taxes are paid by producers	They can absorb the costs or reformulate products to avoid taxation, but the majority pass them to consumers
	Sales taxes	It is less onerous on retailers if the tax has already been collected before the product reach the shelves
Should it be a general or an earnmarked tax?	Governments sometimes choose to earmark the tax, even though few constitutions allow earmarking	Evidence suggests increased public and political support for earmark taxes (when revenues are allocated to a specific aim, rather than being channeled into the government's general tax revenue)

Adapted from: WCRF 2018a.

As taxes should be shaped by context and vary by country and local jurisdiction, specific details about sugar-sweetened beverage tax design and concepts are given in Table 1. To date, it is possible to observe many differences between sugar-sweetened beverage taxes already implemented, and the main possible effects observed post-tax implementation are presented below (WCRF 2018a):

a. increase in sugar-sweetened beverage prices: which can cause the increase of purchases and consumption of untaxed beverages, along with a decrease in the purchases of sugar-sweetened beverages, potentially impacting weight gain and the risk of NCDs;
b. increased public awareness about sugar consumption, which can help decrease the purchases of sugar-sweetened beverages;
c. revenue generation, that can be used to fund programs promoting public health or social good, depending on the local priorities and needs;
d. product reformulation to diminish the sugar content of beverages.

Some positive effects of implemented sugar-sweetened beverage taxes among children and their families are a higher reduction in sugar-sweetened beverage purchases among households with children in Mexico (Colchero, Molina, and Guerrero-López 2017) and greatest decline in sugar-sweetened beverage purchases for lowest income households in Berkeley - USA (Falbe et al. 2016). Although, more studies are needed in this area since tax design is different and the context may determine the outcomes observed (Cawley et al. 2019). Additionally, it is crucial to further address how the combinations of strategies to promote the intake of healthy foods, such as taxation and front-of-package nutrition labeling, for example, may interact and therefore influence consumer behavior (Acton et al. 2019).

FOOD LABELING

The last 2 decades represented a global change on the pattern of eating, that was based on basic food, cooked at home to an Ultra-processed food (UPF) consumption, ready-to-eat food, fast-food and packaged food, and drinks manufactured by global enterprises that sales food products, made with the same ingredients (corn, wheat, fat, salt and sugar) worldwide (Popkin 2017). This kind of food product is presented packed and all of them have food labels, that describes the food composition and other information.

All the global standards for food labeling (FL) are discussed and approved by the *Codex Alimentarius*[1] that defines FL as: "FL is the primary means of communication between the producer and seller of food on one hand, and the purchaser and consumer on the other." The *Codex Alimentarius* standards and guidelines on food labeling are a compact regulation, containing basic information, approved by consensus among its members, that serves as a guide for governments to define their local regulations, regulatory authorities, food industries, and retailers, and consumers (FAO/WHO 2007; FAO/WHO 1985 last revised 2017).

The label of foods was created in the century XIX worried about the expiration date and along the time it incorporated other information as the composition, ingredient list, allergenic ingredients, nutritional profile, and alerts about calories, fats, sugar and other ingredients related with noncommunicable diseases. According to the Codex Alimentarius, food label is "any tag, brand, mark, pictorial or other descriptive matter, written, printed, stenciled, marked, embossed or impressed on, or attached to, a container of food." There are three types of nutrition labeling: nutrient declarations; nutrition and health claims; and supplementary nutrition information (FAO/WHO 1985 last revised 2017). Table 2 describes the Codex Alimentarius Commission principles for nutrition labeling.

Currently, the food package contains more than nutrition information and expiration date, the package is commonly used as a marketing tool, with claims about healthy ingredients, characters, brand symbol among other strategies to improve the sales of these products. The children are one of the most important targets of this marketing strategy, with lots of products designed especially for them. According to the World Health Organization nutrition labeling is an important tool to guide consumers to do better choices and contribute to a healthier diet (WHO 2017a).

The labels are a complex combination of information, delimited by local regulations and the product comparison turns out to be a task with multiple variables ranging from package size, portion size, ingredient names, and the need to perform mathematical calculations for comparison. Different guidelines recommend the improvement of national regulation of food labeling, focusing the trustworthy information on the food labels. Labels can be used to educate and inform consumers.

The supplementary nutrition information is a scheme the improve the capacity of comprehension of nutritional information and to help to clarify the nutrient declaration which includes front-of-pack labeling (FOPL). Different experiences around the world drive in different ways. The chosen model must take account of the level of literacy, education, socioeconomic status among other factors.

[1] The Codex Alimentarius Commission is an intergovernmental body with over 170 members, within the framework of the Joint FAO/WHO Food Standards Programme established by the Food and Agriculture Organization of the United Nations (FAO) and the World Health Organization (WHO), with the purpose of protecting the health of consumers and ensuring fair practices in the food trade.

Table 2. The Codex Alimentarius Commission principles for nutrition labeling

Nutrient declaration	Information supplied should be for the purpose of providing consumers with a suitable profile of nutrients contained in the food and considered to be of nutritional importance. The information should not lead consumers to believe that there is exact quantitative knowledge of what individuals should eat in order to maintain health, but rather to convey an understanding of the quantity of nutrients contained in the product. A more exact quantitative delineation for individuals is not valid because there is no meaningful way in which knowledge about individual requirements can be used in labeling.
Supplementary nutrition information	The content of supplementary nutrition information will vary from one country to another and within any country from one target population group to another according to the educational policy of the country and the needs of the target groups.
Nutrition labeling	Nutrition labeling should not deliberately imply that a food which carries such labelling has necessarily any nutritional advantage over a food which is not so labeled.

Source: FAO/WHO 1985 last revised 2017.

The food labeling advanced along the time and at 1989 Swedish National Food Agency (Swedish Food Agency n.d.) created the Keyhole symbol as a tool to help the consumers to do better choices comparing the UPF. The symbol was developed to promote the products with fewer sugars and salt, more fiber, and whole grain and healthier or less fat than food products of the same type without the symbol. This kind of proposal used to promote the consumption of UPF under the understanding that it is possible a healthy diet based on these products. One positive outcome of this kind of FOPL is the reformulation of products to achieve the seal and be considered healthier than other products in the same category (PAHO 2016).

The WHO on the "Guiding principles and framework manual for front-of-pack labeling for promoting healthy diet" recommends 5 principles on the FOPL (WHO 2019):

- *Principle 1:* The FOPL system should be aligned with national public health and nutrition policies and food regulations, as well as with relevant WHO guidance and Codex guidelines;
- *Principle 2:* A single system should be developed to improve the impact of the FOPL system;
- *Principle 3:* Mandatory nutrient declarations on food packages are a prerequisite for FOPL systems;
- *Principle 4:* A monitoring and review process should be developed as part of the overall FOPL system for continuing improvements or adjustments, as required;
- *Principle 5:* The aims, scope, and principles of the FOPL system should be transparent and easily accessible.

Currently, there is a set of FOPL models, some of them are based on positive aspects of UPF as fiber, unsaturated fat, vitamins and, minerals. On the other hand, in the last decade, the FOPL models started to highlight negative aspects of UPF as excess of calories, free sugar, sweeteners, fats (total, saturated, trans), and sodium, based on limits and thresholds considered high. The models could be categorized into 4 groups: interpretive, semi-interpretive, non-interpretive, and mixed, as described below in Table 3.

In addition to the FOP model, it is also necessary to define which criteria will be adopted to define which products will be labeled according to product categories, ingredients and consumption purposes. The Pan-American Health Organization (PAHO) published in 2016 a guideline to help the countries on America´s Region to determine standards and threshold to classify the UPF aiming the FOPL containing a recommendation to sodium, free sugars, other sweeteners, total fat, saturated fat, and trans-fat (PAHO 2016). The criteria vary among the countries, a product considered high in sodium in Chile could be considered normal in the United Kingdom.

Table 3. Models of FOPL labeling, concept and examples

Models	Concept	Examples
Interpre-tive	They combine several criteria to establish an indication of the healthiness of the food. Provides judgment, opinion or guidance on food without nutrient specific information.	Ranking Models Health claims
Semi- interpre-tive	Provide information about a set of specific nutrients. Uses symbols, qualitative descriptors or colors to aid in understanding the level of each nutrient in the food.	Nutritional Traffic Lights Qualitative alerts
uninter-pretive	Display information about a specific nutrient pool without any kind of judgment, opinion or guidance or qualitative elements to assist in the interpretation of the information.	Guideline Daily Amount (GDA)
Mixed models	Combine attributes of non-template interpretive models interpretative or semi-interpretative.	Colored GDA Health Star Rating (HSR)

Source: ANVISA 2019.

In 2016, Chile implemented the obligatory use of FOPL warning labels (an octagonal black symbol) on packaged foods/beverages high in energy, sugars, saturated fats, and sodium. A study conducted with mothers of children (2-14yo), one year after the FOPL labeling implementation concluded that this kind of rule impacts the opinions about the regulation and the children have influenced the families' choices, changing the pattern of food choice (Correa et al. 2019). Low-income mothers in Uruguay were interviewed about the use of nutritional information the choose the children foods at the market. They stated that the label information was very confusing. When presented with FOPL strategies, the same mothers had more ease in making product choices for their children (Machín et al. 2016) Similar findings were found in a study conducted in Minneapolis (USA) where pairs of parents and children were presented for products with and without FOPL and the classification of products with FOPL was easier (Graham et al. 2017).

A study conducted with Brazilian children, compared products that were FOPL with semi-interpretive (nutritional Traffic Lights and qualitative alerts) versus no-interpretative models (GDA). The alerts showed a better level of accordance to classify the unhealthy products when compared with the two other models (Lima, Ares and Deliza 2018). Similar results were found by Neal et al. (2017) when comparing different types of FOPL.

The food and beverage labeling (food labeling) could influence not only the consumer behaviors but also the industry, that can react with a better nutrient profile. A meta-analysis conducted aimed at the evaluation of food labeling effects on the industry responses showed that labeling decreased product contents of sodium by 8.9% and artificial trans-fat by 64.3% (Shangguan et al. 2019). The report "A qualitative study concerning the Keyhole's influence over 25 years on product development" also describes the improvement of nutrient profile in Swedish industrialized food products, due to the FOPL implementation (Swedish Food Agency n.d.).

Another approach to food labeling is the restaurant menu labeling with a description of calories, fats, sodium, and sugar in the restaurant meals. A study evaluated the impact of parents' (children aged 3–12) demand for fast-food kids when the calories and sodium values are available. They compared 5 different scenarios 1) No Nutrition Information; 2) Calories-Only; 3) Calories + Contextual Statement (CS); 4) Calories, Sodium, + CS; and, 5) Calorie and Sodium in Traffic Lights + CS. The results showed the description of calories plus other information allowed the parents to identify which meal was more caloric and with high levels of sodium. This initiative may influence future purchases and menu choices with better nutritional profiles (Hobin et al. 2016).

Loureiro and Rahmani (2016) found similar behavior of food choice on the controlled environment (questionnaire application) but the opposite was found on the field experiment (shopping experience) alerting to the existence of other factors that can influence fast food consumption, such as advertising. A meta-analysis designed to evaluate the influence of menu labeling on food choices among children and adolescents resulted in three outcomes: the supposed food purchases in controlled settings indicates that menu labeling might be effective in reducing calories purchased for or by children and adolescents but real-life studies are not as incisive about menu labeling, even though school-based studies were commonly positive, reinforcing action on this setting (Sacco et al. 2017).

Currently, there are a dozen of models of FOPL and sometimes a mix of FOP models at the same label. Some countries already have regulations and others, the food industry presents voluntary FOPL as GDA. The development of national rules must define the model of the regulation and the establishment of just one model could prevent the consumer confusion, and make the UPF choice easier, especially for children (Leek, Szmigin, and Baker 2015).

FOPL is one of the strategies that can be adopted to reduce childhood obesity. This measure is effective when it comes to choosing UPF with better nutrient profiles. It has also been shown to impact industry reformulation of products. Children are more beneficiated by simple models as warnings. The ideal is to reduce consumption of UPF, and when consuming them, opt for the least harmful.

Regulatory Controls on the Marketing of Unhealthy Foods and Beverages to Children

Marketing can be defined as “any form of commercial communication or message that is designed to or has the effect of, increasing the recognition, appeal and/ or consumption of particular products and services. It comprises anything that acts to advertise or otherwise promote a product or service” (WHO 2012).

Children are most vulnerable to promotional appeals and advertising. Food marketing is omnipresent and can deeply influence food choices (IOM 2006). It can take on many forms, such as, branding, sponsorship of events, celebrity endorsements, contests and sales promotions, social media posts, commercials, etc (WHO 2010). Additionally, food marketing can involve raising brand awareness, developing new products, promoting them through advertising, and even paying grocery stores for prominent shelf space. Thereby, these different strategies are designed to create food trends, encourage people to buy certain foods or drinks or buy foods in order to get promotional items, as well as, to create links between certain foods or brands and a particular lifestyle (Federal Trade Commission 2012).

It should be also highlighted recent changes in marketing efforts and techniques that mirror changing patterns of media use among children and adolescents. Given the increased role of digital media in the lives of children and adolescents, the potential for marketers to reach these audiences through digital applications and novel marketing techniques is great (Potvin Kent et al. 2019).

Table 4 shows examples of marketing strategies used in food and beverage product marketing.

Table 4. Marketing strategies used in food and beverage product marketing

Marketing Strategies	Examples
Advertising	Broadcast (TV, Radio) Printed media (newspapers, magazines and comic books) Online (on-search engines, social networks, blogs, media clips, programmes, films and media clips watched online, etc.) Outdoor (billboards, posters, vehicles) Cinemas
Direct Marketing	Promotional e-mails Promotional sales by phone Promotional SMS in mobile phones Home catalogues and leaflets (doorstep selling) "Money off" Vouchers Promotional food sampling events
Product Placement and Branding	Promotional placement (TV, Radio, Films, computer games) Branded books Branded toys Branded computer games, interactive web sites
Product Design and Packaging	Product design (Fun and attractive colorings) Packaging design (imagery, colors, playshapes) Product portions (king size, duo packs) On pack/in-pack promotions (gifts, puzzles, vouchers)
Sponsorships	TV and Radio programmes Events, including community and schools Educational material and equipment Programmes (public health campaigns, school breakfasts/lunches) Sport activities and teams, athletes, celebrities
Point of Sale	On-shelf displays Displays in check-outs, pay-points, end-of-aisles Special offers and price incentives Vending machines (including schools) Loyalty schemes Free samples and tastings

Adapted from World Health Organization - A framework for implementing the set of recommendations on the marketing of foods and non-alcoholic beverages to children (WHO 2012).

Food marketing is recognized as an important contributor to the childhood obesity problem, mostly by influencing food preferences and choices (PAHO 2011). Since food preferences are established early in life, it may encourage them to adopt unhealthy dietary practices that persist into adulthood, increasing the likelihood of overweight, obesity and associated health problems such as diabetes and cardiovascular diseases (WHO 2014). Unlike tobacco and alcohol consumption, young people do not need to learn that consuming these foods is rewarding (Harris, Brownell and Bargh 2016). A recent systematic review found a strong body of evidence that exposure to food marketing impacts children's attitudes, preferences, and consumption of unhealthy foods, with detrimental consequences to health (Smith et al. 2019).

Ultra-processed food (UPF) industries are rapidly penetrating emerging global markets, just as the tobacco industry has done (Moodie et al. 2013). These products are described as highly convenient, hyper-palatable products that are attractively packaged and aggressively marketed (Monteiro, Cannon and Levy 2016). Energy-dense foods, high in fat and sugar and low in micronutrients and fiber are promoted extensively, are more visible, and are cheaper and easier to obtain than healthy options (Barquera et al. 2018; Vandevijvere et al. 2018).

The aggressive food marketing practices are working directly against young people's right to adequate food for nutritional health and wellbeing (SNC 2006). Therefore, the public health community has become increasingly concerned about food marketing targeted to children and their potential negative impact on health. One of its key arguments focuses on social responsibility to protect vulnerable age groups who may not be able to understand, or maturely interpret, the persuasive intent of advertising (IOM 2006).

Governments can encourage better choices through regulation, taxation, advertising codes, and informational campaigns. These may restrict individual choices a little, but they also make it easier for individuals to make healthier choices if they wish (Jochelson 2006).

In May 2010, 192 Member States in the World Health Assembly endorsed the "*Set of Recommendations on the Marketing of Foods and Non-alcoholic Beverages to Children*". These recommendations urged Member States to develop appropriate multisectoral approaches to reduce the impact on children of the marketing of foods high in saturated fats, trans-fatty acids, free sugars, or salt - HFSS (WHO 2010). The set of recommendations reiterated the goal of the Global Strategy on Diet, Physical Activity and Health, and complimented the action plan for the global strategy for the prevention and control of noncommunicable diseases.

It was followed up in 2012 by a specific implementation framework. The WHO framework addresses policy development, implementation, monitoring, and evaluation (WHO 2012).

Regarding policy development it is recommended that ministries of health or other designated bodies establish a working group on food marketing to children and include representatives from multiple governmental departments, agencies and bodies. This government-led working group should also dialogue with a broader stakeholder group, including civil society, academia, legislators, the private sector, and the advertising/media industry, while protecting the public interest and avoiding conflicts of interest. The core of the policy development is selecting the comprehensiveness of the policy approach, and the definitions of the terms and scope of the policy. A comprehensive approach means that the Member States should restrict all forms of marketing to children of foods that are high in saturated fats, trans-fatty acids, free sugars, or salt. On the other hand, a stepwise approach implies that some form of risk assessment and prioritization is undertaken in order to identify different forms and types of marketing and the impact of such marketing (WHO 2012).

On policy implementation, WHO recommends that the government should define the policy aim and objectives, and determine the appropriate regulatory approaches, e.g., using statutory regulation, focusing on government led or approved self-regulation of the industry, or other options, such as a combination of legislation and self-regulation or non-binding state guidelines. Another important issue to consider is the need to establish intergovernmental collaboration in order to reduce the impact of cross-border marketing, as well as, global actors that will be required to reduce its impacts (WHO 2012).

Considering a broad range of activities and outcomes necessary to monitor and evaluate, the document recommends prioritizing what information will be most beneficial. It is important to ensure that policies are being implemented according to the original intention, and that they are effective, with no unwanted side effects. Monitoring may, therefore, include surveys to assess whether a policy is indeed being put into practice and adhered to by all relevant parties as well as surveys to assess the policy outcomes, the power of this marketing, and changes in children's food preferences and dietary patterns (WHO 2012).

Other scientific and public health organizations also have issued recommendations aiming to reduce the negative effect of food advertising to children, such as the American Heart Association and World Cancer Research Fund International (AHA 2015; WCRF 2018b).

In 2013, WHO's Regional Office for Europe released data, from monitoring activities in 53 countries, that demonstrated the majority of the EU countries rely on general advertising regulations, which do not specifically address the promotion of HFSS food and beverage products to children, and on self-regulatory mechanisms which may or may not include specific controls to limit the promotion of such products to children (WHO 2013).

Countries around the world have adopted different measures to limit the effects of food marketing to children and adolescents. Although national governments had developed or implemented some relevant statutory measures, the nature and extent of the marketing restrictions differed across countries and regions (Hawkes and Lobstein 2011). In a document, The World Cancer Research Fund Nourishing framework provides examples of the types of policy action that can be taken within this policy area, examples of where these policy actions have been implemented, and a brief description of what the action involves (WCRF 2018b).

Most national legislation relates to advertising restrictions of HFSS foods to children or adolescents in broadcast or non-broadcast media (Chile, Iran, Ireland, Mexico, Norway, South Korea, Sweden, Twain, Turkey, United Kingdom-UK), as well as restriction of food advertising in schools (Costa Rica, Chile, Ecuador, Bulgaria, Lithuania, Poland, Spain, Uruguay, United States of America-USA). Some countries expand mandatory restrictions to advertising across any kind of media (Brazil, Canada, Finland, Peru, Thailand) and marketing techniques such as product placement, sponsorship, and the use of licensed characters (UK, Ireland, USA). Brazil, Latvia, and Lithuania have mandatory regulation of marketing of specific food items and beverages (Brazil bans advertisement and promoting of ultra-processed food). France and Turkey have a mandatory requirement that advertisements must carry a health message or warning. Also, some Governments engage with industry to develop self-regulation to restrict food marketing to children, mostly, via broadcast media (Denmark, Latvia, Malaysia, Norway, Spain), and other governments support voluntary pledges developed by industry (Belgium, European Commission, Hungary, Portugal, Turkey, Malaysia, Switzerland, Thailand, USA) (WCRF 2018b).

A systematic review examined available data on levels of exposure of children to the advertising of less healthy foods since the introduction of the statutory and voluntary codes. The results showed that high levels of such advertising of less healthy foods continue to be found in several different countries worldwide. It was observed only low levels of improvement over the period, although there is stronger evidence for an improvement in the UK and South Korea (Galbraith-Emami and Lobstein 2013). Another review appraising the current literature on food marketing to children in Canada, suggests that current Canadian approaches have not reduced children's exposure to food marketing in different settings, such as homes (via television, or online), public schools, grocery stores, fast food restaurants, except for some positive influences from Quebec's statutory regulations (Prowse 2017).

Additionally, a recent review assessed the effects of environmental interventions on the consumption of sugar-sweetened beverages, anthropometric measures and health outcomes, and on any reported unintended consequences or adverse outcomes. No studies were found regarding advertisement regulation (von Philipsborn 2019). This result highlights the need for studies in the field.

Despite some advances, challenges remain. As noted by WHO's document describing the status of the implementation of the Set of Recommendations in countries across the WHO European Region, existing regulations are designed to limit food marketing targeted to children. However, these regulations could fail since children are exposed to a substantial amount of media elsewhere (WHO 2016). Furthermore, social media influencers became a new source in advertising and, unfortunately, children may fail to recognize influencer content as advertising (De Veirman, Hudders, and Nelson 2019). Therefore, several sources by which food marketing reaches children poses major challenges for any jurisdiction attempting to restrict food and beverage marketing (Potvin Kent 2019).

Conclusion

All strategies discussed in this chapter aim to improve dietary habits and to reduce unhealthy food consumption, consequently, to reduce obesity rates. To effectively advance about protecting children from unhealthy food and beverage, multilateral coordination will likely be required. Interventions focused only on parent's education do not work and can even be detrimental. It is essential raising the awareness and involvement of all the actors - governments, companies, families, educators, researchers and, therefore, of society as a whole to adopt measures to create a less obesogenic environment, making the healthy choice easier and unhealthy choices harder. Efforts are needed to establish more comprehensive and rigorous approaches to monitoring and evaluating these actions that are still incipient.

References

Abarca-Gómez, L., Abdeen, Z. A., Hamid, Z. A., Abu-Rmeileh, N. M., Acosta-Cazares, B., Acuin, C., Adams, R. J., et al. (2017). Worldwide trends in body-mass index, underweight, overweight, and obesity from 1975 to 2016: a pooled analysis of 2416 population-based measurement studies in 128·9 million children, adolescents, and adults. *The Lancet*, 390 (10113): 2627–42.

Acton, R. B., Jones, A. C., Kirkpatrick, S. I., Roberto, C. A., and Hammond, D. (2019). Taxes and front-of-package labels improve the healthiness of beverage and snack purchases: a randomized experimental marketplace. *International Journal of Behavioral Nutrition and Physical Activity*, 16 (1): 46.

ANVISA - Brazilian Health Regulatory Agency. (2019). *Relatório de Análise de Impacto Regulatório sobre Rotulagem Nutricional [Regulatory Impact Analysis Report on Nutrition Labeling].* http://portal.anvisa.gov.br/documents/33880/5313808/Relat%C3%B3rio+de+An%C3%A1lise+de+Impacto+Regulat%C3%B3rio+sobre+Rotulagem+Nutriconal.pdf/31d15194-568c-4862-82ec-97e38202b1a1.

American Heart Association - AHA. (2015). American Heart Association Facts: No 04/2015, *Unhealthy and unregulated: Food advertising and marketing to children.*

Bailey, R. L., Fulgoni, V. L., Cowan, A. E., Gaine, P. C. (2018). Sources of added sugars in young children, adolescents, and adults with low and high intakes of added sugars. *Nutrients,* 10 (1): 102.

Barbosa, R. M. S., Colares, L. G. T., Soares, E. A. (2008). Development of food-based dietary guidelines in several countries. *Revista de Nutrição*, 21 (4): 455-467.

Barquera, S.; Hernandez-Barrera, L.; Rothenberg, S. J.; Cifuentes, E. (2018). The obesogenic environment around elementary schools: Food and beverage marketing to children in two Mexican cities. *BMC Public Health* 2018, 18.

Brazil. Ministry of Health. (2014). *Guia alimentar para a população brasileira [Dietary Guidelines for the Brazilian population]*. 2. ed. – Brasília.

Brazil. Ministry of Health. (2019). *Guia alimentar para crianças brasileiras menores de 2 anos [Dietary Guidelines for Brazilian children under two years of age]*. 1. ed. Brasília.

Bucher Della Torre, S., Keller, A., Laure Depeyre, J., Kruseman, M. (2016). Sugar-sweetened beverages and obesity risk in children and adolescents: a systematic analysis on how methodological quality may influence conclusions. *Journal of the Academy of Nutrition and Dietetics*, 116 (4): 638–59.

Cawley, J., Frisvold, D., Hill, A., and Jones, D. (2019). Oakland's Sugar-Sweetened Beverage Tax: Impacts on Prices, Purchases and Consumption by Adults and Children. *NBER Working Paper No*. 26233, Cambridge, MA.

Charvet, A., and Huffman, F. G. (2019). Beverage intake and its effect on body weight status among wic preschool-age children. *Journal of Obesity*, 16 (2019): 3032457.

Chen, Y. C., Fan, H. Y., Huang Y. T., Huang, S. Y., Liou, T. H., Lee, Y. L. (2019). Causal relationships between adiposity and childhood asthma: bi-directional mendelian randomization analysis. *International Journal of Obesity,* 43 (1): 73–81.

Colchero, M. A., Molina, M., and Guerrero-López, C. M. (2017). After Mexico implemented a tax, purchases of sugar-sweetened beverages decreased and water increased: difference by place of residence, household composition, and income level. *The Journal of Nutrition*, 147 (8): 1552–57.

Correa, T., Fierro, C., Reyes, M., Dillman Carpentier, F. R., Taillie, L. S. and Corvalan, C. (2019). Responses to the chilean law of food labeling and advertising: exploring knowledge, perceptions and behaviors of mothers of young children. *International Journal of Behavioral Nutrition and Physical Activity,* 16 (1): 21.

Crowe, M, O'Sullivan, M., Cassetti, O. and., O'Sullivan, A. (2019). Estimation and consumption pattern of free sugar intake in 3-year-old irish preschool children. *European Journal of Nutrition*. Jul 19.

Damião, J. J., Rotenberg, S. (2019). Amamentação e trabalho feminino: responsabilidade de toda a sociedade [Breastfeeding and women's work: responsibility of the whole society]. *Brazilian Observatory on Food Habits – OBHA*. https://obha.fiocruz.br/?p=397.

de Ruyter, J. C., Katan, M. B., Kuijper, L. D., Liem, D. G., Olthof, M. R. (2013). The effect of sugar-free versus sugar-sweetened beverages on satiety, liking and wanting: an 18 month randomized double-blind trial in children. *PLoS One*, 8 (10): e78039.

de Veirman, M., Hudders, L., Nelson, M. R. (2019). What is influencer marketing and how does it target children? A Review and Direction for Future Research. *Frontiers in Psychology*; 3(10):2685.

Falbe, J., Thompson, H. R., Becker, C. M., Rojas, N., McCulloch, C. E., and Madsen, K. A. (2016). Impact of the berkeley excise tax on sugar-sweetened beverage consumption. *American Journal of Public Health*, 106 (10): 1865–71.

FAO: Food and Agriculture Organization of the United Nations. (2014). *The state of Food-based Dietary Guidelines in Latin America and the Caribbean.* http://www.fao.org/3/a-i3677s.pdf.

FAO/WHO Codex Alimentarius Comission. (1985). *Codex Alimentarius: Guidelines on nutrition labelling:* World Health Organization: Food and Agriculture Organization of the United Nations. Adopted in 1985. Last revised in 2017.

FAO/WHO Codex Alimentarius Comission. (2007). *Codex Alimentarius: Food Labelling*. 5th ed. Rome: World Health Organization: Food and Agriculture Organization of the United Nations.

Farajian, P., Risvas, G., Panagiotakos, D. B., and Zampelas, A. (2016). Food sources of free sugars in children's diet and identification of lifestyle patterns associated with free sugars intake: The GRECO (Greek Childhood Obesity) Study. *Public Health Nutrition,* 19 (13): 2326–35.

Federal Trade Commission. (2012). *A review of food marketing to children and adolescents: follow-up report*. Washington: U.S: Federal Trade Commission.

Fischer, C. G., and Garnett, T. (2016). *Plates, pyramids, planet Developments in national healthy and sustainable dietary guidelines: a state of play assessment.* Rome: FAO/The Food Climate Research Network at The University of Oxford: Oxford.

Frantsve-Hawley, J., Bader, J. D., Welsh, J. A., and Timothy Wright, J. (2017). A systematic review of the association between consumption of sugar-containing beverages and excess weight gain among children under age 12." *Journal of Public Health Dentistry,* 77 (June): S43–66.

Galbraith-Emami, S., Lobstein, T. (2013). The impact of initiatives to limit the advertising of food and beverage products to children: a systematic review. *Obesity Reviews*, 14(12):960-74.

Gibson, S., Francis, L., Newens, K., and Livingstone, B. (2016). Associations between free sugars and nutrient intakes among children and adolescents in the UK. *British Journal of Nutrition*, 116 (7): 1265–74.

Gombi-Vaca, M. F., Sichieri, R. and Verly, E. (2016). Caloric compensation for sugar-sweetened beverages in meals: a population-based study in Brazil. *Appetite* 98 (March): 67–73.

Graham, D. J., Lucas-Thompson, R. G., Mueller, M. P., Jaeb, M., and Harnack, L. (2017). Impact of explained vs. unexplained Front-of-Package Nutrition Labels on parent and child food choices: a randomized trial. *Public Health Nutrition,* 20 (5): 774–785.

Harris, J. L., Brownell, K. D., and Bargh, J. A. (2009). The Food Marketing Defense Model: Integrating Psychological Research to Protect Youth and Inform. *Social Issues and Policy Review*, 3(1): 211–271.

Hawkes, C., and Lobstein, T. (2011). Regulating the commercial promotion of food to children: a survey of actions worldwide. *International Journal of Pediatric Obesity*. 2011; 6(2):83–94.

Hobin, E., Lillico, H., Zuo, F., Sacco, J., Rosella, L., and Hammond, D. (2016). Estimating the impact of various menu labeling formats on parents' demand for fast-food kids' meals for their children: an experimental auction. *Appetite,* 105: 582–590.

Institute of Medicine – IOM. (2006). *Food Marketing to Children and Youth: Threat or Opportunity?* Washington, DC: The National Academies Press.

Jochelson, K. (2006). Nanny or Steward? The role of government in public health. *Public Health,* 120(12):1149-55.

Kumar, S., and Kelly, A. S. (2017). Review of childhood obesity: from epidemiology, etiology, and comorbidities to clinical assessment and treatment. *Mayo Clinic Proceedings*, 92 (2): 251-265.

Leek, S., Szmigin, I. and Baker, E. (2015). Consumer confusion and Front of Pack (FoP) Nutritional Labels. *Journal of Customer Behaviour,* 14 (1): 49–61.

Lei, L., Rangan, A. M., Flood, V. M., and Louie, J. C. (2016). Dietary Intake and Food Sources of Added Sugar in the Australian Population. *British Journal of Nutrition*, 115 (5): 868–77.

Lima, M., Ares, G., and Deliza, R. (2018). How do front of pack nutrition labels affect healthfulness perception of foods targeted at children? Insights from Brazilian children and parents. *Food Quality and Preference,* 64: 111–119.

Lobstein, T., Baur, L., Uauy, R., and IASO International Obesity TaskForce. (2004). Obesity in children and young people: a crisis in public health. *Obesity Reviews*, 5 (Suppl 1): 4-104.

Lobstein, T., Jackson-Leach, R., Moodie, M. L., Hall, K. D., Gortmaker, S. L., Swinburn, B. A., James, W. P., et al. (2015). Child and adolescent obesity: part of a bigger picture. *The Lancet*, 385 (9986): 2510-20.

Loureiro, M. L., and Rahmani, D. (2016). The incidence of calorie labeling on fast food choices: a comparison between stated preferences and actual choices. *Economics & Human Biology,* 22: 82–93.

Luger, M., Lafontan, M., Bes-Rastrollo, M., Winzer, E., Yumuk, V., Farpour-Lambert, N. (2018). Sugar-sweetened beverages and weight gain in children and adults: A systematic review from 2013 to 2015 and a comparison with previous studies. *Obesity Facts* 10 (6): 674–93.

Maani Hessari, N., Ruskin, G., McKEE, M., Stuckler, D. (2019). Public meets private: conversations between coca-cola and the CDC. *Milbank Quarterly* 97 (1): 74–90.

Machín, L., Giménez, A., Curutchet, M. R., Martínez, J., and Ares, G. (2016). Motives underlying food choice for children and perception of nutritional information among low-income mothers in a latin american country." *Journal of Nutrition Education and Behavior,* 48 (7): 478–485.e1.

Martin-Calvo, N., Martínez-González, M. A., Bes-Rastrollo, M., Gea, A., Ochoa, M. C., Marti, A., GENOI Members. (2014). Sugar-sweetened carbonated beverage consumption and childhood/adolescent obesity: a case-control study. *Public Health Nutrition,* 17 (10): 2185–93.

Mialon, M., Swinburn, B., and Sacks, G. (2015). A proposed approach to systematically identify and monitor the corporate political activity of the food industry with respect to public health using publicly available information. *Obesity Reviews,* 16 (7): 519–30.

Monteiro C. A., Cannon G., Levy R. et al. (2016). NOVA. The star shines bright. *World Nutrition*, 7, 28–38.

Monteiro, C. A., Levy, R. B., Claro, R. M., Castro, I. R. R., Cannon, G. (2010). A new classification of foods based on the extent and purpose of the processing. *Cad Saúde Pública*, 26 (11): 2039-49.

Moodie R., Stuckler D., Monteiro C. et al. (2013). Profits and pandemics: prevention of harmful effects of tobacco, alcohol, and ultra-processed food and drink industries. *The Lancet*, 381, 670–679.

Muth, N. D., Dietz, W. H., Magge, S. N., Johnson, R. K.; American Academy of Pediatrics; Section on Obesity; Committee on Nutrition; American Heart Association. (2019). Public Policies to Reduce Sugary Drink Consumption in Children and Adolescents. *Pediatrics*, 143(4). pii: e20190282.

Neal, B., Crino, M., Dunford, E., Gao, A., Greenland, R., Li, N., Ngai, J., et al. (2017). Effects of different types of front-of-pack labelling information on the healthiness of food purchases—a randomised controlled trial. *Nutrients,* 9 (12): 1284.

Oliveira, M. F. B. (2018). *Autonomia culinária: desenvolvimento de um novo conceito [Cooking autonomy: development of a new concept]* (Masters Thesis) State University of Rio de Janeiro, Nutrition Institute. 155p.

Onis, M. (2005). Preventing childhood overweight and obesity. *Journal de Pediatria*, 91 (2): 105-107.

Pan American Health Organization - PAHO. (2016). *Nutrient Profile Model*. Washington, DC.

Pan American Health Organization PAHO. (2011). *Recommendations from a Pan American Health Organization Expert Consultation on the Marketing of Food and Non-Alcoholic Beverages to Children in the Americas*. In. Washington, DC.:130.

Pell, D., Penney, T., Hammond, D., Vanderlee, L., White, M., Adams, J. (2019). Support for, and perceived effectiveness of, the UK soft drinks industry levy among uk adults: cross-sectional analysis of the international food policy study. *BMJ Open,* 3; 9 (3): e026698.

Perry, D. C., Metcalfe, D., Costa, M. L., Van Staa, T. (2017). A Nationwide Cohort Study of Slipped Capital Femoral Epiphysis. *Archives of Disease in Childhood,* 102 (12): 1132–36.

Popkin, B. M. (2017). Relationship between Shifts in Food System Dynamics and Acceleration of the Global Nutrition Transition. *Nutrition Reviews,* 75 (2): 73–82.

Potvin Kent, M., Pauzé, E., Roy, E. A., de Billy, N., Czoli, C. (2019). Children and adolescents' exposure to food and beverage marketing in social media apps. *Pediatric Obesity*, 14 (6): e12508.

Prowse, R. (2017). Food marketing to children in Canada: a settings-based scoping review on exposure, power and impact. *Health Promotion and Chronic Disease Prevention in Canada*, 37 (9): 274-292.

Robinson, S., Marriott, L., Poole, J., Crozier, S., Borland, S., Lawrence, W. et al. (2007). Dietary patterns in infancy: the importance of maternal and family influences on feeding practice. *British Journal of Nutrition*, 98: 1029–1037.

Sacco, J., Lillico, H. G., Chen, E., and Hobin, E. (2017). The influence of menu labelling on food choices among children and adolescents: A systematic review of the literature." *Perspectives in Public Health,* 137 (3): 173–181.

Shangguan, S., Afshin, A. Shulkin, M., Ma, W., Marsden, D., Smith, J., Saheb-Kashaf, M., et al. (2019). A meta-analysis of food labeling effects on consumer diet behaviors and industry practices. *American Journal of Preventive Medicine,* 56 (2): 300–314.

Shore, B. J., Allar, B., Miller, P. E., Yen, Y., Matheney, T. H. and Kim, Y. (2018). Childhood obesity: adverse effects on activity and hip range of motion. *The Orthopaedic Journal at Harvard Medical School*, 19: 24–31.

Simmonds, M., Llewellyn, A., Owen, C. G., and Woolacott, N. (2016). Predicting adult obesity from childhood obesity: a systematic review and meta-analysis. *Obesity Reviews*, 17 (2): 95–107.

Smith, R., Kelly, B., Yeatman, H., Boyland, E. (2019). Food marketing influences children's attitudes, preferences and consumption: a systematic critical review. *Nutrients*, 11 (4): 875.

Smith, A. (1776). Book V: On the revenue of the sovereign or commonwealth. In.: *An Inquiry into the Nature and Causes of the Wealth of Nations*, 5th ed. Random House.

Standing Committee on Nutrition – SCN. (2006). *The human right of children and adolescents to adequate food and to be free from obesity and related diseases: the responsibilities of food and beverage corporations and related media and marketing industries.* http://www.unscn.org/files/Statements/Joint_statement _lifecycle_nehr_ The_human_right_of_children_and_adolescents_to_adequate_food_and_bee_free_fr om_obesity.pdf.

Styne, D. M., Arslanian, S. A., Connor, E. L., Farooqi, I. S., Murad, M. H., Silverstein, J. H., Yanovski, J. A. (2017). Pediatric obesity-assessment, treatment, and prevention: an endocrine society clinical practice guideline. *Journal of Clinical Endocrinology and Metabolism* 102 (3): 709–57.

Swedish Food Agency. (2015). *A qualitative study concerning the Keyhole's influence over 25 years on product development.* https://www.livsmedelsverket.se/globalassets/publikationsdatabas/rapporter/2015/keyholes-influence-on-product-development-2015.pdf.

Swedish Food Agency. (n.d.) *The Keyhole.* https://www.livsmedelsverket.se/en/food-and-content/labelling/nyckelhalet/.

Swinburn, B., Egge, G. (2002). Preventive strategies against weight gain and obesity. *Obesity Reviews.* 3 (4): 289-301.

Teng, A. M., Jones, A. C., Mizdrak, A., Signal, L., Genç, M., Wilson, N. (2019). Impact of sugar-sweetened beverage taxes on purchases and dietary intake: systematic review and meta-analysis. *Obesity Reviews* 20 (9): 1187–1204.

United Nations Children's Fund - UN, World Health Organization - WHO, The World Bank. (2019). *Levels and trends in child malnutrition: key findings of the 2019 edition of the joint child malnutrition estimates.* Geneva: World Health Organization. https://www.who.int/nutgrowthdb/jme-2019-key-findings.pdf?ua=1.

Vandevijvere, S.; Molloy, J.; Hassen de Medeiros, N.; Swinburn, B. (2018). Unhealthy food marketing around New Zealand schools: A national study. *International Journal of Public Health*, 63: 1099–1107.

von Philipsborn, P., Stratil, J. M., Burns, J., Busert, L. K., Pfadenhauer, L. M., Polus, S., Holzapfel, C., Hauner, H., Rehfuess, E. (2019). Environmental interventions to reduce the consumption of sugar- sweetened beverages and their effects on health. *Cochrane Database of Systematic Reviews*, Issue 6. Art. No.: CD012292.

World Cancer Research Fund International. (2018a). Building momentum: lessons on implementing a robust sugar sweetened beverage tax. www.wcrf.org/buildingmomentum.

World Cancer Research Fund International - WCRF. (2018b). *NOURISHING framework: Restrict food advertising and other forms of commercial promotion.* https://www.wcrf.org/sites/default/files/Restrict-advertising.pdf.

World Health Organization - WHO. (2010). *Set of recommendations on the marketing of foods and non-alcoholic beverages to children.* https://apps.who.int/iris/bitstream/handle/10665/44416/9789241500210_eng.pdf?sequence=1, accessed 23 December 2019.

———. (2012). *A framework for implementing The Set of Recommendations on the Marketing of Foods and non-Alcoholic Beverages to Children.* World Health Organization Regional Office for Europe. http://www.euro.who.int/__data/assets/pdf_file/0003/384015/food-marketing-kids-eng.pdf.

———. (2013). *Marketing of foods high in fat, salt and sugar to children: update 2012-2013.* Copenhagen: World Health Organization Regional Office for Europe. http://www.euro.who.int/__data/assets/pdf_file/0019/191125/e96859. pdf.

———. (2014). *Protecting children from the harmful effects of food and drink marketing.* https://www.who.int/features/2014/uk-food-drink-marketing/en/.

———. (2015). *Guideline: Sugars intake for adults and children.* Geneva: World Health Organization. https://apps.who.int/iris/bitstream/handle/10665/149782/9789241549028_eng.pdf?sequence=1.

———. (2016). *Evaluating implementation of the WHO Set of Recommendations on the marketing of foods and non-alcoholic beverages to children.* Progress, challenges and guidance for next steps in the WHO European Region. https://apps.who.int/iris/bitstream/hadle/10665/80148/9789241503242_eng. pdf?sequence=1.

———. (2017a). *Report of the Commission on Ending Childhood Obesity: Implementation Plan: Executive Summary.* Geneva. https://apps.who.int/iris/handle/10665/259349.

———. (2017b). *Best Buys' and Other Recommended Interventions for the Prevention and Control of Noncommunicable Diseases.* https://apps.who.int/iris/bitstream/handle/10665/259232/WHO-NMH-NVI-17.9-eng.pdf?sequence=1.

———. (2019). *Guiding Principles and Framework Manual for Front-Ofpack Labelling for Promoting Healthy Diets.* https://www.who.int/nutrition/publications/policies/guidingprinciples-labelling-promoting-healthydiet.pdf?ua=1.

In: Childhood Obesity
Editor: Roya Kelishadi

ISBN: 978-1-53618-158-6
© 2020 Nova Science Publishers, Inc.

Chapter 14

LIFESTYLE MODIFICATIONS AND DIETARY APPROACHES TO PREVENT OBESITY HYPERTENSION AMONG CHILDREN AND ADOLESCENTS

Farahnak Assadi*, MD
Professor, Department of Pediatrics, Division of Nephrology, Rush University Medical Sciences, Chicago, USA

ABSTRACT

Obesity hypertension (HTN) is serious health problem worldwide and its prevalence has been rising steadily. Obesity HTN is still not being recognized or treated. Effective preventive therapy exists but is inadequately applied. Incidence varies widely by race and ethnicity. Cardiovascular (CV) and chronic kidney diseases (CKD) are leading risk factors of obesity HTH.

Early detection can make a difference. Primary health care providers play a significant role in early diagnosis, treatment, and patient education that can improve patient outcomes. They can maintain blood pressure less than 125/80 mmHg, treat CV risk, especially smoking and metabolic syndrome and refer to dietician for a reduced sodium, low fat and carbohydrate diet. Routine screening with clinic blood pressure (BP) appears to have significant clinical benefit given the high prevalence of childhood HTN. Body mass index (BMI) greater the 85th percentile has a major determinants of the development of HTN. Efforts should be made to prevent obesity and to avoid the development of hypertensive CV and CKD. Preventive strategies should focus on life style modification, dietary intervention, physical activity, and treatment of obesity. The best strategy is to maintain appropriate BMI percentile for age and sex to avoid the development of obesity and HTN. The risk factors are positive family history of HTN, obesity, CKD, and CV events. A DASH-type diet (Dietary approaches to stop hypertension), rich in fruits, vegetables, whole

* Corresponding Author's Email: fassadi@rush.edu

grains, low sodium foods, and low-fat dairy along with decreased calories intake) along with 45 to 60 minutes per day moderate to vigorous physical activity at least 3 to 5 days per week are vital to maintain an appropriate BMI and help to lower BP. Stress reduction and avoidance of tobacco products are also important preventive strategies to reduce CV risk.

Keyword: obesity; hypertension; lifestyle modifications; DASH-diet; prevention

INTRODUCTION

Obesity hypertension (HTN) in children and adolescents is an epidemic and a major health concern worldwide [1, 2]. There has been an increase in the prevalence of obesity-related HTN among children and adolescents over the last four decades [3, 4]. While the rates of obesity HTN have raised in virtually all segments of the population, Hispanic and African have potentially higher rates compared to the non-Hispanic and white population. The prevalence of obesity HTN is also higher among children and adolescents who are overweight and obese (4% to 25%) [1,2]. Studies suggest that childhood obesity and HTN in is associated with development of HTN in adulthood [5-7]. In addition, results of the cross-sectional and longitudinal studies clearly establish an increasing HTN prevalence with increasing BMI percentile [8]. There is a fourfold increase in blood pressure (BP) among children and adolescents with morbid obesity (body mass index (BMI > 99th percentile) versus a twofold increase in in those with overweight (BMI > 95th-98th percentile) compared with normal weight children and adolescents [8-13].

Evidence suggests that sleep-disordered breathing (SDB) including obstructive sleep apnea syndrome occurs more frequently in overweight and obese children with or without hypertension compared with normal weight children and adolescents [14, 15].

Obesity also is an independent risk factor for chronic kidney disease (CKD) and its progression and development of end stage disease [16]. Obesity HTN related kidney disease is characterized by proteinuria and focal glomerulosclerosis as a result of glomerular hyperfiltration and over activity of the renin-angiotensin-aldosterone system (RAS) [17-19].

Childhood obesity and HTN is also known to be associated with cardiometabolic risk factors including dyslipidemia and altered glucose metabolism, insulin resistance, and cardiovascular disease (CVD) [20-25]. Children and adolescents with multiple risk factors, including obesity HTN, dyslipidemia, and insulin-resistant hyperglycemia are at higher prevalence of left ventricular hypertrophy (LVH) (43% vs. 12%), left atrial dilatation (63% vs. 22%; $p < 0.001$) and reduced systolic and diastolic functions compared with those without multiple risk factors [25].

Despite the demonstration of effective therapy, screening of high-risk patients, referral to dietitian and consultation with nephrologists and cardiologist, and even provision of therapy after diagnosis is inadequate.

PREVALENCE OF OBESITY HYPERTENSION AMONG CHILDREN AND ADOLESCENTS

In the last four decades global obesity related HTN among men has tripled from 2.3 in 1985 to nearly15% in 2014 It is now estimated that globally nearly 600 million adults are obese and a further billion are overweight.

It is now estimated that HTN affects approximately 25%, overweight 30% and obesity 15% of population worldwide. The prevalence of HTN increases progressively with increasing BMI from 15% among people with BMI between 85th to 95th percentiles and to 40% among those with a BMI > 95th percentile [26, 27].

Overweight and obesity account for more than 300,000 premature deaths, CVD, CKD, and stroke annually in the United States, second only to tobacco-related deaths.

Approximately 20% obese infants become obese children, 40% obese children become obese teens, and 80% obese teens become obese adults.

The prevalence of HTN, including BP values between the 90th and 94th percentiles in children or from120/80 to 130/80 mmHg in adolescents, is consistently greater in boys (3.5% to 19%) than in girls (2.2%-12%) [28,29].

Unfortunately, approximately 15%-20% of hypertensive patients are not aware hey have and those who are even ware of their conditions, only 50% have controlled BP [10].

WHY DO WE CARE ABOUT OBESITY HYPERTENSION?

We care, because of the increased health risk such as CKD, CVD, stroke, metabolic syndrome, sleep disorders, increased health cost and social inequity of health risks.

RISK FACTORS

The risk factors for obesity and HTN are positive family history of HTN, obesity, CKD, and CVD. Obesity and HTN have their origins during fetal life. Maternal diet and obesity predispose offspring to develop obesity HTN. Placental function is sensitive to women's nutrition during pregnancy and can influence their offspring to develop HTN in adulthood [30]. Environmental chemical exposures and life stressors also play a significant role.

Strategies to Prevent Obesity Hypertension and Cardiovascular Events

Untreated elevated HTN during childhood increases the risk of adulthood HTN and metabolic syndrome [27, 31]. The key contributors to CVD include tobacco exposure, obesity, physical inactivity and unhealthy diet, rich in salt, carbohydrates, and animal fats [32, 33]. Given the prevalence of these key risk factors in children and adolescents, it becomes apparent that adult CVD and CKD have their origins in early childhood. Nearly 50% of US adolescents have elevated BMI (> 99th percentile), over half of teenagers do not meet the goal for ideal physical activity levels and more than 80% of children and adolescents consume a poor diet consisting of more than 3-5 gram per day salt, inadequate fruits and vegetables, and large amount of animal fats [34, 35].

Therefore, routine measurement of BP at well-child clinic visits is vital for early detection and management of primary HTN given its high prevalence and high rates of accompanying CVD and CKD comorbidity risks.

Lifestyle Change and Non-Pharmacologic Interventions

Current treatment recommendation for HTN management in children and adolescents are systolic and diastolic BP levels < 90th percentile or < 125/80 mmHg in adolescents ≥ 13 years old, which results in lower risk of target organ damage and lower risk of adulthood HTN and CVD [36].

Studies in obese children and adolescents have demonstrated that nutritional interventions, including reducing sodium intake, and a diet high in olive oil polyphenols and rich in fruits and vegetables lower BP [37-40]. Weight loss improves BP control, lowers proteinuria, reduces the renin-angiotensin-aldosterone system (RAAS) activity and halts the CKD [41] progression by reducing the glomerular hyperfiltration [42].

Dietary Approaches to Stop Hypertension (DASH Diet)

Population studies suggest that reduced risk of obesity related HTN, and CVD is associated with high consumption of foods rich in sirtuin and butyrate such a fruits, vegetables and grains [43]. Sirtuin is a class of proteins that are involved in regulating much important biological process such as aging, metabolism and acts as histone methyltransferse inhibitor [44]. Butyrate is a short-chain fatty acid, synthesized from non-absorbale carbohydrate by intestinal microorganisms and plays important role in prevention of insulin resistance, dyslipidemia, and ischemic CVD. It acts as histone deacetylase inhibitors [45].

The specific elements of the DASH diet approach include a diet that is rich in whole grains (6 servings/day), fruits and vegetable (4-5 serving/day), legumes and nuts (1 serving /day), fish, poultry and lean red meats (≤ 2serving/day) along with low-fat milk products (2-3 servings/day), limited sweets (≤ 1 serving/day and salt intake < 2.3 g/day [46].

Studies of hypertensive in children and adolescents who are overweight and obese demonstrate relationship between elements of the DASH diet and lowering BP [46, 47]. Lacks of high intake of fruits, vegetables, and legumes and high fat consumption have been associated with HTN in childhood [43-47].

Physical Activity

Clinical studies have shown an association increasing physical activity results in lower BP [48-50]. These studies suggest that 45-60 minutes per session of moderate to vigorous, aerobic physical activity for at least 3 to 5 days per week lowers systolic BP by an average of 7 mmHg and may improve vascular dysfunction [51]. The association of step volume and intensity with over overall lower mortality rates, in a recent cohort study of 16741 women showed averaged 4400 steps/day, significantly reduced mortality rate during a follow-up of 4.3 years and with more steps taken per day, mortality rates decreased leveling off at approximately 7500 steps/day [52]. Life stress reduction and avoidance of tobacco products are also important preventive strategies to reduce CVD risk [53].

Management Strategies

Initiative should be undertaken to make health care providers, policy makers, and the general population more aware of seriousness of obesity HTN epidemic and its risk factors for the development of CKD, CVD and stroke.

Role of Primary Health Care Providers

Primary health care providers remain the cornerstone for early detection and management as well as general team direction that involves nurses, dietitian, and social workers. They can provide a greater emphasis on detecting HTN, and managing it prior to the development of CKD and CVD, can improve patient outcomes. Primary health care providers can improve detection of HTN at its early stage to prevent the development of CKD and CVD. They can improve identification of patients at risk and can promote a multi-disciplinary, coordinated and integrated team approach of care.

Primary care providers, at the time of diagnosis of high BP, should recommend the DASH-type diet and advise moderate to vigorous physical activity for 45 to 60 minutes per session for at least 3-5 days per week. DASH diet reduces and its effects on lowering the BP are comparable to antihypertensive medications used in stage-1HTN. Reduction in systolic BP by 11 mmHg has been reported in patients with mild HTN by adhering to DASH diet alone [45].

They should advise their patients to reduce salt intake to < 3 g/day, reduce dietary intake of, maintain adequate potassium, calcium, and magnesium intake, do aerobic exercise, 45 to 60 minutes at lease 3-5 days per week, and have them to stop using tobacco products, and lose weight if overweight (BMI > 85th percentile). The combine diet and physical activity have shown to prevent childhood obesity and HTN (Table 1) [47, 48].

Table 1. Effects of lifestyle intervention on blood pressure

Modification	Approximate SBP reduction
Weight loss (10 kg)	5-10 mmHg
Adopt DASH eating plan	8-14 mmHg
Dietary sodium reduction	2-8 mmHg
Physical activity	4-9 mmHg
Smoking cessation	2-4 mmHg

SBP, systolic blood pressure; DASH dietary approached to stop hypertension.

Modified from: Moore LL, Bradlee ML, Singer MR, Qureshi MM, Buendia JR, Daniels SR. Dietary approaches to stop hypertension (DASH) eating pattern and risk of elevated blood pressure in adolescent girls. Br J Nutr.2012;108(9):1678-1685; Doring N, Ghaderi A, Bohman B, et al. Motivational interviewing to prevent childhood obesity: a cluster RCT. Pediatrics.2016;137(5):1-10.

SUMMARY

Just as we have been observing in adult patients, overweight and obesity related HTN rates are on the rise among children and adolescents, and accompanied by metabolic syndrome, CKD, and CVD risk.

Early life events during the critical stages in pregnancy can potentially play a powerful role in influencing later susceptibility to obesity and HTN. An adverse embryonic, fetal or neonatal environment is responsible for epigenetic modifications leading to metabolic changes later in life. There is clear association between maternal nutrition and increased risk of Obesity, HTN, dyslipidemia, altered glucose intolerance or vascular endothelial dysfunction in the offspring later in life. Disease risk is higher in those born premature, small for gestational age that become obese and hypertensive as adolescents.

REFERENCES

[1] Sorof JM, Daniels S. Obesity hypertension in children: a problem of epidemic proportions. *Hypertension*. 2002;40(4):441-447.

[2] Sorof JM, Lai D, Turner J, Poffenbarger T, Portman RJ. Overweight, ethinicity,and the prevalence of hypertension in school-aged children. *Pediatrics.* 2004,113(3, p1):475-482.

[3] Koebnick C, Black MH, WU J, et al. High blood pressure in overweight and obese youth. Implications for screening. *J. Clin. Hypertens.* (Greenwich). 2013;5(11):793-805.

[4] Falkner B, Gidding SS. Ramirez-Garnica G, Wiltrout SA, West D, Rappaport EB. The relationship of body mass index and blood pressure in primary care pediatric patients. *J. pediatr.* 2006;148(2):195-200.

[5] Chen X, Wang Y. Tracking of blood pressure from childhood to adulthood: a systemic review and meta-regression analysis. *Circulation.* 2008;117 (25):317-318.

[6] Kit BK, Kuklina E, Carroll MD, OStchega Y, Freedman DS, Ogden CL. Prevalence of and trends in dyslipidemia and blood pressure among US children and adolescents, 1999-2012. *JAMA Pediatr.* 2015;169 (3):272-279.

[7] Theodore RF, Broadbent J, Nagin D, et al. Childhood to early-midlife systolic blood pressure trajectories: early life predictors, effect modifiers, and adult cardiovascular outcomes. *Hypertension.* 2015;66 (6):1108-1115.

[8] Hansen ML, Gunn PW, Kaelber DC. Under diagnosis of hypertension I children and adolescents. *JAMA*. 2007;298 (8):874-879.

[9] Chiolero A, Cachat F, Burnier M, Paccaud F, Bovet P, Prevalence of hypertension in school children based on repeated measurements and associations with overweight. *J. Hypertens.* 2007;25(11)2209-2215.

[10] Mozaffarian D, Benjamin EJ, Go As, et al. Writing Group Members' American Heart Association Statistics Committee. Executive summary-2016 update: a report from the American Hear Association. *Circulation.* 2016;133(4):447-454.

[11] DiPierto A, Kees-Folts D, DesHarnais S, Camacho F, Wassner SJ. Primary hypertension at a single center: treatment, time to control, and extended follow-up. *Prdiatr. Nephrol.* 2009;24(12):2421-2428.

[12] Parker ED, Sinaiko AR, Kharbanda EO, et al. Change in weight status and development of hypertension. *Pediatrics.* 2016;137(3):e20151662.

[13] Rosner B, Cook NR, Daniels S, Falkner B. Childhood blood pressure trends and risk factors for high blood pressure: The NHANES experience 1988-2008. *Hypertension.* 2013;62 (2):247-254.

[14] Archbold KH, Vasquez MM, Goodwin JL, Quan SF. Effects of sleep patterns and obesity on increases in blood pressure in a 5-year period: report from the Tucson Children's Assessment of sleep Apnea Study. *J. Pediatr.* 2012;161(1):26-30.

[15] Li AM, Au CT, Ng C, Lam HS, Ho CKW, Wing YK. A 4-year prospective follow-up study of childhood OSA and its association with BP. *Chest.* 2014;145(6):1255-1263.

[16] Kramer H, Luke A, Bidani A, et al. Obesity and prevalent and incident CKD. The Hypertension Detection and Follow-Up Program. *Am. J. Kidney Dis.* 2005;46:587-594.

[17] Foster MC, Hwang SJ, Larson MG, et al. Overweight, obesity, and the development of stage 3 CKD: the Framingham Heart Study. *Am. J. Kidney Dis.* 2008;52:39-48.

[18] Mathew AV, Okada S, Sharma K. Obesity related kidney disease. *Curr. Diabetes Rev.* 2011.4:41-49.

[19] Saiki A, Ohira M, Endo K, et al. Circulating angiotensin II is associated with body fat accumulation and insulin resistance in obese subjects with type 2 diabetes mellitus. *Metabolism. 2009*;58:708-713.

[20] Kelishadi R, Mirmoghtadaee P, Najafi H, Keikha M. Systemic review on the association of abdominal obesity in children and adolescents with cardiometabolic risk factors. *J. Res. Med. Sci.* 2015;20(3):294-307.

[21] Friedmann C, Heneghan C, Mahyani H, Thompson M, Perera R, Ward AM. Cardiovascular disease risk in healthy children and its associations with body mass index: systemic review and meta-analysis. *BMJ.* 2012;345:e4759.

[22] Lurbe E, Torro I, Aguilar F, et al. Added impact of obesity and insulin resistance in nocturnal blood pressure elevation in children and adolescents. *Hypertension.* 2008;51(3):635-641.

[23] Chagnac A, Weinstein T, Herman M, et al. The effect of weight loss on renal function in patients with severe obesity. *J. Am. Soc. Nephrol.* 2003;14:1480-1486.

[24] Zhang T, Zhang H, Li S, et al. Impact of adiposity on incident hypertension is modified by insulin resistance in adults: longitudinal observation from the Bogalusa Heart Study. *Hypertension.* 2016;67(1):56-62.

[25] De Simone G, Daniels SR, Devereux RB, Meyer RA, et al. Left ventricular mass and body size in normotensive children and adults: assessment of allometric relations and impact of overweight. *J. Am. Coll. Cariol.* 1992;20:1251-1260.

[26] Vernooij JWP, van der Graaf Y, Visseren FL, Spiering W; SWART study group. The prevalence of obesity-related hypertension and risk for new vascular events in patients with vascular disease. *Obesity* (Silver Spring). 2012;20(10):2118-2123.

[27] Nguyen NT, Magno CP, Lane KT, Hinojosa MW, Lane JS. Association of hypertension, diabetes, dyslipidemia, and metabolic syndrome with obesity: findings from the National Health and Nutrition Examination Survey. *J. Am. Coll. Surg.* 2008; 207(6);928-935.

[28] American Academy of Pediatrics Steering Committee on Quality Improvement and Management. Classifying recommendations for clinical practice guidelines. *Pediatrics.* 2004;114(3):874-877.

[29] Din-Dzietham R, Lu Y, Bielo MV, Shamsa F. High blood pressure trends in children and adolescents in national surveys,1963 to 2002. *Circulation.* 2007;116(13):1488-1496.

[30] Eisenberg DL, Stika C, Desaie A, Baker D, Yost KJ. Providing contraception for women taking potentially teratogenic medications: a survey of internal medicine physician's knowledge, attitudes and barriers. *J. Gen. Intern. Med.* 2010;25(4):291-297.

[31] Juhola J, Magnussen CG, Vikari JS, et al. Tracking of serum lipid levels, blood pressure, and body mass index from childhood to adulthood: the Cardiovascular Risk in Young Finns Study. *J. Pediatr.* 2011:159(4):584-590.

[32] Lloyd-Joned DM, Hong Y, Labarthe D, et al. American Heart Association Strategic Planning Task Force and Statistics Committee. Defining and setting national goals for cardiovascular health promotion and disease reduction: The American Heart Association's strategic impact goal through 2010 and beyond. *Circulation.* 2010; 121(4):586-613.

[33] Ning H, Labarthe DR, Shay CM, et al. Status of cardiovascular health in US children up to 11 years of age: The National Health and Nutrition Examination Surveys 2003-2010. *Circ. Cardiovasc. Qual. Outcomes.* 2015;8(2):164-171.

[34] Ogden CL, Carroll MD, Lawman HG, et al. Trends in obesity prevalence among children and adolescents in the United States, 1988-1994 through 2013-2014. *JAMA.* 2016;315(21):2292-2299.

[35] Skinner AC, Skeleton JA. Prevalence and trends in obesity and severe obesity among children in the United States, 1999-2012. *JAMA Pediatr.* /2014;168(6):561-566.

[36] Tuttle KR, Sunwold D, Kramer H. Can comprehensive lifestyle change alter the course of chronic kidney disease? *Semin. Nephrol.* 2009;29:512-523.

[37] DiPierto A, Kees-Folts D, DesHarnais S, Camacho F, Wassner SJ. Primary hypertension at a single center: treatment, time to control, and extended follow-up. *Prdiatr. Nephrol.* 2009;24(12):2421-2428.

[38] Alder AJ, Taylor F, Martin N, Gottlieb S, Taylor RS, Ebrahim S. Reduced dietary salt for the prevention of cardiovascular disease. *Crochrone Dattabase Syst. Rev.* 2014;(12):CD009217.

[39] Moreno-Luna R, Munoz-Hernandez R, Miranda MI, et al. Olive oil polyphenols decreases blood pressure and improve endothelial function in young women with mild hypertension. *Am. J. Hypertens.* 2012:25(12):1299-1304.
[40] Damasceno MM, de Araujo MF, de Freitas RW, de Almeida PC, Zanetti MI. The association between blood pressure in adolescents and the consumption of fruits, vegetables and fruit juice-an exploratory study. *J. Clin. Nurs.* 2011; 20(11-12):1553-1560.
[41] Ladowska-Kozlowska J, Litwin M, Niemirska A, Wierzbicka A, Wawer ZT, Janes R. Change in left ventricular geometry during antihypertensive treatment in children with primary hypertension. *Pediatr. Nephrol.* 2011;26(12):2201-2209.
[42] Morales E, Valero MA, Leon M, Hernandez E, Praga M. Beneficial effects of weight loss in overweight patients with chronic proteinuric nephropathies. *Am. J. Kidney Dis.* 2003;41:319-327.
[43] Seeman T, Gilik J. Long-term control of ambulatory hypertension in children: improving with time but still not achieving new blood pressure goals. *Am. J. Hpertens.* 2013;26(7):939-945.
[44] Yuan WL, Kakinami L, Gray-Donald K, Czernichow S, Lambert M, Paradis G. Influence of diet products consumption on children's blood pressure: results from the QUALITY cohort. *J. Acad. Nutr. Diet.* 2013;113(7(:936-941.
[45] Saks FM, Svetkey LP, Vollmer WM, Apple LJ, Bray GA, Harsha D, et al. Effects on blood pressure of reduced dietary sodium and the Dietary Approaches to Stop Hypertension (DASH) diet. DASH-Sodium Collaborative Research Group. *N. Engl. J. Med.* 2001;344(1):3-10.
[46] Barnes TL, Crandell JL, Bell RA, Mayer-Davis EJ, Dabelea D, Liese AD. Change in DASH diet score and cardiovascular risk factors in youth with type 1 and type 2 diabetes mellitus: The Search for Diabetes in Youth Study. *Nut. Diabetes.* 2013;3:e91.
[47] Moore LL, Bradlee ML, Singer MR, Qureshi MM, Buendia JR, Daniels SR. Dietary approaches to stop hypertension (DASH) eating pattern and risk of elevated blood pressure in adolescent girls. *Br. J. Nutr.* 2012;108(9):1678-1685.
[48] Doring N, Ghaderi A, Bohman B, et al. Motivational interviewing to prevent childhood obesity: a cluster RCT. *Pediatrics.* 2016;137(5):1-10.
[49] Flattum C, Friend S, Neumark-Sztainer D, Story M. Motivational interviewing as a component of a school-based obesity prevention program for adolescent girls. *J. Am. Diet. Assoc.* 2009:109(1):91-94.
[50] Resnicow K, McMester F, Bocian A, et al. Motivational interviewing and dietary counseling for obesity in primary care: an RCT. *Pediatrics.* 2015;135(4):649-657.
[51] Monazavi R, Dreimane D, Geffner ME, et al. Improvement in risk factors for metabolic syndrome and insulin resistance in overweight youth who are treated with

lifestyle intervention. *Pediatrics.* 2006;117(6). Available at: www.pediatrics.org/cgi/content/full/117/6/e1111.

[52] Lee M, Shiroma EJ, Kamada M, et al. Association of step volumes and intensity with all-cause mortality in older women. *JAMA Intern. Med.* 2019;179(8):1105-1112.

[53] Gregoski MJ, Barnes VA, Tingen MS, Harshfield GA, Treiber FA. Breathing awareness mediation and LifeSkills Training programs influence upon ambulatory blood pressure among African American Adolescents. *J. Adolesc. Health.* 2011; 48(1):59-64.

In: Childhood Obesity
Editor: Roya Kelishadi

ISBN: 978-1-53618-158-6
© 2020 Nova Science Publishers, Inc.

Chapter 15

APPROPRIATE PHYSICAL ACTIVITIES FOR CONTROLLING CHILDHOOD OBESITY

***Vazgen Minasian*[1,*] *and Roya Kelishadi*[2,†]**
[1]Department of Exercise physiology, University of Isfahan, Isfahan, Iran
[2]Child Growth and Development Research Center, Research Institute of Primordial Prevention of Non-Communicable Disease, Isfahan University of Medical Sciences, Isfahan, Iran

ABSTRACT

This chapter discusses the importance of designing proper physical activity with the aim of controlling and preventing overweight/obesity in children and adolescents. The main challenge is to increase knowledge related to the negative consequences of inactivity in children that nowadays is one of the main concerns of health organizations worldwide. Increasing awareness of the levels of physical activity in children and adolescents with obesity and their out-of-school activities can help to develop obesity prevention and control strategies.

Development of awareness about physical activity assessment methods in children and adolescents with obesity and their behavioral habits such as driving to school can develop obesity prevention and control strategies. Although it may not be rational for all children to have the same exercise training protocol, providing general principles of exercise training and active lifestyle interventions can help to modify children's physical fitness and obesity and eventually improve children's health status.

* Corresponding Author's Email: vazgenmin@yahoo.com.
† Corresponding Author's Email: kelishadi@med.mui.ac.ir.

INTRODUCTION

Today, almost one-third of children and youth are overweight or obese worldwide [1]. Physical inactivity in children and adolescents and across the lifespan are linked to many chronic conditions, including diabetes, heart disease, cardiovascular and metabolic conditions, and cancer. Childhood obesity is a complex phenomenon that can many risk factors. It is characterized, among other factors, by an imbalance between energy intake and energy expenditure that would increase the body fat mass. Over the last few decades, this worldwide health problem has been becoming increasingly prevalent in the pediatric populations.

Different health organizations have provided scientific guidelines for physical activity (PA) of children and adolescents. For children aged 5–17 years, guidelines consistently recommend participating in moderate-to-vigorous intensity daily PA, and indicate that a greater volume of PA is associated with a greater health benefit [2], and the concept of using exercise as medicine implies that exercise can be used in a dose-dependent manner to positively impact health outcomes for individuals with chronic diseases such as obesity [3]. Pediatric obesity is also a multifactorial condition which is a result of genetic and environmental factors and the complex interactions among these. Medical interventions for the treatment of childhood obesity are very limited, but it is crucial to establish a comprehensive management program that emphasizes appropriate nutrition, exercise, and behavior modification. Lifestyle modification involving nutrition and PA remains the basis of the treatment approach to childhood obesity. It is crucial to involve the children's families in this approach. Behavioral change is needed to improve the energy balance, i.e., to reverse the disproportionately high energy intake compared with energy expenditure.

PHYSICAL ACTIVITY AND CHILDREN'S HEALTH

Nowadays, numerous studies have highlighted the role and importance of PA in improving health-related physical fitness and reducing obesity and related illnesses. PA has a crucial role in prevention and control of childhood obesity. In recent studies, the need for lifestyle changes has been mentioned, but PA for children should be planned in a pleasant setting where children can follow it for a long period and in life span. PA is defined as an intentional, voluntary movement directed toward achieving an identifiable goal. Accordingly, PA is a broad term that comprises training, exercise, sport, dance and leisure activities [4].

Physical educators and coaches have an important role in guiding children and adolescents to perform physical activities appropriate for their age and physical ability, hence this should include trying to maximize PA in educational settings, especially in schools, to contract long periods of sitting, watching TV social media and inactivity due to this behaviors. One of the major negative consequences of childhood obesity and little engagement with fitness is the increase in health-related risk factors. Physical activity in childhood has numerous benefits, and physically active children display healthier values of some indicators of the heart disease risk factors, blood pressure, body composition, and lipid profile in childhood and later in adulthood [5]. The technological advances in developed and undeveloped countries have resulted in reduction in the opportunities for PA; therefore, sedentary lifestyle has become a challenging issue in children [5].

CHILDREN'S PHYSICAL ACTIVITY LEVELS

Primary School

Physical activity during early childhood has been shown to have positive effects on adult health habits. Despite this knowledge, many children are not sufficiently engaged in physical activity to benefit their health. Additionally, it has been shown that PA habits are established at a young age and are often carried into adulthood. Therefore, PA promotion has to start at a young age [6].

The majority of interventions designed to increase children's PA fall into two categories, those that target teaching strategies and those focusing on fitness. Recent studies that have measured PA in primary school children have suggested that less than 50 percent of boys and 25 percent of girls are achieving the recommended amount of daily PA for children. Since the time in physical education is often limited, recess is scheduled more frequently throughout the day and/or daily. Therefore, as these recess periods may represent the only PA children participate in during the school day, how best to organize the recess periods to increase PA behavior in children becomes an important topic of inquiry.

During recess periods, elementary-school children often participate in free play in a gymnasium or an outdoor setting where they are given access to the age-appropriate PA equipment and/or sedentary alternatives (e.g., coloring books, puzzles) in any pattern or amount they want. However, children have been shown to spend less than 50% of a free play period participating in PA. It has also been reported that adding structure to these recess periods may increase the number of physically active children who participate during the recess. Structure during recess could include the provision of equipment and/or games with instruction, prompts or encouragement from teachers as to how to use this equipment or play these games. Therefore, it is possible that providing some structured play during recess periods may foster greater PA in children than an unstructured free-play recess period. While previous evidence suggests that providing structured play during recess may promote PA behavior in elementary school students, there is very little research examining this relationship in preschool-aged children. Investigations focusing on preschool-aged children are crucial because early childhood PA participation has been linked to PA behavior and obesity risk later in life. It is at this point that children are starting to develop habits that they may carry into adulthood.

Secondary School

Children's PA is known to decline as they age, and the transition to adolescence, coinciding with the move from primary to secondary education, is seen as the key point for intervention [7]. Additionally, evidence suggests a decline in young people's cardiorespiratory fitness (CRF), which is an important predictor of overall health status, and there is a strong relationship between obesity and cardiovascular status of children [8, 9].

Physical activity levels have been shown to decline more strongly over these ages at school lunchtimes, during which school grounds are more important locations for PA than other periods of the school day. There is some evidence pointing out that changes in the environmental supportiveness of schools between primary and secondary settings are associated with changes in PA. It has been suggested that young people's weekday step counts increased if the number of schoolyard facilities and equipment was higher at secondary schools than primary schools. Despite this, much work on activity promotion through the design of school grounds has focused on primary schools [7]. A recent review of the role of school playgrounds in children's PA included 33 papers, of which only two were set in secondary schools, following analyses found associations between increases in the number of facilities in the school grounds and increased self-reported PA during recess. Moreover, it has been concluded that further work is needed to explore the possibility and the way secondary school grounds can be adapted to promote PA in older children and adolescents [10].

Physical Activity of Girls

Commonly, girls' participation in all forms of PA, including sport, rapidly declines during their early high school years with approximately 50 percent dropping out between the ages of 10 and 14 years. There was a consistent trend for greater participation in males than females in all age groups, but the difference was marked in the 12–14 and 15–19 age groups. Girls don't like to draw attention to themselves and often withdraw from physical education classes and activities. Many girls prefer activities that allow them to work together to improve or to work as a team to accomplish goals as opposed to participation in individual competitive activities such as fitness testing [11]. School-based interventions are considered the most promising approach for increasing adolescents' PA levels, although it is unclear which types of school-based interventions have the greatest impact on adolescent females as a particular group at risk of declining PA.

Physical Activity out of School Hours

There are relatively few international studies that have examined children's PA and sedentary behaviors in their time spent out of schools. Internationally, most work has been conducted in the USA, and regarding after-school programs, it is found that children spent the majority of their leisure time in sedentary conditions, and only a relatively small amount of the daytime was engaged in regular PA. Given the conflicting evidence, lack of attention paid to screening time practices in after-school programs, and lack of recent data, further research to expand and update our understanding of PA and screen time in out of school care programs is warranted. Most children, in many countries globally, do not get enough PA and get too much screen time, and Out of School Hours Care (OSHC), the setting offers an opportunity to positively impact the daily activity patterns of children [12]. Reviews have identified that current practices regarding PA and screen time in the OSHC setting are highly variable across services and that there is a lack of oversight/guidance from the overarching guidelines and policy. Research in the out of school care setting is scant, and future work examining practice and policy in other jurisdictions will be important to determine the scale of the issue. Development of guidelines and intervention programs to encourage healthful PA and screen behaviors in the out of school care setting are necessary [12].

Active Transport to and from School

A major PA opportunity for many children is active commuting to and from school, walking or cycling in general. However, a commonly identified barrier to this opportunity for increasing PA and reducing travel by car is perceived safety [13]. Unfortunately, in some developed countries more than 50 percent of children are taken to school by car, although it seems that similar patterns of transport to school are evident in most undeveloped countries.

Younger children were more likely to travel by car and boys were more likely to be allowed to walk or cycle than girls, and recently an aspect has been developed that refers to a 'car culture' that views modes of travel such as walking and cycling as less attractive than using cars. Schools that had the most walkers or cyclists were located in the middle of a neighborhood, whereas parents in more affluent areas were more likely to drive children to school [14]. Beginning at age seven, children are progressively socially conditioned into the car culture [15]. Without an established walking and cycling culture at a school, levels of walking and cycling are consistently lower. Recent studies indicate that walking to school holds real promise as a meaningful way of impacting children's overall PA levels [15].

MONITORING AND MEASURING PA LEVELS

Numerous methods have been used to assess PA; these vary in usefulness depending on the desired precision and accuracy of the technique, the intended use for the data, and those responsible for measurement. A general description of a range of methods follows, including the advantages and disadvantages of each method.

The methods most often utilized are questionnaires, heart rate monitoring, accelerometry, and geometry. There are several questionnaires, but only a few of them were normally used frequently [16]. It must be kept in mind that when a questionnaire is being administered, all information is being collected in a self-report, recall-based manner. Therefore, if a 5 or 6-year old child is being questioned, the likelihood of the child giving accurate information is poor. In this case, a parent should be asked to describe the child's activity patterns and answer questions related to an activity history. As children get older, their ability to recall may get better, but it may also be influenced by testers in that the adolescent may report activities that are suspected to be expected of them. While questionnaires may offer a significant amount of information, it is very difficult to translate the qualitative information to quantitative information in a manner that maintains validity and accuracy [16]. Heart rate monitoring allows for a cardiovascular view of PA which indicates elevated heart rates as activity that is not sedentary, and greatly elevated heart rates as moderate-to-vigorous activity.

However, some limitations of this method include that it is time-consuming and requires cooperation from the subject, which in and of itself can be difficult to obtain in a 7- or 8-year old child (who must be sitting still), not to mention in one that is attempting to be active. As already stated, heart rate monitoring is based on the intensity of the activity at hand, and thus for children who are constantly on the move, it may not be the best way to assess PA. However, it may be more applicable in those older adolescents who are beginning a regular exercise routine.

Pedometers and accelerometers offer a physical assessment of activity. Pedometers are not as accurate or as useful as accelerometers. They can only count steps at a fixed stride length; therefore, they do not take into account changes in speed, direction, or activities that do not require walking (i.e., cycling, rowing, etc.). On the other hand, accelerometers are based on the relationship between muscular force and body acceleration that occurs during movement patterns. Unlike pedometers, accelerometers measure activity in all three planes and can distinguish between a multitude of speeds. This means their use in children is practical considering the sporadic nature of children's activity patterns [17].

Assessment of Physical Inactivity

Because PA is considered a time-use behavior, excessive electronic device use within out-of-school settings may lead to increased sedentary or inactivity behavior. Excessive use of screen-based media is linked to lower sports and PA participation in children and adolescents. In adolescents, higher video game use is associated with poorer health status, health-related quality of life, and higher levels of depression and anxiety. In teenagers, the use of nearly every type of technological activity predicts indicators of poor health, and relationships that are inconsistent in other pediatric populations such as preteens and younger children [13].

Assessment of sedentary behaviors is usually done on a self-report basis, using questionnaires or simple intake forms. Again, the recall error is present and parents and children are usually both asked the questions, which will offer some form of comparison, as was the case in a study done by Robinson. Accelerometers can also be a way of measuring inactivity, as all movement is measured.

Trends of Physical Activity

Childhood PA is on the decline in part because of the societal changes that have occurred over the past few decades. Typically, there are now two working parents at home, leaving the parents to rely on media as a distraction so they can tend to their errands without worrying about their child's safety. As a result, children's leisure activity is no longer mostly active, but they are increasingly sedentary and there is a high prevalence of physical inactivity in children and adolescents, with higher rates among girls and older ages [18].

Besides, as more families hire outside help (i.e., housekeepers and nannies), the children's physical activities of daily living, such as walking to and from school and doing chores, are decreasing. Additionally, electronic equipment in the bedroom, consisting of televisions, phones, computers, and videogames, has been shown to negatively associate with MVPA and positively associated with BMI. It has also been shown that a higher number of electronic items in the bedroom correlates with a lower estimated VO_2 Peak in children, an important health-related indicator.

Children now play less outside and focus more on the internet, computers, and television. As a result, approximately 25 percent of children are now classified as overweight and 11 percent are classified as obese. Even more compelling is that 70 percent of these obese adolescents will likely grow up to be obese adults. Public interventions should be implemented to prevent these trends from tracking into adulthood [19].

SELF-REPORT AND RECALL

Self-reports may include diaries completed by the individual, self-administered questionnaires, interviewer questionnaires, and proxy reports completed by parents or teachers. Self-report instruments have the advantages of being cost-effective, user-friendly [20] and easy to administer with minimal participant burden. Both qualitative and quantitative data can be collected; however, there is a heavy reliance on the accuracy of the information provided by the individual. The self-report technique is more useful in adults with reliability and validity concerns such as subject bias and difficulty for many children in recalling physical activities accurately. A further issue is that both adults and children frequently overestimate their actual activity level. Despite these limitations, researchers have shown that several recall instruments have acceptable reliability and validity when they are used with adolescent and adult populations [20].

DIRECT OBSERVATION

Studies suggested that the direct observation technique is highly effective in measuring PA levels. An observer logs both the intensity and type of activity performed during short periodic intervals. Despite being valid and reliable, the approach is labor-intensive and time-consuming even for trained observers. More advanced software programs have helped to enhance data collection, recording, and subsequent analysis. Systematic observation is an effective technique, but much training and observation time are required. Some would argue that it is only useful in a research context; however, when working with obese youngsters in limited numbers, this approach may be very useful [21].

Activity Monitors

Accelerometers are some kind of motion sensors that provide real-time estimates of the frequency, intensity, and duration of free-living PA. Accelerometers have gained widespread acceptance for the measurement of activity. There are numerous activity monitors such as uniaxial, bi-axial or tri-axial modes [22]. The integration of time and activity allows verification of activity level with data stored in the monitor and downloaded to a personal computer for analysis. An advantage of accelerometers is that participants aren't able to change the input; however, a disadvantage is the inability of users to provide immediate feedback and motivation. Another limitation for widespread use of activity monitors in the field is their relative expense. The cost of such devices may limit the number of participants who may participate in activity programs [23].

Pedometers

Pedometers measure the number of steps a person takes when involved in ambulatory activities, and detect movement through a spring-loaded, counter-balanced mechanism that records vertical acceleration at the hip joint. Pedometers are cheaper than accelerometers or heart rate monitors, but provide valid measurements [23]. However, it is important to acknowledge the limitations of pedometers. Pedometers are less accurate when children move slowly or walk with an uneven gait, in other words, they overestimate distance covered at slower speeds and underestimate actual distance at higher speeds [23].

Heart Rate Monitors

Heart rate monitors enable the assessment of PA levels over extended periods with relative ease, and it has long been used to monitor the intensity of PA over time and store data collected in varying time intervals and later downloaded to a computer. Heart rate monitors can be used in both laboratory and field settings and provide safety training zones for users, including in the context of weight control programs [17]. However, PA can cause an increase in heart rate without increased energy expenditure and factors such as increased ambient temperature, emotional stress, age and training state all have the potential to impact heart rate. Heart rate monitors are also unable to distinguish between upper body heart rates compared to lower body aerobic or resistance physical activities.

Heart rate monitors primarily respond accurately to aerobic types of activity. Since they focus on the intensity of aerobic activity, they may not be the precise instrument of choice when working with obese youth. These youngsters may already be opposed to intense activity and perceive it to be quite difficult. In this case, focusing on the movement of all types rather than intensity may be more appropriate [17].

In a school setting, some participants do not like to wear the straps around their chests and see them as intrusive or even uncomfortable when worn for several hours. Additional considerations for the use of this instrument are the cost, which would be prohibitive for a large number of students, as well as the difficulty in gathering information outside school hours.

Physical Activity for Obese Children

Obese children have to work harder than children with normal-weight to accomplish the same task, thus they need adjusted workloads. All children do not and should not have to do the same workload. It is unreasonable to expect obese children to be capable of workloads similar to those of lean youngsters. The basic principles of training are the foundation for all physical exercise programs, and the same should also be applied for PE classes. This concept includes the basic principles of training (overload, progression, specificity, continuity, and individuality), the application of which is facilitated by FITT guidelines (FITT is an acronym for frequency, intensity, time, type) [24].

Activity Frequency

The overall objective when developing an activity program for an overweight or obese child is to set the individual up for success rather than failure. Prescribing too much activity too soon will surely lead the child to experience frustration and failure. Again, the objective is to incorporate regular, daily activity into their lives to increase their daily energy expenditure. In developing such a program, the frequency of activity must carefully be considered. Most instructors recommend that children engage in regular activity the most, if not every day of the week [25]. However, for obese and overweight children, this is very likely to be an unrealistic starting point. Again, the objective is to instill positive activity habits through positive reinforcement. Hence, one must be realistic when prescribing the frequency of activity, starting more slowly with 3 to 5 times per week and building from there. Adopting and reiterating the philosophy that some activity is better than none will help to instill positive activity behaviors and associations. Once the frequency of activity can realistically be established, the intensity of the activity should then be considered [25].

Activity Intensity

The intensity of the activity for children should be carefully predetermined and prescribed. Children with overweight/obesity will reach their prescribed levels of intensity much more quickly than the normal weight persons, simply because of the burden of the extra weight they carry. Once again, prescribing too much too soon will likely set the child up for failure, while also placing them at greater risk for injury [26], instead, it is the total calories burned, rather than the specific intensity of the activity, that should be emphasized.

There are several methods to consider when recommending and monitoring the intensity of an activity, but the most practical approach to prescribing intensity is via the use of perceived exertion. The intensity of the activity prescribed based on a child's "perceived" level of exertion, is an easier way for children to monitor their intensity of activity. Not only is the use of Rating of perceived Exertion (RPE) easier to incorporate and monitor, but researchers have also found that RPE is correlated to physiological parameters, such as heart rate and maximal oxygen uptake [27].

Although using the RPE scale can be effective in prescribing intensity of activity, when working with the obese and overweight children, particularly at the beginning phases of the activity program, it is important to begin the exercise program slowly to avoid injury. Having this in mind, the focus should be placed on low-to-moderate intensity-type activities. There are many obese children in whom the intensity will not be significant enough to improve their cardiovascular fitness level. Yet weight loss and caloric expenditure should be the initial focus, and for that reason, the duration rather than the intensity of the activity should be the starting point of any activity. Higher intensity activities should be promoted as the children and adolescents improve and progress through the exercise regularly. Additionally, the Omni walk/run scale has been indicated as a valid and reliable measure of perceived exertion over a wide range of intensity of dynamic exercise training in children and adolescents. It uses a 0–10 numeric rating with a pictorial descriptor that represents a child at different exertion levels walking/running, and exertion levels range from "not tired at all" to "very, very tired." Before undertaking the assessment, participants were oriented to the perceived exertion definition and the scaling instructions of the OMNI walk/run scale. The term OMNI is a contraction of the word omnibus and refers to a numerical category scale that employs interchangeable sets of mode-specific pictorial descriptors positioned along a visually discernible exertional intensity gradient [27, 28].

Duration of Physical Activity

The duration of the activity, or amount of time per activity session prescribed, is the second most critical component for the obese and overweight child's activity program. As mentioned previously, many children do not participate in the American College of Sports Medicine's (ACSM) recommended 60 min of moderate to vigorous-intensity physical activity (MVPA) each day [25]. The objective is to instill positive activity behaviors with positive reinforcement. Asking a child who carries an extra weight of 35 to 40 kilograms to walk for 30 minutes nearly every day is simply unrealistic [25].

Previous studies suggest that the activity needed to be continuous (i.e., one 30–45-minute session) to reap the benefits of the exercise. However, recent researches have shown that shorter, more frequent bouts of activity are just as effective. For obese or overweight children, this is ideal, as one can prescribe a program with a goal of 20 minutes per day and slowly increase the duration of exercise until 60 minutes has been reached. Notably, this activity can be broken up into several 10-minute bouts with the same activity benefits gained. Furthermore, not only are these shorter bouts more attainable, but they can also be broken down into shorter increments as needed (and increased as the subjects become stronger, more fit, and more confident and capable in abilities). These shorter bouts can also be incorporated into their daily lives with minimal inconvenience. The key is to prescribe a duration that is realistic and attainable for the overweight or obese child [25].

Type of Activity

One of the most important considerations when developing a PA program for an obese or overweight child is the type of activity prescribed. The type of activity is critical, particularly for minimizing the risks of injury and maximizing energy expenditure, but it can also serve as the cornerstone of a potentially successful program.

The type of activity with which an overweight or obese child should initiate a PA program depends on several factors, including his or her medical history, level of fitness, past experiences with activity, and the child's interests and needs [25]. Walking or running, although challenging for the morbidly obese child, can be implemented into virtually every child's daily routine. It is weight-bearing, which maximizes energy expenditure; and it is a familiar form of activity, thereby minimizing the chances of injury. Initially, the emphasis should simply be placed on incorporating walking into a child's daily activities, whether it be a prescribed amount of time daily or simply increasing the amount of walking each day at home. As the child becomes stronger and more confident and capable in his or her abilities, a specific walking or activity program can be prescribed. Once this point has been reached, additional considerations must be made when developing the program, including the frequency, intensity, and duration of the activity to be prescribed.

Aquatic aerobic activities, due to the physical properties of water, especially the fluctuation, can be alternatives of exercises indicated for obese children, by reducing the impact on the joints responsible for the weight support of the body [29]. During aquatic activities, it is emphasized that walking or deep-running, can be executed with or without using floating equipment. Also, the locomotion of the body in aquatic exercises due to the viscosity of water is more difficult. Walking in water, in addition to the reduction of joint stress, provides a higher energy expenditure to overcome the resistance of the water [30].

Exercise Modalities for Prevention and Treatment of Childhood Obesity

Participating in regular exercise training has been shown to have beneficial effects on physical, mental, and social health as well as academic performance. The World Health Organization recommends 60 min of moderate-to-vigorous PA (MVPA) per day for children and adolescents aged 5–17 years (Tremblay et al., 2011). However, based on self-report data, in most European countries, less than 50% of children and adolescents follow these guidelines. An analysis of device-based measured global PA data of 13–15-year-old adolescents, collected from 105 countries, revealed that 80.3% did not meet the recommended activity guidelines [31]. Based on literature most common interventions and modalities consist of different types of aerobic exercise, resistance training, combined aerobic/resistance training and applying different training protocols as follows:

High-Intensity Interval Training (HIIT)

High-Intensity Interval Training, is characterized by brief repetitions of high-intensity exercise (5s-1min) alternated with periods of rest or low-intensity exercise (1-5 min). Although continuous aerobic training is generally included in intervention programs, low volume high-intensity interval training (HIIT) can produce similar or improved responses compared with traditional continuous aerobic training, despite the short amount of time that HIIT requires. Alvarez et al. observed that following an HIIT program for a total of 18 sessions (three times per week) improved the insulin resistance levels as well as the anthropometric, cardiovascular, and physical performance of insulin-resistant school children [32]. A systematic review of children and adolescents reported that HIIT programs are a time-efficient tool for improving the biomarkers of cardiovascular disease [33]. However, there are no exact recommendations regarding the intensity, volume, frequency, mode of the exercise, and rest intervals regarding the application of HIIT in the context of school and PE classes. The review of literature revealed that HIIT resulted in significant improvements in body composition in less time than less intense exercise, cardiorespiratory fitness, and the HIIT protocols also are highly applicable to PE classes due to their short duration and adaptability to the school setting [34].

The main purpose of a weight management exercise training in children with obesity is to make positive changes in body composition in favor of a reduction in fat mass and gaining fat-free mass. Racil et al.1 compared HIIT with moderate-intensity interval training (MIIT) and found that HIIT led to greater improvements on cardiometabolic variables [35], on the other hand, Lau et al. observed a significant decrease in the sum of skinfolds of overweight children who followed HIIT programs in comparison with low-intensity (LI) interval exercises. In another study Racil et al., compared HIIT programs with HIIT-plus-plyometric programs and reported that both approaches produced significant results (BMI, BF%, WC) [36]. Hay et al., however, did not report any differences in adiposity measurements between groups who undertook HIIT and those who followed a moderate-intensity endurance training (ET) program. Lambrick et al. found that the anthropometric parameters of obese children improved significantly compared with the control group through high-intensity discontinuous games [37].

In some studies, similar results were reported for body composition when comparing HIIT with endurance training, although the duration of HIIT sessions was 70% less than endurance training sessions. Still, in another study, HIIT proved to be a more effective approach for weight loss in obese adolescents compared with endurance training [38]. An intervention which employed different exercise methods reported that HIIT groups achieved greater increases in fat oxidation rates and greater decreases in BMI than the LI groups, but concerning waist circumference (WC), the application of HIIT for obese adolescents resulted in a greater decrease than moderate exercise [36].

Individuals engaged in both HIIT and endurance training reported similar energy expenditures, which could explain the similar results for body composition in some cases, despite the lower total volume of training and time commitment of HIIT. According to the review of recent literature, HIIT is a time-efficient tool for increasing cardiorespiratory fitness in adolescents. A further benefit of high-intensity compared with LI training for obesity and cardiovascular health is the improvement of parasympathetic tone and autonomic heart modulation in obese adolescents, and furthermore, it has been suggested that HIIT exercise caused significantly greater improvements in VO_{2max} than ET [34]. The gold standard of cardiorespiratory fitness (CRF) is considered as maximal oxygen uptake (VO_{2max}), which can be measured by using maximal graded cardiorespiratory test or by using an indirect calculating method to estimate maximal oxygen uptake. There is strong and consistent evidence from epidemiological studies that low CRF is associated with higher morbidity and mortality from all causes, including cardiovascular disease (CVD) and cancer. Furthermore, higher levels of CRF in childhood and adolescence are associated with a healthier cardiovascular profile later in life [8, 33].

Besides, an intervention which compared HIIT with LI aerobic training for 6 months showed significant reductions in systolic and diastolic blood pressure of participants in both groups, beneficial changes in HR were only observed in the HIIT group. It is important to consider that while aerobic continuous training is beneficial, its application requires longer session times to achieve similar results to HIIT. On the other hand, HIIT increases stress on metabolic and cardiorespiratory systems, and these results are supported by a recent study conducted on school-age children, which revealed increased VO_2 following 12 intervals of 30s at 90% HRmax, however, maintaining optimal levels of these parameters plays a significant role in limiting the risk factors in overweight adolescents. Also, HIIT methods require less time than low-intensity activities, making them applicable for use in schools as a strategy to prevent and control the childhood obesity. The incorporation of HIIT programs could be carried out alongside existing PE activities within the same lesson or in specific periods during the school day.

HIIT programs can result in improvements in body composition and cardiorespiratory capacity, as well as improvements in health markers. Previous studies suggest that to guarantee HIIT effectiveness, programs should include 2-3 sessions per week, with intervals of 15-30s and passive or active rest periods of 15-30s. For higher volume programs, discontinuous games of up to 6 min work with 4 min rest periods for a total session time of 40 min can be used. Despite some studies highlight the importance and feasibility of HIIT methodology in a school setting, some questions need to be addressed. Future research should identify the optimal duration of HIIT sessions for improving physical, physiological and cognitive health in young children. Likewise, future studies should determine the optimal frequency within the school calendar for this type of program.

Continues Submaximal Intensity Exercise Training

Physical activity is a critical component in managing childhood obesity, and it has been recommended by both the American College of Sports Medicine and WHO that children and adolescents should perform at least 60 minutes of moderate-to-vigorous continues PA (MVCPA) per day, and at least 3 times of high-intensity exercise per week [39]. In the pediatric population, the traditional methods to increase PA have principally used continuous training, which tends to rely on longer-duration sessions involving moderate-intensity continuous training. Although previous studies have examined that moderate-intensity continuous training is associated with significant reduction in body fat and cardiovascular risk factor in obese children and adolescents, studies have shown that the majority of children failed to meet the recommended PA guidelines, such as only 30% of school-aged children met MVCPA recommendations in China [39]. Lacking time has been considered as the main barrier. Therefore, it is necessary to explore more time-efficient exercise modality for obese children and adolescents.

School-Based Exercise

It has been suggested that children spend six hours a day for nearly 40 weeks in one year at school. Therefore, it seems logical to utilize this setting for the promotion of PA as schools provide both an infrastructure and a context for such programs [40]. Also, schools are ideal settings for the delivery of PA programs because they have access to young people as well as the necessary facilities and equipment, and qualified staff. Studies suggest that school-based PA interventions targeting children ageing 5–11 years old and young adolescents have had mixed success [31].

The success and sustainability of PA interventions are largely dependent on agreement and support of school principals and teachers, which may wane over time in the face of competing time demands. As enhancing students' academic performance is the core business of schools, providing evidence for the impact of vigorous PA on cognitive and academic outcomes may provide a novel 'hook' for schools to implement PA interventions. Nevertheless, school-based PA interventions need to be time-efficient because lack of time is the most commonly cited implementation barrier cited by teachers.

Previous studies aimed to identify and evaluate school-based interventions based on their scalability, cost-effectiveness, feasibility, acceptability to children and youth and those delivering the intervention, and their potential to reach the target audience [41]. Furthermore, schools are places where children and youth spend a significant amount of time, making them prime locations for intervention. The World Health Organization's Global Strategy on Diet, PA, and Health identifies schools as a target setting for promoting PA among children and youth. WHO defines school health interventions as a combination of curriculum development, educational policy and guideline development, professional training opportunities for educators, as well as research, evaluation, and knowledge transfer for evidence-based policies, programs, and practices [42].

Although physical education programs offer children and adolescents an opportunity to be physically active, decreased levels of PA in physical education class have been observed, accompanied by lower physical fitness levels in children and adolescents. Strategies to promote PA during physical education classes have shown to increase the overall time spent being physically active as well as participation in PE programs.

School-based PA interventions may have not only positive effects on motor performance, but also benefit health outcomes and exercise knowledge in children and adolescents [31]. A previous study found that the school-based intervention affects PA behavior in part mediated by self-efficacy. A complete evaluation of mediating factors of energy balance-related behavior found evidence for a mediated effect of self-regulation, enjoyment, intrinsic motivation, and autonomy support on PA. Since mediating variables explain the causal sequence between the intervention and the outcome, the identification of relevant mediators can increase the effectiveness of future interventions. Intervention developers should, therefore, disclose the theoretical base of their intervention, including the mediating variables along with the applied intervention strategies, and only then it is possible to determine the effective strategies for changing the mediators of certain behavior.

There are several theoretical frameworks which exercise interventions for promoting physical fitness can be based on. The self-determination theory (SDT) is an appropriate theoretical framework for developing health intervention programs and for understanding the motivations of children and adolescents towards PA [43]. During the implementation of SDT in health intervention studies, the focus is conducting the processes through which a person acquires the motivation for initiating new health-related behaviors and maintaining them during their life span. Within SDT, different types of motivation can be characterized along with the autonomy-control continuum, depending upon the degree to which autonomous or controlled regulations are represented. Autonomous behavior is characterized by the extent to which an individual agrees, and is willing, to engage in a certain behavior, i.e., the degree to which an individual is intrinsically motivated to act. Intrinsically motivated behavior is accompanied by a feeling of effectance and enjoyment. Controlled behavior, on the other hand, is led by a consequence of external reward, social approval, or avoidance of punishment. Extrinsically motivated behavior can also be experienced as autonomous when the behavior is associated with valued or important outcomes. Hence, behavior can be externally regulated (controlled by external forces the individual does not agree with) or can be controlled through introjection, in which case individual acts to receive self or external approval, and avoid feelings of guilt, shame, and disapproval.

A motivation can be described as a state of passiveness, a lack of intentionality and motivation to act, and can be based on a feeling of lack of competence or arise from a lack of interest, relevance, or value in a given action. Concerning a targeted behavior, SDT assumes that the development of intrinsic motivation requires the satisfaction of three basic psychological needs: autonomy, competence, and relatedness [31]. Regarding health behavior, autonomy and competence are crucial for the processes of internalization and integration of health-beneficial behaviors like PA. Organizing an autonomy-supportive environment can increase adherence and health consequences. Furthermore, for individuals to accept health-beneficial behaviors and their values, a sense of belonging is required. The satisfaction of these psychological needs has been associated with better health-related outcomes, such as increased PA and fitness.

Building upon the SDT, the Hierarchical Model of Intrinsic and Extrinsic Motivation (HMIEM) by Vallerand considers intrinsic motivation, extrinsic motivation, and motivation on a situational, contextual, and global level. According to this theoretical model, motivation varies both in its type and in its level of generality. Specifically, situational motivation can be described as motivation during a specific task in physical education classes, while contextual motivation can be described as motivation towards PE in general [31]. Global motivation describes general motivation personality. The different types of motivation exist within the individual at the three different levels of generality [44]. It has been revealed that interventions successful in changing situational motivation could affect contextual motivation (i.e., physical education in general) and finally global motivation, leading to a healthy lifestyle [31].

Another theory, focusing on classroom motivation, is the Achievement Goal Theory, where goal orientations are grouped into performance goal orientation and mastery goal orientation. Performance goal orientation is characterized by being successful without much effort, outperforming others and being judged based upon ability. Mastery goal orientation is characterized by developing new skills, valuing the process of learning and attainment of mastery [45]. Ames and Archer reported that students perceiving an emphasis on mastery goals used effective learning strategies, preferred challenging tasks, and had a more positive attitude towards class. Perception of performance goal orientations was negatively related to attitudes and self-perception of ability [45]. In the context of PE, Goudas and Biddle found that the mastery dimension was present not only when self-improvement was valued and effort was rewarded rather than ability, but also when students felt the teacher took a personal interest in them and were involved in decision-making [46]. Motivational teaching strategies to increase students' motivation in PE have been developed and include amongst others the Task, Authority, Recognition, Grouping, Evaluation, Time (TARGET) approach [47]; the Sport Education Model [48]; and Teaching Games for Understanding (TGfU) approach [49]. Systematic reviews have pointed out that the effects of PA interventions within a school setting on PA behavior are for the most part small, for example, an increase in 2.6 min of PE-related PA. Additionally, the effects on PA behavior may decline in the long term, due to a decrease in motivational constructs [31]. Inconclusive results were found when examining the effects of school-based PA interventions on enjoyment, which is linked to intrinsic motivation. The findings of a meta-analysis indicated significant effects of school-based intervention strategies on PA enjoyment, with a true population effect of small-to-moderate magnitude.

In summary, studies suggest that theory-based PA interventions implementing motivational strategies may have positive treatment effects on PA behavior and outcomes associated with motivation. However, none of these studies evaluated PA intervention effects on the different types of motivation, which are assumed to determine the direction of PA behavior. The poor implementation may explain why so many school-based PA interventions fail to reach their potential. Lack of time has been noted as the greatest barrier to implementation by teachers and providing robust evidence for the positive effects of vigorous PA on cognitive and mental health outcomes may provide the impetus for schools to make a mandatory PA program for older adolescents.

Exercise Prescription and Special Considerations

- As fewer children are prepared to participate in continuous vigorous PA, initially low volume PA should be recommended. The recommendation for at least 60 minutes of daily activity for children and youth is higher than the 30 minutes per day activity recommendation for adults [50].
- Children and adolescents must have experience in all aspects of PA and for all elements of physical fitness, not limited to aerobic/cardiovascular fitness.
- Children in primary school should be engaged in a minimum of 60 minutes up to several hours of proper physical activities based on age and gender on all or most days.
- With an increase in age, children become more inactive, so we could check that children and adolescents receive approximately 60 minutes a day PA to decrease their inactivity levels as they age.
- It is recommended that each day children take part in 10-15-minute moderate to vigorous activity. However, it should be noted that in most children and adolescents short duration all-out activities alternating with periods of rest are dominant.

- In children younger than the age of 13, engaging in a moderate to vigorous continuous PA lasting for more than five minutes without rest periods are not common. This is because children typically participated in a short period of intermittent PA.
- Because typical activities of children involve sporadic bursts of energy, a greater time involvement rather than a greater intensity of continuous exercise is recommended.
- Several (three to six or more) activity sessions programmed throughout the day may be necessary to accumulate adequate activity time for primary school children. Some of these periods should be 10–15 minutes or more in length, alternating intermittent activity and rest within this period.
- For adolescents, the guidelines are similar. The major difference is that longer sessions of moderate to vigorous activity are recommended.
- Adolescents should engage in three or more sessions of weekly activities that last 20 minutes or more and require moderate to vigorous levels of intensity. This is a period of rapid growth and there is evidence to show that alternating aerobic activities with strength and flexibility activities allow youngsters to rest between aerobic intervals and, maybe, more importantly, optimizes growth [5].
- Children and adolescents should be encouraged to participate in various physical activities that are enjoyable and age-appropriate.
- Children should also participate in the unstructured active play, which typically consists of short duration moderate to vigorous-intensity PA, alternating with brief periods of rest. It is important to recognize that these small bouts of PA, however brief, are highly effective to improve fitness.
- Adolescents may safely participate in strength training activities with receive proper instruction and supervision.
- Generally, adult guidelines for resistance training may be applied to adolescents with some considerations.
- Because of immature thermoregulatory systems, adolescents should avoid sustained, heavy exercise in exceptionally hot humid environments, be properly hydrated, and appropriately modify activities.
- Children and adolescents who are overweight or physically inactive may not be able to achieve 60 $min \cdot d^{-1}$ of moderate-to-vigorous intensity PA. These individuals should start with moderate intensity PA as tolerated and gradually increase the frequency and time of PA to achieve the 60-$min \cdot d^{-1}$ goal, and to include vigorous-intensity PA, resistance exercise, and bone loading activity on at least 3$d \cdot wk^{-1}$ [50].
- Children and adolescents should be encouraged to participate in various PAs that are enjoyable and age-appropriate. PA in young children should include

unstructured active play, which typically consists of sporadic bursts of moderate and vigorous-intensity PA, alternating with brief periods of rest. It is important to recognize that these small bouts of PA, however brief, count toward FITT recommendations.

- Children and adolescents with diseases or disabilities such as asthma, diabetes mellitus, obesity, cystic fibrosis, and cerebral palsy should have their exercise prescription tailored to their condition, symptoms, and physical fitness level.
- Efforts should be made to decrease sedentary activities (i.e., television watching, web surfing, and playing video games) and increase activities that promote lifelong activity and fitness (i.e., walking, running, swimming and cycling).

Table 1. A physical activity guide for overweight/obesity in children [50]

Aerobic		Resistance	Flexibility
Frequency	Daily	3d.Wk$^{-1}\geq$	2d.Wk$^{-1}\geq$
Intensity	Moderate to vigorous intensity to increase heart rate.	Use of body weight as resistance or 8-15 repetition.	Stretch to the point of tightness or slight discomfort.
Time	$\geq$ 60min.d^{-1}	$\geq$ 60min.d^{-1}	Hold stretch for 30-60s
Type	Enjoyable and appropriate activities, including running, walking, swimming, bicycling, and sports such as Soccer, Basketball, Badminton or Tennis.	Muscle strengthening physical activities (e.g., playing on playground equipment, climbing trees), lifting weights, exercises with elastic bands, medicine balls and Physioballs.	Any PA that increase flexibility. Using Static and dynamic stretches for each muscle group.

REFERENCES

[1] Cabrera T CI, Oliveira dos Santos D, Pacagnelli F, Prado M, Dias da Silva T, Monteiro C, Fernani D. Analisys of the prevalence of owerwight and obesity and the level of physical activity in chilfren and adolescents of a soudwestern city of São Paulo. *JHGD.* 2014;24(1):66-7.

[2] Saint-Maurice PF, Troiano RP, Berrigan D, Kraus WE, Matthews CE. Volume of light versus moderate-to-vigorous physical activity: similar benefits for all-cause mortality? *Journal of the American Heart Association.* 2018;7(7):e008815.

[3] Ara I, Sanchez-Villegas A, Vicente-Rodriguez G, Moreno L, Leiva M, Martínez-González M, et al. Physical fitness and obesity are associated in a dose-dependent manner in children. *Annals of Nutrition and Metabolism.* 2010;57(3-4):251-9.

[4] Newell KM. Physical Education in Higher Education: Chaos Out of Order. *Quest.* 1990;42(3):227-42.

[5] Pangrazi RP. Promoting physical activity for youth. *Journal of science and medicine in sport.* 2000;3(3):280-6.

[6] Kobel S KS, Dreyhaupt J and Steinacker MJ. Objectively Determined Physical Activity Levels in German Primary School Children after a One Year School-based Health Promoting Intervention. *Journal of Childhood Obesity.* 2017;2(2:8):1-10.

[7] De Meester F, Van Dyck D, De Bourdeaudhuij I, Deforche B, Cardon G. Changes in physical activity during the transition from primary to secondary school in Belgian children: what is the role of the school environment? *BMC public health.* 2014; 14(1):261.

[8] Minasian V, Marandi SM, Kelishadi R, Abolhassani H. Correlation between aerobic fitness and body composition in middle school students. *International journal of preventive medicine.* 2014;5(Suppl 2):S102.

[9] Francesquet M, Silva PTd, Schneiders LdB, Silveira JFdCd, Soares SS, Tornquist D, et al. Youth overweight/obesity and its relationship with cardiovascular disease and parental risk factors. *Archives of endocrinology and metabolism.* 2019;63(4):411-6.

[10] Harrison F VE, Corder K, Jones A. School groundsand physical activity: Associations at secondary schools, and over the transition from primary to secondary schools. *Health & Place.* 2016;39:34-42.

[11] Lubans DR, Morgan PJ, Dewar D, Collins CE, Plotnikoff RC, Okely AD, et al. The Nutrition and Enjoyable Activity for Teen Girls (NEAT girls) randomized controlled trial for adolescent girls from disadvantaged secondary schools: rationale, study protocol, and baseline results. *BMC Public Health.* 2010;10(1):652.

[12] Maher C VR, Okely T, Stanley R, Watson M and Lewis L. Physical activity and screen time in out of school hours care: an observational study. *BMC Pediatrics.* 2019;19(283):2-10.

[13] Burns RD, Pfledderer CD, Brusseau TA. Active Transport, Not Device Use, Associates with Self-Reported School Week Physical Activity in Adolescents. *Behavioral Sciences.* 2019;9(3):32.

[14] Brown V, Moodie M, Mantilla Herrera AM, Veerman JL, Carter R. Active transport and obesity prevention – A transportation sector obesity impact scoping review and assessment for Melbourne, Australia. *Preventive Medicine.* 2017;96:49-66.

[15] Vanwolleghem G, D'Haese S, Van Dyck D, De Bourdeaudhuij I, Cardon G. Intervention study to promote active transport to school in children. *Assessing, understanding and changing active transport in children and adolescents: the role of the physical environment.* 2017;11:205.

[16] O'Neill B, McDonough SM, Wilson JJ, Bradbury I, Hayes K, Kirk A, et al. Comparing accelerometer, pedometer and a questionnaire for measuring physical activity in bronchiectasis: a validity and feasibility study. *Respiratory Research.* 2017;18(1):16.

[17] Zeng N, Gao X, Liu Y, Lee JE, Gao Z. Reliability of using motion sensors to measure children's physical activity levels in exergaming. *Journal of clinical medicine.* 2018;7(5):100.

[18] Kelishadi R, Qorbani M, Djalalinia S, Sheidaei A, Rezaei F, Arefirad T, et al. Physical inactivity and associated factors in Iranian children and adolescents: the Weight Disorders Survey of the CASPIAN-IV study. *Journal of cardiovascular and thoracic research.* 2017;9(1):41.

[19] Brusseau TA, Hannon JC, Fu Y, Fang Y, Nam K, Goodrum S, et al. Trends in physical activity, health-related fitness, and gross motor skills in children during a two-year comprehensive school physical activity program. *Journal of Science and Medicine in Sport.* 2018;21(8):828-32.

[20] Sallis JF, Saelens BE. Assessment of physical activity by self-report: status, limitations, and future directions. *Research quarterly for exercise and sport.* 2000;71(sup2):1-14.

[21] McKenzie TL, Sallis JF, Prochaska JJ, Conway TL, Marshall SJ, Rosengard P. Evaluation of a two-year middle-school physical education intervention: M-SPAN. *Medicine & Science in Sports & Exercise.* 2004;36(8):1382-8.

[22] Plasqui G, Westerterp KR. Physical activity assessment with accelerometers: an evaluation against doubly labeled water. *Obesity.* 2007;15(10):2371-9.

[23] Mitre N, Lanningham-Foster L, Foster R, Levine JA. Pedometer Accuracy in children: Can we recommend them for our obese population? *Int J Ther Rehabil.* 2012;19(7):387-93.

[24] Ayers SF, Sariscsany MJ. Physical education for lifelong fitness: the physical best teacher's guide: *Human Kinetics;* 2011.

[25] Ruch N, Melzer K, Mäder U. Duration, frequency, and types of children's activities: Potential of a classification procedure. *Journal of Exercise Science & Fitness.* 2013;11(2):85-94.

[26] Lu KD, Cooper DM, Haddad F, Radom-Aizik S. Four Months of a School-Based Exercise Program Improved Aerobic Fitness and Clinical Outcomes in a Low-SES Population of Normal Weight and Overweight/Obese Children with Asthma. *Frontiers in pediatrics.* 2018;6:380.

[27] Elnaggar RK, Elshazly FA, Abdelbasset WK, Ahmed AS. Cardiovascular risk profile, oxygen uptake, and perceived exertion rate in children with obesity: the interactive effect of exercise intensity and duration. *Diabetes, metabolic syndrome and obesity: targets and therapy.* 2019;12:527.

[28] Robertson RJ, Goss FL, Andreacci JL, Dube JJ, Rutkoweski JJ, Snee BM, et al. Validation of the children's OMNI RPE scale for stepping exercise. *Medicine & Science in Sports & Exercise.* 2005;37(2):290-8.

[29] Chu KS, Rhodes EC. Physiological and cardiovascular changes associated with deep water running in the young. *Sports Medicine.* 2001;31(1):33-46.

[30] Honorio SAA DMP, Batista M, Serrano J, Miguel Duarte R, Oliveira J, Petrica J. Effects of swimming and water walking on body composition and spirometric values in young children. *Journal of Human Sport & Exercise.* 2019;14(proc1):S47-S58.

[31] Demetriou Y, Reimers AK, Alesi M, Scifo L, Borrego CC, Monteiro D, et al. Effects of school-based interventions on motivation towards physical activity in children and adolescents: protocol for a systematic review. *Systematic Reviews.* 2019;8(1):113.

[32] Alvarez C, Ramírez-Campillo R, Ramírez-Vélez R, Izquierdo M. Effects of 6-Weeks High-Intensity Interval Training in Schoolchildren with Insulin Resistance: Influence of Biological Maturation on Metabolic, Body Composition, Cardiovascular and Performance Non-responses. *Frontiers in Physiology.* 2017;8(444).

[33] Cao M QMaZJ. Effect of High-Intensity Interval Training versus Moderate-Intensity Continuous Training on Cardiorespiratory Fitness in Children and Adolescents: A Meta-Analysis. *Int J Environ Res Public Health.* 2019;16(1533):1-13.

[34] Delgado-Floody P, Latorre-Román P, Jerez-Mayorga D, Caamaño-Navarrete F, García-Pinillos F. Feasibility of incorporating high-intensity interval training into physical education programs to improve body composition and cardiorespiratory capacity of overweight and obese children: A systematic review. *Journal of Exercise Science & Fitness.* 2019;17(2):35-40.

[35] Racil G, Ounis OB, Hammouda O, Kallel A, Zouhal H, Chamari K, et al. Effects of high vs. moderate exercise intensity during interval training on lipids and adiponectin levels in obese young females. *European journal of applied physiology.* 2013; 113(10):2531-40.

[36] Racil G, Zouhal H, Elmontassar W, Abderrahmane AB, De Sousa MV, Chamari K, et al. Plyometric exercise combined with high-intensity interval training improves metabolic abnormalities in young obese females more so than interval training alone. *Applied physiology, nutrition, and metabolism.* 2016;41(1):103-9.

[37] Lambrick D, Westrupp N, Kaufmann S, Stoner L, Faulkner J. The effectiveness of a high-intensity games intervention on improving indices of health in young children. *Journal of sports sciences.* 2016;34(3):190-8.

[38] Boutcher SH. High-intensity intermittent exercise and fat loss. *Journal of obesity.* 2010;2011.

[39] Liu J-X, Zhu L, Deng J-M. The effects of high-intensity interval training versus moderate-intensity continuous training on fat loss and cardiometabolic health in pediatric obesity: A protocol of systematic review and meta-analysis. *Medicine* (Baltimore). 2019;98(10):e14751-e.

[40] Cohen KE, Morgan PJ, Plotnikoff RC, Hulteen RM, Lubans DR. Psychological, social and physical environmental mediators of the SCORES intervention on physical activity among children living in low-income communities. *Psychology of Sport and Exercise.* 2017;32:1-11.

[41] Leahy AA, Eather N, Smith JJ, Hillman C, Morgan PJ, Nilsson M, et al. School-based physical activity intervention for older adolescents: rationale and study protocol for the Burn 2 Learn cluster randomised controlled trial. *BMJ Open.* 2019;9(5):e026029.

[42] Van Dongen BM, Ridder MAM, Steenhuis IHM, Renders CM. Background and evaluation design of a community-based health-promoting school intervention: Fit Lifestyle at School and at Home (FLASH). *BMC public health.* 2019;19(1):784.

[43] González-Cutre D, Sierra AC, Beltrán-Carrillo VJ, Peláez-Pérez M, Cervelló E. A school-based motivational intervention to promote physical activity from a self-determination theory perspective. *The Journal of Educational Research.* 2018; 111(3):320-30.

[44] MacKelvie KJ, Khan KM, Petit MA, Janssen PA, McKay HA. A School-Based Exercise Intervention Elicits Substantial Bone Health Benefits: A 2-Year Randomized Controlled Trial in Girls. *Pediatrics.* 2003;112(6):e447.

[45] Vaquero-Solís M, Gallego DI, Tapia-Serrano MÁ, Pulido JJ, Sánchez-Miguel PA. School-based Physical Activity Interventions in Children and Adolescents: A Systematic Review. *International Journal of Environmental Research and Public Health.* 2020;17(3):999.

[46] Rudisill ME, Johnson JL. Mastery Motivational Climates in Early Childhood Physical Education: What Have We Learned over the Years? *Journal of Physical Education, Recreation & Dance.* 2018;89(6):26-32.

[47] Morgan K. Applying Mastery TARGET Structures to Cooperative Learning in Physical Education. *Journal of Physical Education, Recreation & Dance.* 2019; 90(3):27-32.

[48] Segovia DG, Díaz-del-Campo. Teachers' and students' perceptions of the HIIT application in Physical Education. Sport Education Model vs traditional approach. *ÁGORA para la Educación Física y el Deporte.* 2018;20(2/3):133-61.

[49] Robertson S. *Investigating the Relationship between Teaching Games for Understanding and High School Physical Education Students' Enjoyment, Self-Efficacy, and Intentions to Enroll.* 2016.

[50] Riebe D, Ehrman JK, Liguori G, Magal M, Medicine ACoS. *ACSM's guidelines for exercise testing and prescription*: Wolters Kluwer; 2018.

In: Childhood Obesity
Editor: Roya Kelishadi
ISBN: 978-1-53618-158-6
© 2020 Nova Science Publishers, Inc.

Chapter 16

AN OVERVIEW OF INTERVENTIONS FOR CONTROLLING OBESITY IN PRE-SCHOOL CHILDREN

Golgis Karimi[1], PhD, Seyede Shahrbanoo Daniali[2], PhD and Roya Kelishadi[2,*], MD
[1]Department of Nutritional Sciences & Toxicology, University of California at Berkeley, Berkeley, California
[2]Child Growth and Development Research Center, Research Institute for Primordial Prevention of Non-Communicable Disease, Isfahan University of Medical Sciences, Isfahan, Iran

ABSTRACT

Childhood obesity has increased at an alarming rate worldwide and has become as one of the major public health problems with challenges in its management. The potential origin of obesity is suggested to be in early life, mainly because of a sedentary lifestyle and unhealthy eating. Therefore, interventions used to control obesity in preschoolers mainly targeting mothers during pregnancy, breastfeeding, family education, and preschool programs by focusing on promoting nutrition and physical activity strategies. Various results are reported about the outcomes of these interventions. Some concluded that multidisciplinary and intensive intervention is effective in reducing body fat in preschoolers, while others found that the best approach is lifestyle modification by improving diet quality and physical activity. In addition, some interventions mainly focus on family and home strategies in which parents are considered as the main target for change. In fact, as parents play a crucial role in the establishment of lifestyle, family-based interventions are reported to be successful. Interventions on maternity hospitals by focusing on training breastfeeding did not show considerable effect in preventing obesity. This failure can be due to the lack of focus on social and environmental determinants, or

* Corresponding Author's Email: kelishadi@med.mui.ac.ir; roya.kelishadi@gmail.com.

suboptimal implementation of interventions. Controversy in the results of studies suggests an urgent need to provide successful interventions to control obesity among young children. Therefore, in this chapter, we aim to provide an overview of selected interventions for obesity control in preschool aged children.

Keywords: childhood obesity, preschool age, intervention, prevention

INTRODUCTION

Childhood obesity is one of the most challenging global public health problems in the 21st century. In addition to developed countries, it has increased at an alarming rate in many low- and middle-income countries, particularly in urban areas [1]. The number of overweight or obese infants and young children (aged 0 to 5 years) increased from 32 million globally in 1990 to 41 million in 2016 [2]. It is reported that by such trend, the number of obese infants and young children will increase to 75 million by the year 2025 [3]. The period between age 2 and 6 years is important for the development of excess weight in older ages [4]. Obese children are more likely to have metabolic, cardiovascular, and psychosocial illnesses, e.g., eating disorders, depression, and low self-esteem than their normal-weight counterparts despite being at greater risk of premature illness and mortality in later life [5].

The exact underlying causes of the escalating trend of overweight and obesity are still uncertain; however, as a multifactorial disease, several underlying factors are proposed in this regard. The role of genetic background is notable; some earlier studies indicate that inheritance can explain more than 50% of body weight status (overweight/obesity) incidences [6]. According to the Ecological systems theory (EST), to address and explore the exact underlying mechanisms in developing certain characteristics, the context and situation where an individual situated on in should be considered. EST states that a combination of individuals' characteristics and social environment make the ecological niche. In terms of young children, although the family would be the important parts of the ecological niche, the environment where children live there, as well as child characteristics and child care centers, should be taken into consideration. Therefore, to address the childhood overweight/obesity based on the EST, all the parts of children's ecological niche including their gender, genetics, as well as risk factors including behavioral habits like dietary intakes and dietary patterns, sedentary lifestyle, prolonged screen time, psychosocial aspects, and leisure time activity, as well as the parental behaviors and factors such as stress and anxiety, and siblings interaction should be taken into account [7, 8]. Therefore, to determine the efficacy of interventions for the prevention and management of childhood obesity, all the children's characteristics, risk factors, and parental behaviors and characteristics should be measured [9, 10]. Data show that early childhood obesity tracks into adulthood [3]. Therefore, successful earlier prevention and intervention may potentially be more clinically effective and cost-effective [11]. Therefore, the main objective of this chapter is to identify, synthesize, and evaluate the quality of family-based, school-based, primary care-based, and multi-level multi-component for prevention and control of obesity in preschool-aged children.

METHODS AND MATERIALS

Search Strategy and Selection Criteria

A literature search from inception to January 2020, was conducted using the following databases: MEDLINE (https://www.ncbi.nlm.nih.gov/pubmed/), ScienceDirect (www.sciencedirect.com/science/journals), Embase (https://embase.com/), and Google Scholar (https://scholar.google.com/). The following keywords were used to find relevant articles: "preschool child" OR "children, preschool" OR "preschool children" OR "preschoolers" AND "obesity" OR "body mass index," AND "obesity in childhood," "child obesity," "obesity, child," "childhood obesity," "obesity, childhood," "young-age obesity," AND "school based" OR "school-based" AND "home-based intervention" OR "parental programs" AND "environmental intervention" OR "intervention study."

Table 1. Study selection criteria

	Inclusion criteria	Exclusion criteria
Populations	Healthy children <6 years old	Children with a history of chronic disease, disability or any significant medical condition
Interventions, Policies, or Practices	Any intervention, program or policy aimed at treating or preventing childhood obesity	-
Comparisons	usual care, within the same aged children and in a similar setting	No relevant comparator group
Outcomes	Change in BMI, BMI-z score and other relevant anthropometric measurements	No BMI and anthropometric measurements data

Search results were updated until February 2020, using PubMed's email alert service. Moreover, the reference lists of retrieved articles and reviews were screened to prevent missing any relevant study. We looked for weight management as a primary outcome. Two independent reviewers (GK and SD) screened titles and abstracts of all articles identified by the search strategy, and selected relevant articles according to the inclusion and exclusion criteria, and reviewed by an expert in this field (RK). As presented in Table 1, the inclusion criteria were: 1) the interventional, experimental, and clinical trial studies among children 2) outcomes assessed by anthropometric measures including BMI, waist circumference, skin fold thickness, body fat percentage (BFP), (3) full-text is available.

The studies were excluded if: (1) interventions aimed to treat the obesity complications such as diabetes, 2) interventions involved drug treatments or any clinical operations or treatments (3) the interventions or statistical methods were not described clearly 4) studies were systematic, or protocol or pilot ones, and 5) duration of intervention was less than 12 weeks. Finally, the full texts of relevant articles were assessed.

Data Extraction

Two reviewers (GK and SD) independently extracted the necessary information from the identified eligible studies. In the case of disagreement between reviewers, a consensus was considered with the senior researcher (RK). The following characteristics were extracted from articles: first author, publication year and country, study population, study design, sample size, and the average age of participants, duration and component of the intervention, duration of follow-up, as well as anthropometric components. Studies which reported statistically significant improvement in body mass index (BMI) or BMI-z score between the intervention and control groups were considered as effective.

RESULTS

The search strategy identified 1048 articles and 25 additional ones from reference lists of full texts, of which 50 were duplicates, and 874 were excluded based on titles and abstract reviewing (Figure 1). Of the remaining 149 articles for full-text screening, articles were excluded since anthropometric measurements were not the primary outcome of the study (n=17), or because they were conducted among older school children and adolescents (n=55), or were protocol (n=37) or pilot study (n=9), or duration of intervention was less than 3 months (n=9). Ultimately, 22 articles published since 2000 were included in this systematic review. The majority of the studies used a randomized control trial design. Of the 22 included studies, sixteen were conducted in North America, i.e., US and Canada [12-27], five in Europe [28-32], and one in the Middle-East [33]. The interventions used in the included studies were categorized into four following groups: i) family-based; ii) school-based; iii) primary or clinical-based, and iv) multi-level intervention. Of 22 included studies, six were family-based intervention [12, 19-21, 32, 33], six were school-based intervention [14, 17, 18, 24, 30, 31], two were primary or clinical-based intervention [22, 29], seven consisted of multi-level interventions [15, 16, 23, 26-28, 34], and one study was conducted at both primary or clinical-based alone and multi-level intervention [13]. The findings are presented in Table 2.

Table 2. Characteristics of included studies

Author (year)	Study design	Country	Subjects (n, age)	Intervention type	Intervention duration	Follow-up duration	Primary outcomes	Main findings
Van Grieken et al. (2013), [32]	Cluster RCT	Netherland	Intervention group=349 Control group=288 Mean age=5.7 ± 0.4y	Family-based	2 years	2 years	BMI Waist circumference	-Children with a baseline BMI of 17.25 and 17.50 had a smaller increase in BMI at follow-up compared to control condition (estimated adjusted mean difference 20.67 [se: 0.30] and 20.52 [se: 0.36]). - The mean change in waist circumference from baseline to follow-up was 7.20 [sd: 5.49] centimeter in the intervention condition and 7.33 [sd: 5.30] centimeter in the control condition. -There was no overall difference between intervention and control condition
Taveras et al., 2011 [22]	RCT	USA	Intervention group=1916 Control group=1337 Age=2-6 years	Primary-care based intervention (Multi-component)	1 year	2 years	BMI BMI for age-z score BMI for sex-z score	-Compared with usual care, the intervention group had a smaller, nonsignificant change in BMI (-0.21, 95%CI: -0.5-0.07, p=0.17) -After one year the intervention was not effective in reducing BMI

Table 2. (Continued)

Author (year)	Study design	Country	Subjects (n, age)	Intervention type	Intervention duration	Follow-up duration	Primary outcomes	Main findings
								-In post hoc analyses, the intervention significantly improved BMI among girls and those living in lower-income households.
Quattrin et al., (2012), [12]	RCT	USA	Intervention group=46 Control group=50 2-5 years old	Family-based intervention	Over 6 months	3 and 6 months	BMI z-BMI	-Model-adjusted mean estimates of child %BMI in the intervention were 30.66 ± 9.7, 26.06 ± 9.9, and 24.26 ± 10.1 at baseline, three months, and six months, compared with the control group:30.5±9.3, 28.76 ± 9.4, and 28.36 ± 9.5 respectively. -Children in the intervention group had greater %BMI and z-BMI decreases at 3 and 6 months compared to the control group ($p=0.021$)
Bocca et al., (2014), [28]	RCT	Netherland	Intervention group=40 Control group=35 Age= 3-5 years old	Family-based multidisciplinary intervention	16 weeks	18 and 36 months	Anthropometry Body composition	-The multidisciplinary intervention group showed a greater decrease in BMI-z score: (0.2 ±0.1) and waist circumference-z score (0.3 ± 0.1) than usual care. -After 36 months of follow-up, a significant overall treatment effect of the multidisciplinary intervention program was demonstrated at BMI-z

Author (year)	Study design	Country	Subjects (n, age)	Intervention type	Intervention duration	Follow-up duration	Primary outcomes	Main findings
								(0.28, 95%CI 0.03-0.54), and abdominal subcutaneous fat (0.23, 95% CI 0.01-0.45) compared with the usual care program.
Adamo et al., (2017), [13]	3 arm, cluster-randomized controlled trial	Canada	Childcare intervention group (CC)=59 Childcare and home intervention group (CC +HOM) = 94 Control group (COM) =62 Age=3-5 years old	Childcare intervention alone or in combination with parents (Multi-level based)	6 months	At month 6	Body composition Physical activity	An affordable and easily scalable preschool intervention program delivered in licensed childcare settings, with or without the addition of a parent-driven home physical activity promotion, seems to have no significant effect on physical activity, sedentary time, or body composition BMI Mean (95%CI): CC vs. COM: 0.1(-0.3-0.5, p=0.56) CC+HOM vs. COM: 0 (-0.2-0.2, p=0.87) CC vs. CC+HOM: 0.1(-0.3-0.5, p=0.51)
Buscemi et al., (2015), [14]	RCT	US	N=729 Intervention group=376 Control group=353 Age=3-5 years old	School-based program	14 weeks	1 year	BMI z-BMI	Although baseline parent BMI and child z-BMI were correlated, final path model did not reveal any significant relations between change in parent BMI and child z-BMI from baseline to postintervention or from postintervention to 1-year follow-up.

Table 2. (Continued)

Author (year)	Study design	Country	Subjects (n, age)	Intervention type	Intervention duration	Follow-up duration	Primary outcomes	Main findings
Crespo et al., (2012), [49]	2 × 2 factorial design randomized controlled community trial	US	G1: 198 G2=165 G 3=218 G4=227	Multi-level intervention G1: Family G2: Community G3: G1+G2 G4: Control	1-3 years	1, 2, and 3 years G1:1 year G2, G3, and G4: 3 years	BMI-z score	There were no intervention effects on children's BMI z-score. (family only: p value=0.26, Community only p value=0.92, community and family p value=0.49)
Davis et al., (2016), [16]	RCT	US	Intervention= 500 control= 480 Age: primary population:< 4 years in the fall 2008. -Additional cohorts: a) 4- <6 years in the fall 2008. b) 4- <6 years in the fall of 2009 c) <4 years in the fall of 2009	Multi-level intervention including: Classrooms, teachers and food service training, family, grocery stores, healthcare providers	5 years	For the primary study population: 2 years For additional study populations: 1 year	BMI-z score	-BMI-z increased from baseline by 0.18 ($SE = 0.025$, $p < 0.001$) for children with baseline BMI percentile < 85% but did not increase for children with baseline BMI percentile ≥ 85% (mean = −0.02, $SE = 0.036$, $p = 0.57$). -Change in BMI-z for intervention group with baseline BMI percentile ≥ 85% was 0.03 ($SE = 0.073$, $p = 0.65$) more than in the comparison group. -change for intervention group with baseline BMI percentile < 85% was −0.01 ($SE = 0.049$, $p = 0.83$) was lower than in the comparison group
French et al., (2018), [19]	RCT	US	Intervention=265 Control=269 Age: 2-4 years	Family-based intervention (multi-component including:	18 months	2 and 3 years	Adjusted BMI	- Compared with usual care, the intervention group showed no significant difference in BMI change at 24 (−0.12 kg/m2; 95%CI −0.44, 0.19) or 36 months

Author (year)	Study design	Country	Subjects (n, age)	Intervention type	Intervention duration	Follow-up duration	Primary outcomes	Main findings
				Home visits, telephone check-in, and parenting class)				(–0.19 kg/m2; 95% CI=–0.64, 0.26). -Children with baseline overweight or obesity had lower BMI in the intervention group than those in usual care at 36 months (–0.71 kg/m2; 95% CI= –1.30, –0.12)
Mustila et al., (2018), [29]	Control pragmatic trial	Finland	Intervention group= 71 Control group=76 Age= 2-6 years	Clinical-based intervention (Lifestyle counseling intervention)	6 years	Yearly up to 6 years	BMI SDS	-No significant difference in obesity proportions between the groups at 6 years of age, but the proportion of children with obesity in both groups was high intervention vs. control: 9.9% (95%CI 4.9%-19%, p value=0.7) vs 11.8% (95%CI 6.4%-21%, p value=0.96) The BMI-SDS slopes did not differ significantly between the intervention and the control group (the p-values for linear and quadratic interactions were 0.89 and 0.81)
Niedere et al., (2013), [30]	Cluster randomized controlled single-blinded trial	Switzerland	Intervention group= 342 Control group=310 Age= 5.1 ± 0.7 years	School-based intervention including: Physical activity, nutrition, media use and sleep (collaboration between school and family)	1 year	1 year	BMI	- The intervention effects on adiposity outcomes were modified by BMI-group with a more beneficial effect on waist circumference in OW compared to normal-weight children (P for interaction 0.001), but no significant interactions for BMI

Table 2. (Continued)

Author (year)	Study design	Country	Subjects (n, age)	Intervention type	Intervention duration	Follow-up duration	Primary outcomes	Main findings
								(P for interaction 0.5) and the sum of four SF (P for interaction 0.08) Overweight children had more beneficial effects on waist circumference (p for interaction = 0.001) and all adiposity outcomes (p for interaction 0.03). Average intervention effect sizes for BMI were -0.12, -0.05, -0.26 and -0.02 kg/m^2.
Puder et al., (2011), [31]	Cluster randomized control trial	Switzerland	Intervention group= 342 Control group=310 Age: 5.2 ± 0.6 years old	School-based intervention including: Physical activity, nutrition, media use, and sleep (collaboration between school and family)	1 year	1 year	BMI Aerobic fitness	No significant differences were observed in BMI between intervention and control group (−0.07kg/m2, −0.19 to 0.06; P=0.31). Children in the intervention group had beneficial effects in percentage body fat (−1.1%,−2.0 to−0.2; P=0.02), and waist circumference (−1.0 cm, −1.6 to−0.4; P=0.001).
Paul et al., (2018), [20]	single-center randomized clinical trial	USA	Intervention group=140 Control group= 139 Age=0-3 years	Family-based intervention including feeding, sleep, interactive play, and emotion regulation	3 years	3 years	BMI-z score	At age 3 years, children in the intervention had a lower BMI z-score than control (−0.13 vs. 0.15; absolute difference, −0.28 [95%CI, −0.53to−0.01]; P=0.04).

Author (year)	Study design	Country	Subjects (n, age)	Intervention type	Intervention duration	Follow-up duration	Primary outcomes	Main findings
								Mean BMI percentiles did not differ significantly (47th in the responsive parenting group vs. 54th in the control group; reduction in mean BMI percentiles of 6.9 percentile points [95%CI, −14.5to0.6]; P=.07).
Tucker et al., (2019), [21]	RCT	USA	Intervention group=93 Control group=72 Age= 2-5 years old	Family-based intervention including: Feeding habits and health behaviors	6 months	6 months	BMI-z score $\%BMI_{p95}$	BMI decreased by−0.2 kg/m2 (CI:−0.4,−0.0) (p = 0.028) among participants as a whole, but BMI changes did not differ between groups Overall, BMI z-score decreased, on average, among all patients (mean: −0.09 (CI: −0.17, −0.02)) and among intervention (mean: −0.13 (CI: −0.23, −0.02), but not among control (mean: −0.05 (CI: −0.16, 0.06)). Differences in BMI z-score changes between intervention and control groups were not significant (p = 0.332). %BMIp95 did not significantly change during the intervention (mean: −0.6 (CI:−1.5, 0.4), and%BMIp95 changes did not differ between treatment

Table 2. (Continued)

Author (year)	Study design	Country	Subjects (n, age)	Intervention type	Intervention duration	Follow-up duration	Primary outcomes	Main findings
								(mean: −0.8(CI:−2.1,0.5)) and control groups (mean: −0.3 (CI:−1.6, 1.0)).
Stark et al., (2017), [23]	RCT	USA	Home+ clinic intervention= 47 Parents only=50 Control=54 Age: 2-5 years old	Multi-level intervention including: Clinic and home	6 months	6 months	BMI-z score	Home + clinic intervention group demonstrated a significantly greater decrease in BMI z (mean=−0.32, SD= ±0.33) compared with parents only intervention group (mean=−0.05, SD= ±0.27), $P < .001$, ω2 = 0.74 and compared with control group (mean=−0.13, SD= ±0.31), $p < 0.004$, ω2 = 0.75
Alkon et al., (2014), [27]	RCT	USA	Intervention group=260 Control group=292 Age: 3-5 years old	Multi-level intervention including: Parents and child care	7 months	NA	BMI-z score	Results of HLM by controlling for states, parent education and family poverty showed a significant difference in the mean child-level BMI-z changes between intervention and control group coeff (SE) -0.14(0.06); 95%CI (-0.26, -0.02); t-statistic (df) (-2.54); p=0.02)
Kong et al., (2015), [50]	RCT	USA	Intervention group= 325 Control group=293 Age: 3-5 years old	School-based intervention	14 weeks	1 year	BMI-z score	BMI z-score change in the intervention arm was +0.08 (SE=0.04) and +0.10 (SE=0.04) among controls; however, the between-group difference was not significantly different (−0.01, SE=0.06, p=0.83;

Author (year)	Study design	Country	Subjects (n, age)	Intervention type	Intervention duration	Follow-up duration	Primary outcomes	Main findings
Natale et al., (2017), [24]	RCT	USA	Intervention group=754 Control group= 457 Age: 2-5 years old	School-based intervention	2 years	2 years	BMI percentile (PBMI)	Children in the intervention group had a negative slope (β=-1.95, SE = 0.97, P = .04), indicating that they had less of an increase in PBMI over time than the control group.
Esquivel et al., (2016), [18]	RCT	USA	Intervention group= Control group= Age: 2-5 years old	School-based intervention	7 months	Not stated	BMI-z score	mean BMI *z*-score (z-BMI) increased at postintervention for both intervention (mean = 0.60; standard deviation [SD], 1.16; $n = 114$) and delayed-intervention groups (mean = 0.35; SD, 1.17; $n = 132$), change in z-BMI was not significantly different between the groups ($p = 0.50$; $p = 0.48$).
Fitzgibbon et al., (2006), [17]	RCT	USA	Intervention group=202 Control group=199 Age: 3-5 years old	School-based intervention	14 weeks	1 and 2 years	BMI and BMI-z score	Post-intervention changes in BMI and BMI *z* score were not significantly different between intervention and control groups (0.11 vs. 0.13 kg/m2, *p* _ 0.89 for BMI; and 0.07 vs. 0.05, *p* _ 0.85 for BMI *z* score).
Woo et al., (2017), [26]	Quasi-experimental trial	USA	Intervention group 1= 198 Intervention group 2 (healthcare+ schools) =637 Control group=626 Age: 2-4 years old	Multi-level intervention including: Families, health cares, schools	2 years	At least 6 months	BMI- z score	Results of multivariate linear mixed models did not show any significant differences in BMI-z score between intervention groups and comparison one. (20.02 units/y, [95% CI: 20.11 to 20.07], P=0.61; and 20.05 [20.11 to 20.07], P=0.09.

Table 2. (Continued)

Author (year)	Study design	Country	Subjects (n, age)	Intervention type	Intervention duration	Follow-up duration	Primary outcomes	Main findings
								In sensitivity analyses excluding Asian children, a small decline was observed in BMI z score (20.08 units/y [95% confidence interval: 20.14 to 20.02], P=0.01) in intervention group 2 versus comparison.
Kelishadi et al., (2009), [33]	Randomized clinical trial	Iran	Intervention group1 (dairy rich diet DR) = 40 Intervention group 2 (Energy restricted diet ER)=40 Control group=40 Age: 5-6 years old	Family-based intervention	6 months	3 years	BMI-SDS Waist circumference	BMI-SDS and WC declined significantly in all participants. 3 years later, mean WC increased less in DR group and body fat percentage had a significant decrement in all groups but kept on lower than the baseline measurements

G1= group1, G2=group2, G3=group3, G4=group4, HLM: hierarchical linear model, WC: waist circumference, RCT: randomized controlled trial, OW: overweight.

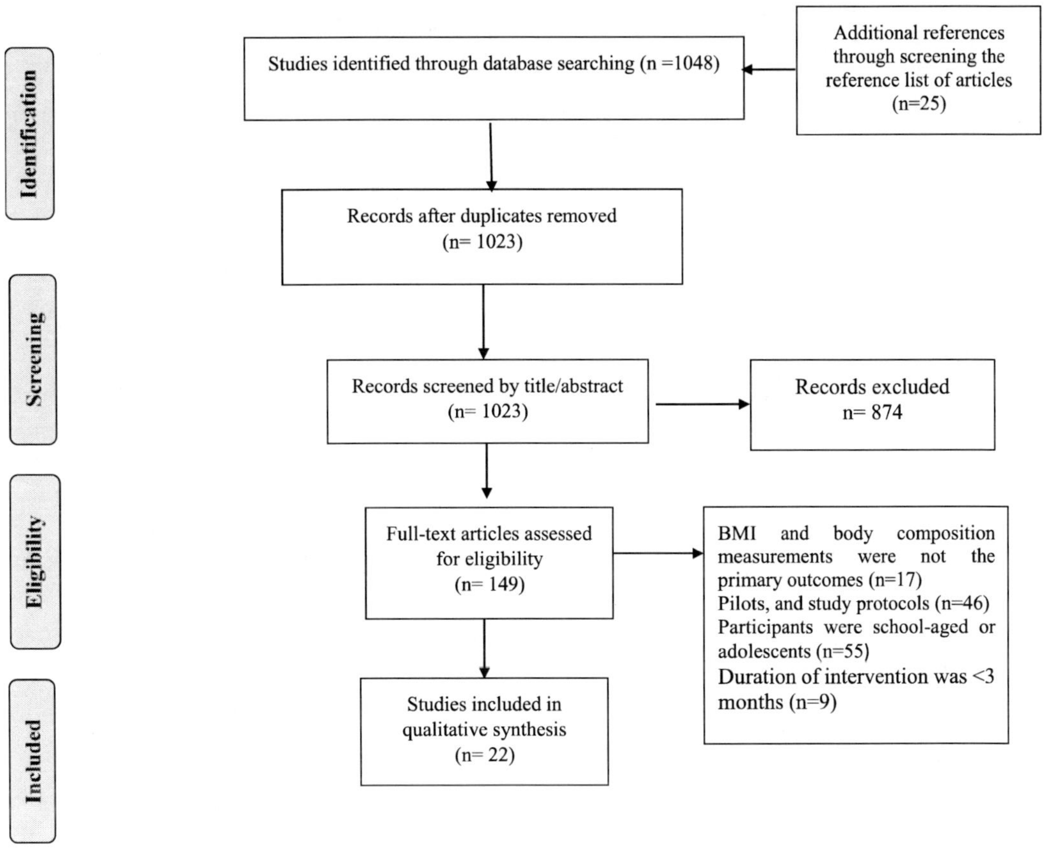

Figure 1. Flow diagram of the study.

DISCUSSION

Family-Based Intervention Studies

One of the most applicable targets for health intervention studies is family. Children in particular preschoolers spend a large number of hours at home with their parents. In fact, children will not reach a healthy weight and lifestyle habits unless their supporters, i.e., parents would provide them healthy behavior choices. According to the literature, one of the most successful ways for prevention and control of childhood obesity is the family-based intervention. In the current review, five out of seven family-based intervention studies showed a positive effect of this kind of intervention in reducing either BMI or BMI-z score of children or both [12, 19, 20, 28, 33] in comparison with control groups. Although two studies did not show significant usefulness of this kind of intervention on improving child's weight status [21, 32], they reported that the obesogenic behaviors of family, as well as the parents' feeding habits and children screen time were significantly improved at the end of the intervention compared to the baseline. An inverse association was reported between screen time and adiposity, which suggests that the screen time of preschoolers is a predictor for their current and future BMI [35-38]. Moreover, family nutrition and physical activity (FNPA) are associated with BMI, which means that by improving the FNPA score, health behaviors would improve, and if this improvement is maintained, it would result in a reduction of adiposity [21, 39]. Another possible explanation for non-significant results of these studies can be because the researchers could not motivate parents enough to participate in interventional sessions. In fact, it is so hard for parents to admit that their children have excess weight and following the new lifestyle and dietary patterns would not have adverse effects on their children's health and growth [40, 41]. According to the results of the current review and earlier literature, it seems that as parents construct their children's lifestyle behavior and are role models for their children, they have the most important role in their children's health, including their weight status. Therefore, more focus on programs involving families can be an effective way to control and treat overweight/obesity in children. In addition, starting these interventions for younger age children is more beneficial as they are still under the control of their parents and do not become independent in choosing their lifestyle. Some of the limitations for family-based intervention studies that should be taken into account by future studies are the high rate of drop-out because of weak motivation families in participating, the small sample size of participants in studies, and lack of long-term follow-up data.

School or Childcare Center-Based Intervention Studies

Although it seems that intervention through childcare centers can be effective because children spend a bulk of their waking time in such places, in the current review four studies that were conducted in childcare centers did not show any significant effect on BMI changes of overweight/obese children at post-intervention or follow-up [14, 17, 18, 31]. There are several factors that may influence these insignificant findings. First, each component of the program such as parental, or teachers may not have been intensive enough. As addressed in this review and some earlier studies, researches that mainly focus on familial factors related to weight status including dietary habits and physical activity underscored the importance of parents' involvement and addressing the family environment in interventions for obesity of young children. Another possible factor that should be considered is the ethnicity of the participants. Results of a study found that Mexican-American children compared to Anglo-Americans spent less time outdoors and made fewer requests for activity, and received fewer prompts from parents. They also report that scores of familial recreations in Mexican-American families were lower than Anglo-American ones. Given that, the more parents are active, the more children have a healthy weight. Besides, ethnic foods and cultural eating habits are other factors that may affect the results of an intervention [42]. Overall, cultural differences may affect the efficacy of health risk reduction programs [43-45]. On top of this, in the current review, studies that show the positive effect of a school-based intervention on body weight management of children had been lasted for at least 1 year while those with no significant effect were less than a year. Therefore, the duration of the intervention is another plausible factor that should be considered in this regard.

Primary or Clinical-Based Intervention Studies

All three included studies in this systematic review did not show any significant effect of the primary care-based intervention on reducing BMI-z score among preschoolers [13, 22, 29]. One of the studies focused on maternity care and prenatal intervention, including nutrition and physical activity for pregnant mothers at risk of gestational diabetes mellitus (GDM). After six years of follow-up, no significant change was observed in overweight/obesity proportions in children of the trial group as compared to the controls. This finding can be because the power of the study resulted into failure to identify differences between groups [29]. Results of a physical activity intervention program showed a significant effect neither on BMI changes of children, nor on their sedentary and physical activity level. Thus, it suggested that physical activity interventions do not have measurable effects on the body composition of preschoolers. They also report that the involvement of parents as a part of intervention makes better results in terms of children's physical activity because parents influence the health habits of young children [13]. A randomized controlled trial at primary-care settings worked on multiple components, including nutrition, physical activity, and screen time. However, it did not find any significant effect of this intervention because of various factors. First, being in the primary-care setting and not involving the children's communities or environment seems to be not effective in changing BMI while it can complement and enhance more comprehensive efforts in multiple settings. Second, low adherence to intervention activities should be considered; it seems that the "dose" of the intervention was not sufficient to make a change in BMI. Third, they provide parents a choice of behaviors to work on in a non-representative way, and this can be one of the possible reasons that parents selected the method that was less effective in BMI changes. Fourth, maybe the effectiveness was lagged behind the behavioral changes, so they need to follow-up for a longer period of time.

Multi-Level Intervention Studies

At the multi-level intervention, of six included studies, four showed that intensive behavioral treatment is necessary and effective in controlling excess weight among preschoolers [16, 23, 26, 27]. Results of these studies are in line with earlier ones at primary-care and school-based level, which found that just motivating parents to change their children dietary habits is not sufficient to overcome the barriers parents face in terms of child behaviors to effectively implement dietary changes [13, 17, 22, 31]. Principally, for prevention and control of childhood obesity, multi-level multi-component interventions providing all aspects of physical activity, nutrition, educating, counseling and motivation programs together at school, home, and clinics setting are more effective than single-component or community-based ones; besides, their results are lasting for a longer period of time [34, 46-48]. Two studies did not show efficacy of the multi-level intervention on reducing BMI or BMI-z score of children. This can be because of different factors such as differences in race/ethnicity of participants or heterogeneity of their BMI at baseline. They reported an improvement in the behavior of intervention groups, including their dietary patterns in terms of consuming less sugar-sweetened beverages, and more fruits and vegetables, as well as physical activity and screen time. These results suggest that multi-level multi-component interventions can positively influence the behavior of children, therefore, in order to assess such effects on BMI and body fat, longer and more intense interventions are needed [13, 15].

Conclusion

Results of the current systematic review show that changes in dietary intake and physical activity for prevention and control of obesity in preschoolers are necessary but not enough. The best result reached out by training parents about the skills of child behavior management. Targeting parent motivation or overcoming ambivalence about dietary changes is not sufficient in this regard. Controlling the obesogenic factors at home appears to be an effective way to assist parents in the acquisition and generalization of these skills as they provide an opportunity for in-vivo practice of these skills with long-term supervision and modeling.

References

[1] Organization WH. *Global Strategy on Diet, Physical Activity and Health, Childhood overweight and obesity.*

[2] Orgaziation WH. *Commission on Ending Childhood Obesity, Facts and figures on childhood obesity.*

[3] Wen LM, Rissel C, He G. The effect of early life factors and early interventions on childhood overweight and obesity 2016. *Journal of obesity.* 2017;2017.

[4] De Kroon ML, Renders CM, Van Wouwe JP, Van Buuren S, Hirasing RA. The Terneuzen birth cohort: BMI changes between 2 and 6 years correlate strongest with adult overweight. *PloS one.* 2010;5(2):e9155.

[5] Hamid MSA, Sazlina SG. Interventions for obesity among schoolchildren: A systematic review and meta-analyses. *PloS one.* 2019;14(1):e0209746.

[6] Wardle J, Carnell S, Haworth CM, Plomin R. Evidence for a strong genetic influence on childhood adiposity despite the force of the obesogenic environment. *The American journal of clinical nutrition.* 2008;87(2):398-404.

[7] Davison KK, Birch LL. Childhood overweight: a contextual model and recommendations for future research. *Obesity reviews.* 2001;2(3):159-71.

[8] Koch FS. *Stress and obesity in childhood*: Linköping University Electronic Press; 2009.

[9] Önnerfält J, Erlandsson LK, Orban K, Broberg M, Helgason C, Thorngren-Jerneck K. A family-based intervention targeting parents of preschool children with overweight and obesity: conceptual framework and study design of LOOPS-Lund overweight and obesity preschool study. *BMC public health.* 2012;12(1):879.

[10] Khashayar P, Kasaeian A, Heshmat R, Motlagh ME, Mahdavi Gorabi A, Noroozi M, et al. Childhood overweight and obesity and associated factors in iranian children and adolescents: A multi-level analysis; the CASPIAN-IV study. *Frontiers in pediatrics.* 2018;6:393.

[11] Foster BA, Farragher J, Parker P, Sosa ET. Treatment interventions for early childhood obesity: a systematic review. *Academic pediatrics.* 2015;15(4):353-61.

[12] Quattrin T, Roemmich JN, Paluch R, Yu J, Epstein LH, Ecker MA. Efficacy of family-based weight control program for preschool children in primary care. *Pediatrics.* 2012;130(4):660-6.

[13] Adamo KB, Wasenius NS, Grattan KP, Harvey ALJ, Naylor PJ, Barrowman NJ, et al. Effects of a Preschool Intervention on Physical Activity and Body Composition. *J Pediatr.* 2017;188:42-9.e2.

[14] Buscemi J, Berlin KS, Rybak TM, Schiffer LA, Kong A, Stolley MR, et al. Health Behavior and Weight Changes Among Ethnic and Racial Minority Preschoolers and Their Parents: Associations Across 1 Year. *J Pediatr Psychol.* 2016;41(7):777-85.

[15] Crespo NC, Elder JP, Ayala GX, Slymen DJ, Campbell NR, Sallis JF, et al. Results of a multi-level intervention to prevent and control childhood obesity among Latino children: the Aventuras Para Ninos Study. *Ann Behav Med.* 2012;43(1):84-100.

[16] Davis SM, Myers OB, Cruz TH, Morshed AB, Canaca GF, Keane PC, et al. CHILE: Outcomes of a group randomized controlled trial of an intervention to prevent obesity

in preschool Hispanic and American Indian children. *Preventive medicine.* 2016; 89:162-8.

[17] Fitzgibbon ML, Stolley MR, Schiffer L, Van Horn L, KauferChristoffel K, Dyer A. Hip-hop to health Jr. for Latino preschool children. *Obesity.* 2006;14(9):1616-25.

[18] Esquivel M, Nigg CR, Fialkowski MK, Braun KL, Li F, Novotny R. Head Start wellness policy intervention in Hawaii: a project of the children's healthy living program. *Childhood Obesity.* 2016;12(1):26-32.

[19] French SA, Sherwood NE, Veblen-Mortenson S, Crain AL, JaKa MM, Mitchell NR, et al. Multi-component obesity prevention intervention in low-income preschoolers: primary and subgroup analyses of the NET-Works randomized clinical trial, 2012–2017. *American journal of public health.* 2018;108(12):1695-706.

[20] Paul IM, Savage JS, Anzman-Frasca S, Marini ME, Beiler JS, Hess LB, et al. Effect of a Responsive Parenting Educational Intervention on Childhood Weight Outcomes at 3 Years of Age: The INSIGHT Randomized Clinical Trial. *Jama.* 2018; 320(5):461-8.

[21] Tucker JM, DeFrang R, Orth J, Wakefield S, Howard K. Evaluation of a Primary Care Weight Management Program in Children Aged 2(-)5 years: Changes in Feeding Practices, Health Behaviors, and Body Mass Index. *Nutrients.* 2019;11(3).

[22] Taveras EM, Gortmaker SL, Hohman KH, Horan CM, Kleinman KP, Mitchell K, et al. Randomized controlled trial to improve primary care to prevent and manage childhood obesity: the High Five for Kids study. *Arch Pediatr Adolesc Med.* 2011;165(8):714-22.

[23] Stark LJ, Spear Filigno S, Bolling C, Ratcliff MB, Kichler JC, Robson SM, et al. Clinic and Home-Based Behavioral Intervention for Obesity in Preschoolers: A Randomized Trial. *J Pediatr.* 2018;192:115-21.e1.

[24] Natale RA, Messiah SE, Asfour LS, Uhlhorn SB, Englebert NE, Arheart KL. Obesity prevention program in childcare centers: two-year follow-up. *American Journal of Health Promotion.* 2017;31(6):502-10.

[25] Kong A, Buscemi J, Stolley MR. Hip-Hop to Health Jr. Randomized Effectiveness Trial. *American journal of preventive medicine.* 2015.

[26] Woo Baidal JA, Nelson CC, Perkins M, Colchamiro R, Leung-Strle P, Kwass JA, et al. Childhood obesity prevention in the Women, Infants, and Children Program: outcomes of the MA-CORD study. *Obesity.* 2017;25(7):1167-74.

[27] Alkon A, Crowley AA, Neelon SEB, Hill S, Pan Y, Nguyen V, et al. Nutrition and physical activity randomized control trial in child care centers improves knowledge, policies, and children's body mass index. *BMC Public Health.* 2014;14(1):215.

[28] Bocca G, Corpeleijn E, van den Heuvel ER, Stolk RP, Sauer PJ. Three-year follow-up of 3-year-old to 5-year-old children after participation in a multidisciplinary or a usual-care obesity treatment program. *Clinical nutrition.* 2014;33(6):1095-100.

[29] Mustila T, Raitanen J, Keskinen P, Luoto R. A pragmatic controlled trial to prevent childhood obesity within a risk group at maternity and child health-care clinics: results up to six years of age (the VACOPP study). *BMC Pediatr.* 2018;18(1):89.

[30] Niederer I, Burgi F, Ebenegger V, Marques-Vidal P, Schindler C, Nydegger A, et al. Effects of a lifestyle intervention on adiposity and fitness in overweight or low fit preschoolers (Ballabeina). *Obesity* (Silver Spring). 2013;21(3):E287-93.

[31] Puder JJ, Marques-Vidal P, Schindler C, Zahner L, Niederer I, Burgi F, et al. Effect of multidimensional lifestyle intervention on fitness and adiposity in predominantly migrant preschool children (Ballabeina): cluster randomised controlled trial. *Bmj.* 2011;343:d6195.

[32] van Grieken A, Veldhuis L, Renders CM, Borsboom GJ, van der Wouden JC, Hirasing RA, et al. Population-based childhood overweight prevention: outcomes of the 'Be active, eat right' study. *PloS one.* 2013;8(5):e65376.

[33] Kelishadi R, Zemel MB, Hashemipour M, Hosseini M, Mohammadifard N, Poursafa P. Can a dairy-rich diet be effective in long-term weight control of young children? *Journal of the American College of Nutrition.* 2009;28(5):601-10.

[34] Hu Y, He JR, Liu FH, Li WD, Lu JH, Xing YF, et al. Effectiveness of a Kindergarten-Based Intervention for Preventing Childhood Obesity. *Pediatrics.* 2017;140(6).

[35] Ariza AJ, Chen EH, Binns HJ, Christoffel KK. Risk factors for overweight in five-to six-year-old Hispanic-American children: a pilot study. *Journal of Urban Health.* 2004;81(1):150-61.

[36] Müller MJ, Koertzinger I, Mast M, Langnäse K, Grund A. Physical activity and diet in 5 to 7 years old children. *Public Health Nutrition.* 1999;2(3a):443-4.

[37] Jago R, Baranowski T, Baranowski JC, Thompson D, Greaves K. BMI from 3–6 y of age is predicted by TV viewing and physical activity, not diet. *International journal of obesity.* 2005;29(6):557-64.

[38] Janz KF, Burns TL, Levy SM. Tracking of activity and sedentary behaviors in childhood: the Iowa Bone Development Study. *American journal of preventive medicine.* 2005;29(3):171-8.

[39] Tucker JM, Howard K, Guseman EH, Yee KE, Saturley H, Eisenmann JC. Association between the Family Nutrition and Physical Activity Screening Tool and obesity severity in youth referred to weight management. *Obesity research & clinical practice.* 2017;11(3):268-75.

[40] Warschburger P, Kröller K. Childhood overweight and obesity: maternal perceptions of the time for engaging in child weight management. *BMC Public Health.* 2012;12(1):295.

[41] Kelishadi R, Azizi-Soleiman F. Controlling childhood obesity: A systematic review on strategies and challenges. *Journal of research in medical sciences: the official journal of Isfahan University of Medical Sciences.* 2014;19(10):993.

[42] Sallis JF, Nader PR, Broyles SL, Berry CC, Elder JP, McKenzie TL, et al. Correlates of physical activity at home in Mexican-American and Anglo-American preschool children. *Health psychology.* 1993;12(5):390.

[43] Flores R. Dance for health: improving fitness in African American and Hispanic adolescents. *Public health reports.* 1995;110(2):189.

[44] Kumanyika SK. Special issues regarding obesity in minority populations. *Annals of Internal Medicine.* 1993;119(7_Part_2):650-4.

[45] Stevens J, Kumanyika SK, Keil JE. Attitudes toward body size and dieting: differences between elderly black and white women. *American journal of public health.* 1994;84(8):1322-5.

[46] Bluford DA, Sherry B, Scanlon KS. Interventions to prevent or treat obesity in preschool children: a review of evaluated programs. *Obesity.* 2007;15(6):1356-72.

[47] Khambalia A, Dickinson S, Hardy L, Gill Ta, Baur L. A synthesis of existing systematic reviews and meta-analyses of school-based behavioural interventions for controlling and preventing obesity. *Obesity Reviews.* 2012;13(3):214-33.

[48] De Bourdeaudhuij I, Van Cauwenberghe E, Spittaels H, Oppert JM, Rostami C, Brug J, et al. School-based interventions promoting both physical activity and healthy eating in Europe: a systematic review within the HOPE project. *Obesity Reviews.* 2011;12(3):205-16.

[49] Crespo NC, Elder JP, Ayala GX, Slymen DJ, Campbell NR, Sallis JF, et al. Results of a multi-level intervention to prevent and control childhood obesity among Latino children: the Aventuras Para Niños Study. *Annals of Behavioral Medicine.* 2012; 43(1):84-100.

[50] Fitzgibbon ML, Stolley MR, Schiffer LA, Braunschweig CL, Gomez SL, Van Horn L, et al. Hip-Hop to Health Jr. Obesity Prevention Effectiveness Trial: postintervention results. *Obesity (Silver Spring).* 2011;19(5):994-1003.

In: Childhood Obesity
Editor: Roya Kelishadi

ISBN: 978-1-53618-158-6
© 2020 Nova Science Publishers, Inc.

Chapter 17

EFFECT OF SCHOOL PROGRAMS FOR HEALTHY EATING AND ACTIVE LIVING TO PREVENT CHILDHOOD OBESITY

Behnaz Abiri[1]***, PhD and Mohammadreza Vafa***[2,*]
[1]Department of Nutrition, Faculty of Paramedicine,
Ahvaz Jundishapur University of Medical Sciences, Ahvaz, Iran
[2]Department of Nutrition, School of Public Health,
Iran University of Medical Sciences, Tehran, Iran

ABSTRACT

Childhood obesity has emerged as a serious public health concern all over the world. The increasing prevalence of childhood obesity is related to emergence of comorbidities including type 2 diabetes mellitus, hypertension, cancers, nonalcoholic fatty liver disease, obstructive sleep apnea, and dyslipidemia. Furthermore, obesity in childhood is known to be an independent risk factor for adult obesity. Inadequate physical activity and unhealthy nutrition due to the consumption of calorie-dense foods are established as primary mechanisms underlying the increase in excess body weight. Hence, physical activity and healthy eating are the primary emphasis of health promotion initiatives aimed at preventing or decreasing childhood obesity. The impacts of childhood obesity on morbidity and mortality, demonstrate that effectual prevention or treatment during childhood, are likely to have an important influence on immediate health, as well as adult diseases. In contrast to clinical interventions, school programs can be provided at little or no cost to families and can reach low income children who otherwise may not receive treatment. There is some evidence demonstrating school-based obesity prevention programs can elevate physical activity and ameliorate dietary habits. Such interventions also ameliorate weight state when implemented for long times. The school cafe can provide an environment where

* Corresponing Author's Email: vafa.m@iums.ac.ir.

children are exposed to and learn healthy eating patterns. Schools also have other resources, including equipment and outdoor playing fields, and physical education programs. The combination of classroom health education, physical education programs, and food service, make schools a practical and appropriate setting for providing obesity interventions in a cost-effective manner. As a whole, school based obesity prevention interventions that involve both nutrition and physical activity seem more beneficial than single component programs. This review summarizes the effects of school-based programs on childhood obesity.

Keywords: school programs, childhood obesity, physical activity, healthy eating

INTRODUCTION

Childhood obesity has emerged as one of the most important public health issues all over the world [1]. Excess body weight has a negative influence on self-esteem and leads to a wide range of comorbidities, including cardiovascular disease, hypertension, type 2 diabetes mellitus, and several cancers, that result in decreased quality of life and life expectancy and account for billions of dollars in health care system spending [2-7]. Moreover, obesity in childhood follows into adulthood, especially in those with severe obesity and/or a strong family history of obesity [8, 9]. Hence, it would appear that small reducing in childhood obesity prevalence leads to large costs savings at the population level, and hence school programs and other interventions that can more reduce overweight prevalence rates will further result to program efficacy and cost savings.

Inadequate physical activity and poor nutrition due to the intake of calorie-dense foods are established as primary mechanisms underlying the increase in excess body weight [10]. Physical activity and diet are therefore the primary emphasis of health promotion initiatives aimed at preventing or decreasing childhood overweight and obesity [10].

The influences of childhood obesity on morbidity and mortality, demonstrate that effective prevention and treatment throughout childhood, are probably to have a significant influence on immediate health status, as well as adult diseases [11]. In addition, due to the refractory nature of obesity, preventing childhood obesity, may be an effectual way to prevent adult obesity [12]. Most obesity interventions have occurred in clinical settings, however schools can provide an excellent chance for preventing and treating obesity. In contrast to clinical interventions, school programs can be provided at little or no cost to families and can reach children with low income families who otherwise may not receive treatment program. Because children eat one or two meals per day in school, the school cafe can provide a natural environment where children are exposed to and learn healthy eating patterns [13]. Schools also have other important resources, including gyms, apparatus and outdoor playing fields, and physical education programs. The combination of classroom health education, physical education programs, food service and health services, as well as qualified personnel, make schools a practicable forum for providing obesity prevention and treatment programs in a cost-effective manner.

The Centers for Disease Control and Prevention (CDC) has published guidelines for school programs aimed at elevating physical activity and healthy eating [14, 15]. The CDC guidelines for healthy eating programs consist of recommendations regarding school policies, curriculums, instructions for students, integration of school food services and nutrition education, staff training, family and community involvement, and program assessment [14]. However, school programs differ substantially as a result of differences in content, community involvement, financial support, and delivery. Hence, the efficacy of such programs differs and is not well established at present [16, 17]. To support evidence-based health policies elevating broader implementation of successful programs, it is important to establish the efficacy of school programs. This chapter reviews the research on school-based interventions to prevent or treat obesity.

Etiology of Childhood Obesity

Childhood obesity is the result of an interaction between a complex set of factors that are associated to the environment, genetics, and ecological impacts including the family, community, and school.

Environmental Factors for Childhood Obesity

The etiological factors for childhood obesity are very complex [18]. Psychosocial and emotional distress lead to surplus weight gain in children through maladaptive coping strategies such as eating to suppress negative emotions, appetite up-regulation, and low-grade inflammation [18, 19]. Eating behaviors in children and risk of childhood obesity have been demonstrated to be related to parental feeding styles, stress, and depression [20]. Other important proposed influences include perinatal factors [21], birth size [22], catch-up growth [23], breast-feeding state [24], antibiotic use [25], environmental chemicals [26], microbiota [27], and unfavorable life experiences [28].

Numerous factors in the present "obesogenic" environment have resulted in elevated calorie intake, such as increasing consumption of sugar-sweetened beverages, sweet snacks, fast foods containing excess fat, large portion sizes, and high glycemic foods [29-32]. Intake of sugar-sweetened beverages has been suggested as an important contributor to the development of obesity in childhood [33]. In nationally representative surveys of children in the United States, sugar-sweetened beverages provided an average of 270 kcal/day, representing 10-15% of the total calorie intake [32]. Fast food consumption has also been claimed to contribute to the rising prevalence of obesity [34].

The alterations in the environment leading to elevated calorie intake have been accompanied by factors predisposing to reduced calorie expenditure such as decreased levels of physical activity and elevating time spent in sedentary activities such as using computers, tablets, television, and phones [35, 36]. The amount of time spent watching television and the presence of a television in a child's bedroom have been reported to be directly associated with the prevalence of obesity in children and adolescents [37, 38]. This relationship can be justified by numerous potential mechanisms such as displacement of physical activity and unfavorable impacts on the quality and quantity of foods consumed [39, 40]. The use of electronic games has also been related to obesity throughout childhood [41]. Since children spend a considerable amount of time and consume a substantial proportion of their daily calories at school, the school environment has an impact on the development of childhood obesity [42].

School-Based Obesity Prevention Programs

School-based obesity prevention programs encompass educational, environmental, and behavioral activities and typically address both physical activity and healthy nutrition before, during, or after school. School-based interventions typically include healthy living and nutrition education classes, enhanced physical education and elevated physical activity opportunities, school-wide promotion of healthy food options and food environment ameliorations, capacity building and professional support for teachers and staff, and family education and support. Specific components may differ by program [43, 44].

A Comprehensive Model for Obesity Prevention and Treatment

Two key interventions for preventing or treating obesity are, increasing physical activity and consuming a healthy, lower fat and calorie diet. Within schools, attempts to elevate physical activity and healthy eating between students, should be part of a coordinated, comprehensive program for school health. The comprehensive health program model for schools, developed by Allensworth and Kolbe [45], includes eight interacting components: school health instruction, school-health services, school-health environment, school food service, school-site health promotion programs for staff, school counseling and psychology programs, school physical education, and integrated and connected community and school health-promotion attempts. Implications of the model for obesity prevention and treatment are discussed below.

Health Instruction

The primary aim of health instruction for obesity prevention should be to help children and adolescents adopt healthy eating behaviors and participate in regular physical activity. Foci should be on helping students develop the knowledge, attitudes and behavioral skills they require, to construct and maintain healthy eating and a physically active lifestyle [46, 47]. Important learning concepts consist of the physical, social and mental health advantageous of physical activity and healthy eating, social impacts on eating and physical activity, components of health-associated fitness and a healthful diet, portion-size estimation, healthy and safe weight management strategies, and the development of safe and effectual individualized physical activity programs. Students should also be taught how to apply behavioral skills, such as how to evaluate and monitor diet and exercise behaviors, how to set aims for alteration, and techniques for initiating and maintaining behavior alteration [48]. Characteristics of teaching methods found to be most effectual in school health education instruction include, use of discovery learning, use of student learning stations, cooperative groups, situation analysis, cross-age and peer teaching, use of personal commitment to alter and goal setting, and provision of opportunities to elevate self-efficacy in modifying health behaviors [49]. Teacher training is required on the key eating and physical activity concepts, and active learning and behavior change strategies. Teacher training is probably to result in promoted time spent on teaching nutrition and physical activity in the class [46].

Health Services

School health services for obesity prevention and treatment, potentially consist of screening for overweight, preventive counseling, weight management evaluations and treatment or referral. The school nurse could serve as a central figure to organize programs in the school, and serve as the link with the child's family and health care providers. Schools that have school-based clinics or school-linked health centers, may have access to a multi-disciplinary team that could provide services to overweight students and also provide preventive counseling services. However, the reality is that few schools have the personnel to carry out such interventions [50].

School Food Service

In 1993, the National School Nutrition Dietary Assessment Study [51] reported that school lunches were high in fat, with the average percentage of calories from fat being 38%, compared with the recommended aim of 30%. In addition, only 1% of schools provided lunches with an average of 30% calories from fat. This study, coupled with research on the association between diet and chronic disease risk, spurred drastic alterations in the national school meal program. In 1994, the US Congress passed legislation [52], which needed that meals served through the National School Lunch Program and National School Breakfast Program, adhere to the Dietary Guidelines for Americans [53]. Hence, meals provided through these programs are needed to meet the guidelines for fat and saturated fat.

Nutrition Environment

The school environment offers several food and nutrition activities, experiences and exposures. These involve not only school meals and classroom curricula, but also food sold in school stores and snack bars, fund-raising events, classroom snacks and parties, use of food to reward or discipline, corporate-sponsored nutrition education materials, and in-school advertising of food products. Wolfe and Campbell [54] reported that the nutrition and food experiences offered in schools are fragmented, multi-component and often un-planned, with numerous people involved in decisions about them. The result can be discrepant nutritional messages and messages that are in direct conflict with the aims of healthy eating.

School Physical Education

Physical activity and nutrition must be integrally connected to achieve and maintain healthy weights. Physical education classes could be a major resource for elevating energy expenditure in students, as well as creating expectations and social norms for prevalent and regular physical activity [48]. Concern has been revealed about the quality and quantity of physical education in schools [47]. While progress is slowly changing the focus of physical education away from sports and athletic ability, toward the aim of health-associated fitness, relatively little time is devoted to moderate or vigorous physical activity.

Children and adolescents, who are overweight or obese, may require instruction and programs in which they can develop motor skills, ameliorates fitness and experience enjoyment and success. Young people who are obese or who have other disorders are often clearly or unintentionally discouraged from participating in regular physical activity [47].

By providing modified physical activity programs and extracurricular sports programs, schools can help these young students obtain the benefits and delights of physical activity. Research is required to show the impacts of intensive activity physical education programs on body fat percentage and the weight state [48].

School Worksite Health Promotion

A 1992 USDA national survey of worksite health promotion activities, reported that 78% of large worksites (with more than 750 employees) and 22% of small worksites (with 50 ± 100 employees) provided nutrition education [55]. Almost 24% of worksites provided weight control programs. The literature on school-based worksite interventions for school personnel is scant [55]. A health promotion program for school staff that includes healthy eating, engaging in physical activity and weight management strategies, may have numerous advantageous.

School Commitment and Support

The development of effectual comprehensive school-based programs for prevention and treatment of obesity needs administrative support and commitment, at the school site and at the district level. Price et al. [56] reported a relatively low level of interest among elementary school principals, with only 28% strongly consenting to the statement that schools would be an ideal environment to prevent weight problems between children and 35% strongly consenting to that schools are not doing enough to help improve childhood obesity. However, in another survey [57] of administrators and school nurses in Minnesota, 66% of the administrators and 82% of the school nurses demonstrated that they felt it was the role of the school to offer weight management services. Barriers to providing school-based weight management education and services recognized by the nurses were: lack of time, lack of training, lack of education materials and lack of administrative support. The top barriers recognized by administrators were lack of trained personnel, lack of equipment, lack of budget, lack of classroom time, and lack of staff time. This study affirms there are multiple barriers to developing and implementing obesity prevention and intervention programs.

Integrated Community and School Attempts

The successfulness of obesity interventions, is dependent to the degree to which the intervention incorporates different individuals in the child's environment (for example parents, peers, teachers and health professionals), as well as all the environments in which the child functions (for example school, home and community) [48]. Hence, effectively altering the eating and physical activity behaviors of children will need parental and community involvement. Involvement of community agencies may lead to school program efficacy, via providing a support base of prevention and treatment services, initiatives, campaigns, and sharing of resources. For example, collaborations could be developed between health departments or managed care organizations and schools in providing services to overweight or obese individuals [48].

Parental involvement in obesity prevention and treatment programs is important for the development of a psychosocial environment that elevating healthy eating and physical activity between young people. Epstein and Wing [58] mention 3 reasons for having parents engaged in obesity interventions: 1) obesity runs in families and it may be unrealistic to intervene with one member of a family, while other family members are modeling and supporting behaviors that may impede the interventions' efficacy; 2) specific parental behaviors, such as prompting overeating and low exercising, may be critical in the development and maintenance of unhealthy behaviors; and 3) to produce maximal behavior alteration in children, it may be important to include specific behavior-change strategies for parents to use. While it seems family engagement is crucial, specifically for young children, challenges observed for recruiting and sustaining parent involvement in school-based programs. Perry et al. [59] showed that a home-based correspondence approach for children and parents was effectual in alterations of eating and exercise behaviors between third grade children.

EVIDENCE OF EFFICACY

There is growing evidence that school-based obesity prevention programs elevate physical activity [60], and ameliorate dietary habits [61]. Such programs also ameliorate weight state when performed with high intensity and for long durations [43, 44]. However, there is significant differences in program design and impact [62, 63]. Additional evidence is required to establish long-term impacts.

In general, multi-component school-based obesity prevention programs are more effective than single-component programs [43, 64]. Multi-component school-based obesity prevention programs that consist of both a nutrition and physical activity focus seem more effectual than single-component programs [64].

Multi-component school-based interventions with durations for a year or more, high levels of intensity, and parent and community engagement have the greatest impacts on weight-associated outcomes [64, 65, 66]. Such interventions may also be more effectual between children and adolescents who are overweight or obese [66]. Multi-component school-based obesity prevention programs' impacts on body mass index differ based on duration and intensity of program. Many programs indicate significant positive influences [43, 65], others demonstrate no significant impact [60, 62, 63]. The influence on weight outcomes of multi-component interventions that concentrate on physical activity also associated with the duration and intensity of the intervention [67]. Ameliorations in the school food environment, implemented as part of multi-component nutrition education interventions, have been indicated to decrease or maintain the rate of overweight/obese children [62, 63].

School-based physical activity interventions, as a part of an obesity prevention program, can be advantageous to executive functions of children with overweight or obesity [68]. School-based dietary components of multi-component interventions with a particular focus on self-esteem can ameliorate self-esteem in overweight or obese adolescents [68].

Researches propose that obesity prevention programs are not related to promotions in unhealthy weight control behaviors such as fasting. Programs that particularly include the topic of eating disorders in their curricula are related to a decrease in the percentage of students reporting using unhealthy or extreme weight control behaviors [69].

DISCUSSION

School-based healthy eating and physical activity programs provide an important opportunity to elevate the future health and well-being of children because they can reach almost all children and may 1) elevate learning and provide social advantageous, 2) elevate health during critical periods of growth and maturation, 3) reduce the risk of chronic diseases in adulthood, and 4) help to establish healthy behaviors at an early age that will result to lifelong healthy habits [70]. The efficacy of school-based healthy eating and physical activity programs is important for evidence-based health policy and to justify more extensive implementation of successful programs. However, because only a limited number of studies have been carried out, and results have differed, so, the efficacy of these programs is not well established [16, 17]. For example, in a systematic review of intervention studies, Campbell et al. reported only 7 studies on prevention of childhood obesity, 4 of which showed programs that were effectual and 3 of which indicated programs that were not successful [16]. Additional research is needed to evaluate the efficacy of these programs.

Conclusion

Childhood obesity has emerged as one of the most important medical and public health issues of our day. The etiology of the disorder is multifactorial and complex, resulting from an interaction among genetic and biological agents, environmental factors, and ecological impacts. The multitude of serious comorbidities related to childhood obesity necessitates effective treatment interventions. The key interventions for preventing and treating obesity are enhancing physical activity and consuming a healthful diet. Within schools, attempts to enhance physical activity and healthful eating, should be a part of a comprehensive, coordinated school health program. Both primary and secondary obesity prevention and treatment interventions fit into a comprehensive program of school health. However, the role of the school in preventing and treating childhood obesity must be conceptualized as only one part of more wide community and health care system interventions [48]. Parents of school children also require to be engaged in obesity intervention attempts to make healthy alterations in the home, and reinforce and support healthy eating and regular exercise. The challenge of helping young individuals adopt healthy eating patterns and regular physical activity to achieve and maintain healthy weights cannot be effectually met by the sole attempts of the school or any other organization, it needs a multi-faceted community-wide attempt, but schools are in a unique position to have a critical role in elevating healthy lifestyles and helping to prevent obesity.

References

[1] Kumar S, Kelly AS. Review of Childhood Obesity: From Epidemiology, Etiology, and Comorbidities to Clinical Assessment and Treatment. *Mayo Clin Proc.* 2017 Feb; 92(2):251-265. doi: 10.1016/j.mayocp.2016.09.017.

[2] Calle EE, Thun MJ, Petrelli JM, Rodriguez C, Heath CW. Body-mass index and mortality in a prospective cohort of U.S. adults. *N Engl J Med.* 1999;341: 1097-1105.

[3] Manson JE, Bassuk SS. Obesity in the United States: a fresh look at its high toll. *JAMA.* 2003;289: 229-230.

[4] Calle EE, Rodriguez C, Walker-Thurmond K, Thun MJ. Overweight, obesity, and mortality from cancer in a prospectively studied cohort of U.S. adults. *N Engl J Med.* 2003;348:1625-1638.

[5] Fontaine KR, Redden DT, Wang C, Westfall AO, Allison DB. Years of life lost due to obesity. *JAMA.* 2003;289:187-193.

[6] Peeters A, Barendregt JJ, Willekins F, Mackenbach JP, Mamun AA, Bonneux L. Obesity in adulthood and its consequences for life expectancy: a life-table analysis. *Ann Intern Med.* 2003;138:24-32.

[7] Caterson ID, Franklin J, Colditz GA. Economic costs of obesity. In: Bray GA, Bouchard C, eds. *Handbook of Obesity.* New York, NY: Marcel Dekker Inc; 2004:149-156.

[8] Whitaker RC, Wright JA, Pepe MS, Seidel KD, Dietz WH. Predicting obesity in young adulthood from childhood and parental obesity. *N Engl J Med.* 1997; 337(13):869-873.

[9] Juonala M, Magnussen CG, Berenson GS, et al. Childhood adiposity, adult adiposity, and cardiovascular risk factors. *N Engl J Med.* 2011;365(20):1876-1885.

[10] Nicklas T, Johnson R. Position of the American Dietetic Association: dietary guidance for healthy children ages 2 to 11 years. *J Am Diet Assoc.* 2004;104: 660-677.

[11] Dietz WH. Prevalence of obesity in children. In: Bray GA, Bouchard C, James WPT (eds). *Handbook of Obesity.* Marcel Dekker, Inc: New York, 1996, pp 93-103.

[12] Institute of Medicine. *Weighing the options. Criteria for evaluating weight-management programs.* National Academic Press: Washington, 1998, pp 210-233.

[13] Resnicow K. School-based obesity prevention population versus high-risk interventions. *Ann NY Acad Sci* 1993; 699: 154-166.

[14] Centers for Disease Control and Prevention. Guidelines for school health programs to promote lifelong healthy eating. *MMWR Recomm Rep.* 1996; 45(RR-9):1-41.

[15] Centers for Disease Control and Prevention. Guidelines for school and community programs to promote lifelong physical activity among young people. *MMWR Recomm Rep.* 1997;46(RR-6):1-36.

[16] Campbell K, Waters E, O'Meara S, Summerbell C. Interventions for preventing obesity in childhood: a systematic review. *Obes Rev.* 2001;2:149-157.

[17] Wilson P, O'Meara S, Summerbell C, Kelly S, Effective Health Care Review Team. The prevention and treatment of childhood obesity. *Qual Safety Health Care.* 2003;12:65-74.

[18] Incledon E, Wake M, Hay M. Psychological predictors of adiposity: systematic review of longitudinal studies. *Int J Pediatr Obes.* 2011;6(2-2):e1-e11.

[19] Hemmingsson E. A new model of the role of psychological and emotional distress in promoting obesity: conceptual review with implications for treatment and prevention. *Obes Rev.* 2014;15(9):769-779.

[20] El-Behadli AF, Sharp C, Hughes SO, Obasi EM, Nicklas TA. Maternal depression, stress and feeding styles: towards a framework for theory and research in child obesity. *Br J Nutr.* 2015;113(suppl):S55-S71.

[21] Lau EY, Liu J, Archer E, McDonald SM, Liu J. Maternal weight gain in pregnancy and risk of obesity among offspring: a systematic review. *J Obes.* 2014;2014: 524939.

[22] Yu ZB, Han SP, Zhu GZ, et al. Birth weight and subsequent risk of obesity: a systematic review and meta-analysis. *Obes Rev.* 2011;12(7):525-542.

[23] Taveras EM, Rifas-Shiman SL, Sherry B, et al. Crossing growth percentiles in infancy and risk of obesity in childhood. *Arch Pediatr Adolesc Med.* 2011;165(11):993-998.

[24] Grummer-Strawn LM, Mei Z; Centers for Disease Control and Prevention Pediatric Nutrition Surveillance System. Does breastfeeding protect against pediatric overweight? Analysis of longitudinal data from the Centers for Disease Control and Prevention Pediatric Nutrition Surveillance System. *Pediatrics.* 2004;113(2):e81-e86.

[25] Schwartz BS, Pollak J, Bailey-Davis L, et al. Antibiotic use and childhood body mass index trajectory. *Int J Obes (Lond).* 2016; 40(4):615-621.

[26] Warner M, Wesselink A, Harley KG, Bradman A, Kogut K, Eskenazi B. Prenatal exposure to dichlorodiphenyltrichloroethane and obesity at 9 years of age in the CHAMACOS study cohort. *Am J Epidemiol.* 2014;179(11):1312-1322.

[27] Chang L, Neu J. Early factors leading to later obesity: interactions of the microbiome, epigenome, and nutrition. *Curr Probl Pediatr Adolesc Health Care.* 2015;45(5):134-142.

[28] Fuemmeler BF, Dedert E, McClernon FJ, Beckham JC. Adverse childhood events are associated with obesity and disordered eating: results from a U.S. population-based survey of young adults. *J Trauma Stress.* 2009;22(4):329-333.

[29] Banfield EC, Liu Y, Davis JS, Chang S, Frazier-Wood AC. Poor adherence to US Dietary Guidelines for children and adolescents in the National Health and Nutrition Examination Survey population. *J Acad Nutr Diet.* 2016;116(1):21-27.

[30] Ford CN, Slining MM, Popkin BM. Trends in dietary intake among US 2- to 6-year-old children, 1989-2008. *J Acad Nutr Diet.* 2013;113(1):35-42.

[31] Nicklas TA, Hayes D. American Dietetic Association. Position of the American Dietetic Association: nutrition guidance for healthy children ages 2 to 11 years. *J Am Diet Assoc.* 2008; 108(6):1038-1044, 1046-1047.

[32] Wang YC, Bleich SN, Gortmaker SL. Increasing caloric contribution from sugar-sweetened beverages and 100% fruit juices among US children and adolescents, 1988-2004. *Pediatrics.* 2008;121(6):e1604-e1614.

[33] Malik VS, Pan A, Willett WC, Hu FB. Sugar-sweetened beverages and weight gain in children and adults: a systematic review and meta-analysis. *Am J Clin Nutr.* 2013;98(4):1084-1102.

[34] Mancino L, Todd JE, Guthrie J, Lin BH. Food away from home and childhood obesity. *Curr Obes Rep.* 2014;3(4):459-469.

[35] Taber DR, Chriqui JF, Powell L, Chaloupka FJ. Association between state laws governing school meal nutrition content and student weight status: implications for new USDA school meal standards. *JAMA Pediatr.* 2013;167(6):513-519.

[36] Nelson MC, Neumark-Stzainer D, Hannan PJ, Sirard JR, Story M. Longitudinal and secular trends in physical activity and sedentary behavior during adolescence. *Pediatrics*. 2006; 118(6):e1627-e1634.

[37] Falbe J, Rosner B, Willett WC, Sonneville KR, Hu FB, Field AE. Adiposity and different types of screen time. *Pediatrics.* 2013; 132(6):e1497-e1505.

[38] Gilbert-Diamond D, Li Z, Adachi-Mejia AM, McClure AC, Sargent JD. Association of a television in the bedroom with increased adiposity gain in a nationally representative sample of children and adolescents. *JAMA Pediatr.* 2014;168(5): 427-434.

[39] Epstein LH, Roemmich JN, Robinson JL, et al. A randomized trial of the effects of reducing television viewing and computer use on body mass index in young children. *Arch Pediatr Adolesc Med.* 2008;162(3):239-245.

[40] Lipsky LM, Iannotti RJ. Associations of television viewing with eating behaviors in the 2009 Health Behaviour in School-aged Children Study. *Arch Pediatr Adolesc Med.* 2012;166(5): 465-472.

[41] Stettler N, Signer TM, Suter PM. Electronic games and environmental factors associated with childhood obesity in Switzerland. *Obes Res.* 2004;12(6):896-903.

[42] Welker E, Lott M, Story M. The school food environment and obesity prevention: progress over the last decade. *Curr Obes Rep.* 2016;5(2):145-155.

[43] Waters E, de Silva-Sanigorski A, Burford BJ, Brown T, Campbell KJ, Gao Y, Armstrong R, Prosser L, Summerbell CD. Interventions for preventing obesity in children. *Cochrane Database of Systematic Reviews.* 2011; (12):CD001871.

[44] Mozaffarian D, Afshin A, Benowitz NL, Bittner V, Daniels SR, Franch HA, Jacobs DR Jr, Kraus WE, Kris Etherton PM, Krummel DA, Popkin BM, Whitsel LP, Zakai NA. American Heart Association Council on Epidemiology and Prevention, Council on Nutrition, Physical Activity and Metabolism, Council on Clinical Cardiology, Council on Cardiovascular Disease in the Young, Council on the Kidney in Cardiovasc. Population approaches to improve diet, physical activity, and smoking habits: a scientific statement from the American Heart Association. *Circulation.* 2012 Sep 18;126(12):1514-63. doi: 10.1161/CIR.0b013e318260a20b. Epub 2012 Aug 20. PMID: 22907934; PMCID: PMC3881293.

[45] Allensworth DD, Kolbe LJ. The comprehensive school health program. Exploring an expanded concept. *J School Health* 1987; 57: 409-412.

[46] United States, Department of Health and Human Sciences (USDHHS), Public Health Service, Centre for Disease Control and Prevention (CDC). Guidelines for school health programs to promote lifelong healthy eating. *MMWR* 1996; 45: 1-40.

[47] United States, Department of Health and Human Sciences (USDHHS), Public Health Service. Guidelines for school and community programs to promote lifelong physical activity among young people. *MMWR* 1997; 46: 1-36.

[48] Parcel GS, Green LW, Beetes BA. School-based programs to prevent or reduce obesity. In: Krasnegor NA, Grave GD, Kretchmer N (eds). *Childhood Obesity: A Biobehavioural Perspective.* Jedfor Press, Incl: Caldwell, 1988, pp 143-157.

[49] Seffrin J. Why school health education? In: Wallace HM, Patrick K, Parcel G, Igbe JB (eds). *Principles and Practices of Student Health (Vol 2).* Third Party Publishing: Oakland, 1992, pp 393-422.

[50] Small ML, Majer LS, Allensworth DD, Farquhar BK, Kann L, Pateman BC. School health services. *J School Health* 1995; 65: 319-326.

[51] Burghardt J, Devaney B. *The School Nutrition Dietary Assessment Study.* Mathmatica Policy Research: Princeton, 1993.

[52] National school lunch program and school breakfast program: nutrition objectives for school meals (7 CFR 210, 220). *Fed Regist* 1994; 59: 30218-30251.

[53] US Depts of Agriculture and Health and Human Services. Nutrition and your health: Dietary guidelines for Americans (4th edn*). Home and Garden Bulletin No.* 232. Washington, 1995, US Court Printing Office.

[54] Wolfe WS, Campbell CC. *Nutritional health of school-aged children at Upstate New York: What are the problems and what can schools do?* Cornell University: New York, 1991.

[55] Contento I, Balch G, Bronner YL, Lytle LA, Maloney SK, Olson CM, Swadenei SS. The effectiveness of nutrition education and implications for nutrition education policy, programs and research: A review of research. *J Nutr Educ* 1995; 27: 277-380.

[56] Price J, Desmond S, Stelzer C. Elementary school principals' perceptions of childhood obesity. *J School Health* 1987; 57: 367-370.

[57] Stang JM, Story M, Kalina B. School-based weight management services: perceptions and practices of school nurses and administrators. *Am J Health Prom* 1997; 11: 183-185.

[58] Epstein LH, Wing R. Behavioural treatment of childhood obesity. *Psychol Bull* 1987; 101: 331-342.

[59] Perry CL, Luepker RV, Murray DM, Durth C, Mullis R, Crockett S, Jacobs DR. Parent involvement with children's health promotion: The Minnesota Home Team. *Am J Public Health* 1988; 78: 1156-1160.

[60] Dobbins M, Husson H, DeCorby K, LaRocca RL. School-based physical activity programs for promoting physical activity and fitness in children and adolescents aged 6 to 18. *Cochrane Database of Systematic Reviews.* 2013; (2), CD007651.

[61] Van Cauwenberghe E, Maes L, Spittaels H, van Lenthe FJ, Brug J, Oppert JM, De Bourdeaudhuij I. Effectiveness of school-based interventions in Europe to promote healthy nutrition in children and adolescents: systematic review of published and 'grey' literature. *British Journal of Nutrition.* 2010: 103 (6): 781-797.

[62] Brown T, Summerbell C. Systematic review of school-based interventions that focus on changing dietary intake and physical activity levels to prevent childhood obesity: an update to the obesity guidance produced by the National Institute for Health and Clinical Excellence. *Obes Rev.* 2009 Jan;10(1):110-41. doi: 10.1111/j.1467-789X.2008.00515.x.

[63] Harris KC, Kuramoto LK, Schulzer M, Retallack JE. Effect of school-based physical activity interventions on body mass index in children: a meta-analysis. *CMAJ* 2009; 180(7):719-26.

[64] Shirley K, Rutfield R, Hall N, Fedor N, McCaughey VK, Zajac K. *J Primary Prevent* (2015) 36: 1. https://doi.org/10.1007/s10935-014-0370-3.

[65] Bleich SN, Vercammen KA, Zatz LY, Frelier JM, Ebbeling CB, A PeetersInterventions to prevent global childhood overweight and obesity: a systematic review. *Lancet Diabetes Endocrinol,* 6 (2018), pp. 332-346, 10.1016/S2213-8587(17)30358-3.

[66] Henrique P, Roberto M, Nobre C, Augusto J, Augusto J, Carrazedo A. School-based physical activity and nutritional education interventions on body mass index: a meta-analysis of randomised community trials—project PANE. *Prev Med,* 61 (2014), pp. 81-89, 10.1016/j.ypmed.2014.01.005.

[67] Russ LB, Webster CA, Beets MW, Phillips DS. Systematic Review and Meta-Analysis of Multi-Component Interventions Through Schools to Increase Physical Activity. *Journal of Physical Activity and Health.* 2015; 12(10):1436-1446.

[68] Martin A, Booth JN, Laird Y, Sproule J, Reilly JJ, Saunders DH. Physical activity, diet and other behavioural interventions for improving cognition and school achievement in children and adolescents with obesity or overweight. *Cochrane Database of Systematic Reviews* 2018, Issue 3. Art. No.: CD009728. doi: 10.1002/14651858.CD009728.pub4.

[69] Larson N, Davey CS, Caspi CE, Kubik MY, Nanney MS. School-Based Obesity-Prevention Policies and Practices and Weight-Control Behaviors among Adolescents. *Journal of the Academy of Nutrition and Dietetics.* 2017; 117(2): 204-213.

[70] Baranowski T, Mendlein J, Resnicow K, Frank E, Weber-Cullen K, Baranowski J. Physical activity and nutrition in children and youth: an overview of obesity prevention. *Prev Med.* 2000; 31:S1-S10.

In: Childhood Obesity
Editor: Roya Kelishadi
ISBN: 978-1-53618-158-6
© 2020 Nova Science Publishers, Inc.

Chapter 18

SURGERY TO TREAT OBESITY IN CHILDREN AND ADOLESCENTS

Beheshteh Olang**, MD, PhD, Aliakbar Sayyari, MD, Farid Imanzadeh, MD, Bahareh Amirkalali, PhD, Masoud Khorshidi, PhD and Zahra Fazeli, Mph

PATIENT SELECTION CRITERIA

Surgery to treat obesity is only recommended if:

1 The patient has reached the age of 1 or 2 Tanner from puberty or is more than 5% of adult height. This issue should only be addressed to girls 3 years old or boys 3 years old.

2 A patient with a BMI $\geq$ 1 kg / m 2 associated with serious comorbidities (such as type 2 diabetes, moderate to severe sleep apnea, false-positive brain tumor or non-alcoholic fatty liver disease) or body mass index $\geq$ ٤٠ Concomitant (such as hypertension, insulin resistance, glucose intolerance, significant impairment in daily activities or poor quality of life, dyslipidemia, sleep apnea with an apnea-hypopenia index> 1) or when severe obesity and comorbidities It has been failing for 6 months or more despite having the right lifestyle change plan (with or without medication). (Inability to maintain weight loss by -5% or more)

* Corresponding Author: Beheshteh Olang, MD, Pediatrician, PhD, Assistant Professor in Pediatric Nutrition, Pediatric Gastroenterology, Hepatology and Nutrition Research Center, Research Institute for Children's Health, Shahid Beheshti University of Medical Sciences, Tehran, Iran, Email: beheshteholang@gmail.com.

3 Most guidelines presently suggest that adolescent mental disorder is associated with body mass index - indication of surgery.
4 Full understanding of lifestyle changes: Good candidates should have the understanding and commitment to lifestyle changes, including eating habits that are needed after surgery to prevent unwanted side effects and maintain weight loss.
5 The patient and his or her family must have sufficient power to make decisions, understand the risks and benefits of surgery, and have realistic expectations of weight loss. Having strong family and other social support, such as close friendships and minimizing social isolation, results in better outcomes.
6 Obesity surgery in pre-adolescent children, pregnant or lactating adolescents, or those who plan to become pregnant within 2 years of surgery, and if there are no amenable medical causes, is not recommended. It is also not recommended for patients who do not adhere to the principles of healthy eating and physical activity or who suffer from drug abuse, eating disorders or untreated psychiatric disorders (other than depression).
7 It is strongly recommended that the patient not use nicotine for six weeks before surgery.
8 Percentage of weight loss is independent of primary body mass index, so people who are severely obese will still remain obese after surgery. But even when obesity persists, most obesity-related illnesses improve dramatically after surgery.
9 Because adolescents appear to have a higher rate of diabetes and other obesity-related disorders than adults, early surgery may be beneficial in obese adolescents and subsequently reduce the risk of vascular injury to the elderly.

Patient Preparation Before Obesity Surgery

The following are usually routine:

- Complete blood cell count
  Complete renal testing
  Complete liver test
- Fasting blood glucose and insulin
- Glycosylated hemoglobin (HbA1c)
- Lipid profile
- Vitamin D
- Parathyroid hormone
  Thyroid function test
- ACTH
  Cortisol

- blood group
- Coagulation profile

Radiological examinations include:

- Abdominal ultrasound to see gallstones
- Pelvic ultrasound may be performed on girls over the age of 5 years.
- Skeletal puberty should be evaluated using bone age determined by X-ray of the left wrist.
- Bone Mineral Density Measurement It is important to consider bone mineral density after obesity surgery.
- Polysomnography is recommended if you have a history of sleep apnea.
- If there is a high risk of deep vein thrombosis (DVT) after surgery, prevention with medication and socks is recommended.
- Psychological evaluation including:
    - Assessment of family environment and stressors.
    - Assessment of emotional maturity, cognitive function, and understanding of surgery and related recommendations.
    - Adherence to treatments for other disabilities and obesity-related illnesses.
- His knowledge and expectations of surgery in terms of lifestyle changes and weight loss rates.
    - History of trying to lose weight based on diet and activity.
    - Nutritional habits and disorders such as eating too much or binge eating.
    - Obstacles to doing business, including financial constraints or lack of time.
- Nutritional Assessment:

Minimum preoperative laboratory studies include evaluation of the most common deficiencies, including vitamin D and calcium, complete blood cell count (CBC), iron, transferrin, ferritin, erythrocyte folate levels (in some centers, homocysteine levels for control of status). Vitamins B12, B6, 1B and ۲۵hydroxyvitamin D). Zinc, magnesium and copper may also be evaluated. If a teenager is diagnosed with a micronutrient deficiency, deficiency correction should be performed prior to surgery.

Using a food frequency questionnaire or dietary supplement completed by the adolescent may provide more nutritional information to the patient. Evaluating dietary habits may be valuable in assessing perceptions, attitudes, and conditions that lead to successful nutrition and dietary choices. Compared to restrictive surgical procedures, pre-operative nutritional assessment of the procedures leading to malabsorption should be more precise.

PRE-SURGICAL NUTRITION MANAGEMENT

Nutrition management should begin six months before surgery with the cooperation and coordination of the family. A balanced, healthy diet containing adequate amounts of protein, fruits, vegetables, and whole grains during the pre-operative period is recommended to help maintain weight or lose weight. In addition, it is recommended to use behavioral strategies to control the volume of meals, such as encouraging the use of plates, spoons and small forks when eating. Learning self-control techniques such as daily intake or healthy food registrations are used. Helps maintain weight gain. Estimates of energy intake, protein, and fluid intake, as well as the frequency of meals, should be examined. It is very important for the family to provide an encouraging and supportive environment. The family should provide an environment that will help the teen lose weight nutritionally. This means limiting high-calorie foods with low nutrient densities and replacing them with micronutrient-rich foods.

Days before surgery, calorie restriction to 5kg is achieved by using a carbohydrate-restricted liquid diet that reduces liver glycogen levels, thereby reducing its size and facilitating surgical procedures. It is recommended to take vitamin B12, BD, iron, folate supplements if needed. Because of the high prevalence of micronutrient deficiencies in obese patients and the correction of pre-existing micronutrient deficiencies, a multivitamin supplement is recommended for all adolescents prior to surgery.

PRE-OPERATIVE WEIGHT LOSS COUNSELING AND TRAINING

Advice on Long-Term Diet and Post-Operative Supplements with Particular Regard to Bone Health

Training on a soft and regular diet plan should be better postponed because post-operative training may prevent the adolescent from remembering it well.

The dietitian may want to examine the adolescent's acceptance of the taste or protein supplements that he or she will be offered prior to surgery.

It is recommended that educational information be provided verbally and in writing. A pre-operative nutrition appointment of at least 2 sessions is recommended to complete the nutrition assessment and training sessions for adolescent preparation.

POSTOPERATIVE NUTRITION MANAGEMENT

The post-operative diet focuses on weight loss along with maintaining lean body mass through a protein-rich diet restricted to simple carbohydrates, with no added sugars and moderate fat intake.

Post-Operative Dietary Improvement

Diet improvement protocols vary in different surgical procedures, in terms of number of meals per day, consistency, texture and amount of nutrients consumed per meal.

Surgical Procedure

1 Ice patches, Water, liquids without sugar residucs
2 Full liquids with High protein
3 Fatty foods and smoothies
4 Soft foods
5 All healthy foods With any texture Roux-en Y 1 oz / hour for the first 24 to 48 hours, Then it can be continued for 3-7 days, depending on the patient's wishes and conditions. 2-4 weeks 6-4 weeks 7-9 weeks starting from week 9 and on.

For All Life Gastric band 1 ounce per hour for the first 48-24 hours.

The first 2 weeks after surgery 4-3 weeks 6-5 weeks starting from week 7 and on

For All Life

Sleeve gastrectomy 1 oz / hour for the first 48 to 24 hours,

Then, depending on the patient's condition and condition, it can continue for 3-7 days 5-1 weeks 8-5 weeks 12-9 weeks starting from week 13 and on

For All Life

Goals per day

Step 1

No Liquid Sugar Free 4-6 oz Drinking Water or No Liquid Sugar Free Hour (48-64 oz / day)

Acceptable non-sugar smoothies include: water, smooth meat juice, sugar-free gelatin, fruit-flavored drinks, and non-frozen liquid or frozen sugars, Sugar-Free Liquids Prohibitions: Carbonated drinks, caffeine-containing, red

Step 2

High-Protein Full-Fluid Diet Calories: 500-600 Calories

Protein: 50-60 g

Fluids: 90-80 oz or as estimated

New foods: 1% lean or low-fat milk, low-fat soy milk or lactose-free milk, high-protein drinks, lean yogurt (plain or vanilla) with diluted milk

Food pattern: 3-6 meals a day

Size: Half a glass per serving for solid foods

Step 3

High Protein Smooth Tissue Calories: 700-500 kcal

Protein: 60 g

Fluids: 90-80 ounces (or estimated as needed

New dishes: stir-fried egg, egg, minced turkey or turkey, fully skinned fish meat, tofu puree, tuna, low-fat melted cheese (just a little crumbly), low ricotta cheese Greasy

Food texture: smooth

Try a quarter glass of new food every 2-3 days.

Food pattern: 4-3 meals a day

Size: For solid foods half a glass or 6-5 ounces of high protein drinks per serving

Step 4

Soft foods. Other protein foods, fruits, vegetables and grains Calories: 800-700 kcal

Protein: 60 g

Fluids: 90-80 ounces (or estimated as needed

New foods:

Protein foods: Bearded beef, low-fat cheese, cooked beans

Fruit: Soft or canned in its juice, without skin

Vegetables: Soft cooked or canned

Cereals: Crackers, Oatmeal, Rice, Pasta, Baked Potatoes (Select Whole Grains Only)

Food pattern: 3-6 meals a day

Size: 0.5-5 cups of solid foods per serving or 1 glass (8 oz) high protein drink

Step 5:

Healthy foods for the whole calorie life of 900-800 kcal

Protein: 60 g

Fluids: 90-80 ounces (or estimated as needed)

New foods: All healthy food choices

Food pattern: 6-3 meals a day

Size: Up to three quarters or 1.5 glasses per serving

After adjusting for laparoscopic adjustable gastric banding, which is usually performed 2 weeks after surgery and then every 2 weeks until satiety, a complete fluid regimen is administered for 1 to 2 days after adjustment and then progressed to solid foods. Soft for 2 to 3 days thereafter depending on patient tolerance.

Nutrition Tips for Adolescents Undergoing Weight Loss Surgery

Avoid high-fat foods or simple sugars to avoid dumping syndrome. Symptoms may include abdominal pain, cold sensation, sweating, palpitations, vomiting, and / or diarrhea. Delayed dumping may occur up to two hours after eating foods high in sugar or fat.

] The meal time should be about 5 minutes.

ج Adolescents should be encouraged to refrain from drinking liquids 2 minutes before meals and 2 minutes after meals

] Eating and drinking at the same time may reduce satiety or increase the incidence of vomiting.

] Encourage the patient to eat slowly and eat small snacks. Make sure the food is cut into small pieces. Continue to cook until the mash is completely puree.

Avoid eating and drinking after the first feeling of fullness. When you feel full, skip meals or throw away what is left.

] To prevent water shortages, it is important to encourage the patient to take a sip of fluids (preferably water) during the day. Limit caffeine-containing products.

Do not lie down for 7-8 hours after a meal.

1. Energy

Estimation of total energy should be based on a method previously used in the treatment center to reduce weight.

The energy requirement should be estimated at or below 1% below basal metabolism to achieve maximum weight loss. This value should be reassessed by the occurrence of severe changes in weight or when no expected weight loss occurs.

2. Protein

Since the goal of weight loss surgery is preferably to reduce fat mass, adequate protein intake is essential to prevent lean mass loss. Although the exact amount of protein needed after surgery is unclear, a high-protein diet (-1.5 g / kg ideal body weight) is usually recommended. According to current practices, 4-6 grams of protein a day is recommended in adolescents undergoing RYGB, lap band, and gastric sleeve surgeries. Since it is difficult for many patients to get enough protein, they use high-protein, low-calorie, and low-sugar protein supplements to get the protein they need.

Protein intake should be periodically determined by the medical team to ensure proper training and dietary compliance. Intravenous supplements are used in patients with severe protein malnutrition who do not respond to oral protein supplements. Donor can be used.

3. Hydration

Loss of body dehydration can be due to inadequate fluid intake, secondary diarrhea due to dumping syndrome or high sugar intake (honey, jelly, or candy).

/2 Daily consumption of 2.3 liters of water per day for girls ages 4-5 is recommended, which increases to 2.7 liters per day for children over 5 years.

Boys need more fluids. Boys 3 to 5 years need 3.3 liters a day and boys over 3 years need 3.7 liters a day.

Due to the limiting nature of weight loss surgeries, many patients are not able to consume large amounts of water at one time but must consume water in small amounts throughout the day. The need for fluids varies from patient to patient and one must pay attention to the patient's thirst. However, total fluid intake of at least 1 to 2 ounces per day in adult patients is recommended. This volume is about 2 to 3 ounces of liquid, plus 1 to 2 ounces of whole liquids, such as skim milk, lactose-free milk, soy milk or low-fat yogurt.

All fluids should be caffeine-free and sugar-free with low levels of sorbitol. To maintain hydration, strategies for treating post-operative vomiting in the patient are provided, such as following the instructions in the volume of food at each meal, chewing the food before swallowing, avoiding fluid intake 5 minutes before and after meals. Diarrhea associated with dumping syndrome may lead to water deficiency in patients. Avoiding sugar, candy, honey, jelly, and other foods high in sugar (which may cause diarrhea by increasing the osmolality of the contents of the small intestine) can prevent diarrhea.

4. Need for Micronutrients

The use of a full multivitamin supplement is recommended for all patients. For those who have a specific micronutrient deficiency, correcting that deficiency should be done before surgery. Considering the type of supplement is important because studies have reported differences in the vitamin and mineral content of various supplements. Regular screening is mandatory during the first 6 months (once every 6 months and then annually) and supplements containing vitamins B12, B6, B1, D, folate and iron are required. The most common deficiencies are vitamin D and iron. Replacing iron and folate is especially important in young girls who have menstruation and their chances of pregnancy improve with weight loss.

- Vitamin B1 (thiamin)

After surgery, thiamine deficiency is most likely to occur in patients with persistent vomiting or overweight. Symptoms of thiamine deficiency include weakness, hyperflexia, and vomiting. In adolescents, thiamine deficiency in girls after gastric bypass surgery has been reported to occur in the lower extremities with stocking distribution, nystagmus, and hearing loss 2 to 6 months after surgery. The recommended intake of thiamine is currently for girls in the age group of 3 to 5 mg / day and for boys in the same age group is 1.8 mg / day. Teens undergoing weight loss surgery should receive at least 2 mg of thiamine per day, which can be supplemented by an additional B-complex supplement. In patients with severe and prolonged vomiting, the addition of thiamine to intravenous nutrition during the postoperative period is recommended.

- Vitamin B6 (pyridoxine)

It is recommended that the multivitamin used for people undergoing weight loss surgery contain vitamin B6.

- Vitamin B9 (folic acid)

Among adolescents, the recommended folic acid intake for both sexes is 2 micrograms daily. Based on the experience of postoperative gastric bypass or biliopancreatic diversion in adults, the rate is between 1 and 2 mg / day.

- Vitamin B12 (cobalamin)

Vitamin B12 deficiency occurs in restrictive surgeries or surgery that results in malabsorption, but rarely occurs after banding or gastroplasty unless it is reduced. The recommended intake for cobalamin is 2.4 μg / day for boys and girls ages 14-14. For those who have used restrictive surgeries or surgeries that lead to malabsorption, the use of the supplemental form of 12B supplementation of 1mg or its monthly injection is recommended. The recommended treatment for vitamin B12 deficiency in adults undergoing weight loss surgery is 2 μg orally or 2 μg every 2 to 3 months by intramuscular injection or 6 μg / week nasal spray.

- Vitamin A

Deficiency of fat-soluble vitamins has been reported after weight loss surgery, especially after biliopancreatic diversion. The recommended dose (DRI) of vitamin A for boys is 18-18 yrs / μg / day and for girls 14-18 years / yl / day. The amount of vitamin A administered after weight loss in adolescents is also consistent with DRI values, which are usually found in the daily multivitamin that the patient receives. For those whose surgical procedures lead to more severe malabsorption, such as a duodenal switch or long-limb gastric bypass, additional supplementation may be required.

- Calcium / Vitamin D

DRIs for vitamin D and calcium for men and boys are 2 to 4 years, 4 units / day and 2 mg / day, respectively. After weight loss surgery, the minimum recommended dose of calcium is 2 mg daily and the minimum vitamin D intake should be 3 units per day. Some child treatment protocols prescribe up to 1 vitamin D per day. If vitamin D deficiency is diagnosed, a supplement of 2 to 4 units of vitamin D may be considered to correct the deficiency.

- Iron

Iron deficiency rarely occurs after gastroplasty or bonding, but for a long time mild iron deficiency has been reported due to meat intolerance. In adolescents who have undergone restrictive surgery and have mild meat intolerance, the amount of iron in the routine multivitamin mineral supplement will be sufficient. Adolescents undergoing restrictive surgery and consuming good dietary iron sources (eg, liver, beef, whole grain breads, cereals, eggs and dried fruits) do not need iron supplements.

To prevent iron deficiency in gastric bypass or biliopancreatic diversion, use of 2 mg ferrosulfate daily with vitamin C is recommended. It is important to remember that vitamin C can increase iron absorption by up to 3%. Often the ferritin concentration decreases initially when iron intake is inadequate. However, ferritin is not recommended as an iron deficiency screening tool because it may be affected by other issues (such as inflammatory process).

Hemoglobin Target Group

(g / dL) Hematocrit
(%) MCV *
(fL) TIBC ** sat
(%) Ferritin
(mg / L)
Girl 15-12 years old 8/11> 7/35> 81> 16> 18>
Boy 15-12 years old 5/12> 3/37> 82> 16> 15>
Girl> 15 years 12> 7/35> 85> 16> 15>

Boy> 15 years 3/13> 7/39> 85> 16> 15>

* mean corpuscular volume; ** TIBC:total iron binding capacity

Reference: Centers for Disease Control and Prevention.

ZINC AND MAGNESIUM

Zinc DRIs for boys and girls ages 3 to 5 are 2 and 3 mg, respectively. There is little report of zinc deficiency after weight loss surgery except alopecia following gastric bypass surgery and zinc deficiency among bypass patients who had severe energy protein malnutrition. Because zinc uptake is dependent on lipid uptake, patients who use biliopancreatic diversion or duodenal switch methods are at risk for zinc deficiency. Zinc deficiency is unlikely to occur in surgeries using only restrictive procedures. Low magnesium levels have been reported in 4% of patients after biliopancreatic diversion, but no significant clinical complications have been documented. It should be noted, however, that hypomagnesemia may be the cause of uncontrolled hypocalcemia. The US Food and Drug Administration has issued a statement on the association between long-term use of proton pump inhibitors and hypomagnesa. This issue should be taken into consideration when evaluating patients undergoing weight loss surgery who are heavily using acid blocking drugs.

Zinc and magnesium supplements are recommended based on clinical need and serum level.

Copper

5 micrograms daily for boys and girls between 2 and 4 years. Myelopathy following gastric bypass, anemia and neutropenia after weight loss surgery has been reported in some cases due to copper deficiency. Teenagers may need to consider multivitamin minerals to make sure they contain copper, especially if iron deficiency is not readily corrected in the patient, which may be indicative of copper deficiency.

Omega 3 Fatty Acids

The current recommendation of the American Heart Association is to consume at least 5 ounces of fatty fish per week for adults. There are concerns about the contamination of fish or supplements with mercury, but the benefits are believed to outweigh the potential risks.

Due to the limiting nature of most operations for the treatment of obesity, the consumption of fatty fish in these patients may be limited. Careful analysis of the adolescent's diet may be needed to ensure adequate omega-3 intake and omega-rich food selection training or supplementation to improve her nutritional quality.

Other Nutrients

Daily intake of a complete multivitamin mineral supplement is sufficient to get enough of other nutrients.

Micronutrient Laboratory Parameter Natural Range of Symptoms of Deficiency

Thiamine (B1)

Erythrocyte ketolase stimulation < 15.

Barbarism, neuritis, edema, heart failure, anorexia, hoarseness, numbness, dysfunction and mute

Plasma pyridoxine (B6) PLP < 20 nmol / liter neuropathy, light sensitivity

Folic acid (B9)

Serum folate

RBC folate

Homocysteine> 6 ng / ml,

> 160 ng / ml megaloblastic anemia, irritability, paranoid behavior

Cobalamin (B12)

B12 * Urine / Serum

< 3.60 mmol / mol creatinine

Or

900-200 pg / ml parenchymal anemia, neurodegeneration

Vitamin A

Plasma Retinol

20-72 mg / dL

Night blindness, Xerophthalmia, Dermatomalacia, Weakening of resistance to infection, Follicular

Hyperkeratosis, poor bone growth

Calcium

Ionized calcium

4.92 - 4.48 mg / dl

Numbness and tingling, muscle cramps, seizures, anorexia fatigue and abnormal heart rhythm

25-Hydroxyvitamin D Vitamin D Serum < 50 nmol / liter Rickets, Osteomalacia Vitamin C Vitamin C Plasma 2-0.2 mg / dl Bleeding gums, diarrhea, perifollicular bleeding, scurvy

Plasma vitamin E alpha-tocopherol 10-0.7 mg / dL spinocerebellar hypertrophy and retinal analysis

Zinc zinc 1.2-0.75 mg / liter anorexia, decreased taste sensation, growth retardation or sexual maturity, wound healing

Magnesium Magnesium Serum 2.0 - 1.5 mg / dL Seizure, Neuropsychiatric Disorders, Hypomagnesemia

Serum Copper Copper 1.45-1.10 mg / L Micro-Hypochromic Anemia,, Growth Delay, Osteoporosis, Neutropenia

Supervision of nutrition after weight loss surgery Complete blood cell count control (CBC), iron, ferritin, thiamine, vitamin 12B, methyl malonic acid, 2-hydroxy vitamin D, albumin, calcium, magnesium, phosphorus, serum folate or erythrocyte levels every 6 months or once a year.

Nutrition tests should be performed every 6 months for those who have severe weight loss.

If there is concern about osteomalacia, DEXA scans before and after surgery may be helpful. It is important to ensure that the patient's weight does not exceed the capacity of the device, as many DEXA scans can only cover up to 3 pounds.

Hunger Assessment One way to teach hunger / satiety is to use the Hunger Scale. The patient is asked to rate their hunger / satiety on a scale of 1 to 2 before and in the middle of the meal. The number 1 indicates severe hunger and the number 1 indicates severe satiation. If he registers more than 1 in the middle of the meal, he should be asked to finish the meal.

School Environment

It is recommended that:

Have a bottle of water with them at school to use fluids throughout the day.

- Lunch is between 9:00 and 9:30.
- Consider a snack or protein supplement for school time.
- Prefer eating lunch at home to consume healthier foods.

Reproductive HealthThe American College of Obstetrics and Gynecology recommends avoiding pregnancy for 2 to 6 months after surgery. To date, 3 neonates with neural tube defects, from spina bifida to encephalopathy, have been born to mothers who underwent gastric bypass surgery for more than 6 months.

Since studies show that people do not follow the vitamin supplementation guidelines for a long time after surgery, special attention should be given to girls after weight loss surgery, especially those who have used abusive methods. Is essential. Postoperatively, patients should continue to be monitored for micronutrient deficiencies, especially in the case of folic acid, vitamin 12B, and iron replacement in girls who are seeking pregnancy. After childbirth, proper dietary supplementation with vitamin and mineral supplements in weight loss surgeons is important to ensure proper growth of the infant.

Inappropriate weight gain in a newborn born after gastric bypass surgery has been reported due to inadequate protein intake, which has been resolved by the formula. Congenital vitamin B12 deficiency associated with pan-cytopenia, developmental delay, and atrophy of the cortex have been reported in infants born to mothers several years after gastric bypass surgery.

Predictors of success The purpose of this surgery is to lose weight. None of the surgical treatments for obesity, such as a lap band or a combination of malabsorbing, limiting agents such as RYGB, weight loss will achieve an ideal body weight. Often the percentage of weight loss that a patient has over their ideal weight is used to describe success after surgery.

In obesity surgery, weight loss percentages vary from 58-64%. In restrictive methods, such as band lap, the percentage of overweight is lower (40-54%), whereas those with malabsorption such as RYGB are higher (56-74%). Changes in body mass index are also used to describe weight loss after surgery.

Finally, improving or decreasing the severity of obesity-related diseases is another method of defining successful surgery. Improvements in type 2 diabetes, hyperlipidemia, hypertension, and obstructive sleep apnea can be seen.

Editor's Contact Information

Roya Kelishadi, MD
Professor of Pediatrics, Faculty of Medicine
Founder & Chair, Research Institute for Primordial Prevention of Non Communicable Disease
Founder & Chair, Child Growth and Development Research Center
Isfahan University of Medical Sciences, Isfahan, Iran
Founder & Editor-in-Chief, International Journal of Preventive Medicine

INDEX

B

C

D

E

F

G

H

I

J

K

L

Q

R

S

T

U

V

W

Y